DENTAL PUBLIC HEALTH
AN INTRODUCTION
TO COMMUNITY DENTISTRY

Dental Public Health

An Introduction to Community Dentistry

Edited by
GEOFFREY L. SLACK
Community Dentistry Unit
The London Hospital Medical College
Dental School
in collaboration with
BRIAN A. BURT
Community Dentistry Unit
The London Hospital Medical College
Dental School
University of London

JOHN WRIGHT & SONS LTD.
BRISTOL 1974

ISBN 0 7236 0351 0

Printed in Great Britain by Butler & Tanner Ltd., Frome and London

Preface

by Geoffrey L. Slack OBE, TD, DDS (N. WESTERN), FDS, FACD, DIP BACT
Professor of Dental Surgery
The London Hospital Medical College Dental School

The development of dental public health in the United Kingdom has its origins in the local treatment services established long ago. As far back as 1885, Mr. W. M. Fisher of Dundee called for legislation to secure compulsory attention to the teeth of schoolchildren, and the first few school dentists were appointed soon after. Widespread concern over the poor health of British youth followed the Boer War, where many recruits were found to be dental invalids. The School Dental Service slowly began to emerge after the passage of the Education Act of 1907, which set up the School Medical Service, and the Maternity and Child Welfare Act of 1918 brought in the concept of priority-group treatment. The Local Authority Dental Services, as we now know them, began to take shape from their previously embryonic form.

The British tradition in the development of social services is one of adapting and modifying from the existing framework rather than beginning again; evolution rather than revolution. The National Health Service was therefore not introduced as something completely different; it was an extension of the existing health services available free of charge, and the eligible population was broadened to cover all citizens. It came as some surprise, therefore, that when the General Dental Service of the National Health Service came into being in 1948 the dental profession was overwhelmed by the demand for dental treatment. The measures introduced to regulate the flow were crude and not always in the best interests of the needy. However, the dental profession in the United Kingdom forged itself into an instrument of dental public health in that dental care of a kind became available to every individual of the population. The concept of 'dental public health' at that time was almost completely that of treatment of dental disease. Mass prevention, education, and administration were still undeveloped.

The response of the dental educators under pressure to produce more dentists was mainly to increase the size of their existing departments and staff; in some cases new departments were created. In the latter category the dental care of children in particular became a case of special pleading. *But, somehow the main point was missed, namely that the concept of adequate dental care for children, though a worthy cause in itself, is to make possible the protection of the dental health of the individual throughout his life.*

This failure to appreciate the vital necessity of continuing care for the whole community has resulted in a piece-meal provision, the long-term effects of which are extremely difficult to assess and impossible to remedy.

A further factor of significance was that the specialists in some disciplines in dentistry did not appreciate the public health implication of their work. It is now recognized that there is a basic element of community dentistry in every discipline.

Every dental disease condition poses the question as to its frequency in the population as a whole, the cost of its treatment, the knowledge and attitudes of people about it, the types of personnel who should be involved in its treatment, how it may be prevented or minimized most efficiently, and where it should rank in the priority for treatment.

The reorganization of the National Health Service scheduled for 1974 is especially important in the planning of dental care for the community. This reorganization comes at a time when there has been a substantial increase in the teaching of Community Dentistry in the dental schools. In postgraduate dental education new diplomas and degrees in dental public health have been established during the past four years. This welcome development is long overdue for it will take many years to develop the required skills and expertise in those staff who will occupy key positions in the reorganized service.

The current emphasis on the rediscovered need for good management and leadership in the health services will undoubtedly reveal deficiencies in the education and training of dental surgeons in this field. It is to be hoped that the arrangements now being made will lead to the development of such postgraduate education as will fit the staff for their future role. It is important for the future development of the profession as a whole that a basic understanding of Community Dentistry should be acquired by all students as a part of their wider training in general dentistry. Furthermore, several years of general experience in a variety of fields will enable the dentist dedicated to dental public health to devote himself more effectively to the study in depth of this subject.

This book is intended to provide an overall view of dental public health as affecting the United Kingdom against the background of selected examples of systems used in other countries. Special chapters are devoted to a review of the methods employed in dental public health such as the use of epidemiology, the assembly of statistics, the use of computers, a view of the future, and the way in which the dental team and the use of auxiliaries may be employed.

The contributors bring to their chapters a wide range of experience. Each chapter must be regarded as the author's own views even though they may conflict with those expressed elsewhere. This is desirable for it should encourage students to formulate their own ideas in this rapidly developing subject.

My sincere thanks are due to all my colleagues who have so kindly contributed to this book. They have accepted editorial alterations and amendments with the utmost good humour for which I am most grateful.

In particular I wish to acknowledge the valuable help given by Professor D. S. Berman and my thanks go to Mrs. Margot Smart and Miss Irene Rayner who have helped so much in the production of this book.

September 1973 GEOFFREY L. SLACK

Contents

Chapter 1

Dental Health and the Changing Society

Arthur J. Willcocks BCOM, PHD
Professor of Social Administration, University of Nottingham

Beliefs about health and health care are integrally bound into the culture of any society. Dr. Willcocks provides a general view of the way in which health care services have evolved from early times to the present day, when the successful delivery of health care involves an elaborate inter-relationship of numerous specialities. He gives us some insight into the complex motivating forces which decide whether individuals will utilize a health care service, and he indicates that the attitudes of the consumers is a key factor in determining whether a service reaches its objectives.

Dental illness, like all forms of illness, does not exist as a separate phenomenon—it is a feature of people and their suffering. To begin with a truism like this is to risk a measure of ridicule: not to begin so is to miss both the point of this chapter, and of the book as a whole. Indeed, it is to miss the basic starting point of all dental services. Like medicine, dentistry exists to meet the needs of people for dental health at best, or the amelioration of dental pain and the improvement of oral functioning at least. It continues to deserve to exist only so long as it continues, or aspires, to meet these needs. This chapter is, therefore, to remind the reader of, and to put into perspective, the people who need and use the dental services. Its first theme will be about these people, the societies to which they belong, and the attitudes they have towards health care in general and dental health in particular.

After a brief review of the societies in which dental patients live, reference will be made to the developing role of the state in the provision of medical and dental care. This will, of necessity, be brief and will seek for international generalization rather than detailing the history of any one country.

Finally, in this chapter, the services in England and Wales, their costs and methods of operation will, again briefly, be touched on. The aim throughout will be to sketch in a background to what follows, a background which is not to be taken as an embellishment, or a form of decoration. Instead it is a background, a full understanding of which is essential if the working of the dental health services are to be fully appreciated and evaluated.

THE CHANGING SOCIETY

Our first theme then is the changing society: man and his societies have come a long way since the days when nomadic bands roamed the countryside gathering food wherever they could find it. Life was hazardous and hard; the mere task of survival was a full-time one leaving no time for developing any specialized or luxury skills. At some point in time, man began to settle in fixed geographical locations: he became able to cultivate food rather than gather from the wild plants and bushes. As his ability to cultivate food grew, two inter-related things happened. In the first place he became able, with the increasing power available from rudimentary tools and later from domesticated animals, to grow more food than he required for his own and his family's needs. The excess amount of food so produced made the need for the second development: a system of exchange. He became able to exchange, at first on a barter system, and later using a rudimentary form of money, his 'surplus' to 'purchase' other commodities such as clothes. As the surpluses grew and the system of exchange improved it became possible for some men to specialize on making commodities other than food and yet still survive: the producer of clothes exchanging his products for 'money', or directly for food.

Once this rudimentary exchange and specialization began, man began a historical trend which still continues today. At first the release of more and more men from the business of growing food enabled more directly productive specialisms to develop: the blacksmith, the maker of implements, and so on. But available power has greatly increased even more in recent centuries, especially since what in Britain has come to be called the 'industrial revolution' in the early nineteenth century, we have seen a new kind of specialism develop. Specialisms, which are not themselves directly productive of goods or commodities, have developed to support the productive system and those who work in it. Out of this wave of specialization, late in man's presently recorded history, have come occupations like the school teacher, the administrator, the manager, the banker, and the medical man, among many others. The care of people, rather than the production of goods, is a late form of specialization, but the process has not finished there. At first, those who cared for the sick, for example, were all similarly qualified or unqualified. Today, however, caring for the sick is becoming specialized and fragmented between many occupations, and it is in this period that we can see the development of dentistry as a specialized activity. But, still this is not the end of the growth of specialization: there are those who know more and more about smaller and more technical aspects of dental care. As is implied in later chapters, the question which emerges from this rapid review of history is quite clear: where, if at all, will specialization end?

This trend to ever increasing specialization, or division of labour, which is common to all societies, points to one great comment on modern societies. No longer is any one man independent or master of his own destiny: he cannot live off the product of his own labour until someone engages in exchange. If he is playing a part in the production of motor cars, his future will depend on the willingness and ability of others in the process to play their part (a strike of a few paint sprayers can soon bring a vast assembly line employing thousands of workers to a halt), on the willingness and ability of others to buy motor cars, and on society to let them go on buying motor cars. All societies are made up of people increasingly interdependent one on the others; the dentist depends on his supporting ancillaries, on dental manufacturers who make his equipment and materials, and so on. Furthermore, he can only earn his living if people are willing to come to him for treatment, a point we look at later, and are able to afford his treatment. *The health professions are as much a part of man's interdependence as everyone else.*

This growing interdependence arising from the increasing division of labour can be linked to two other aspects of the changing society: urbanization and the rising standards of living. As the nature of agriculture changes and the new form of the working situation, industrialization, grows, so it is more and more necessary for people to live closer together in greater and greater numbers. A country like Britain where a century and a half ago less than a third of its population lived in towns, today finds itself with all but a small minority living in towns, which are themselves getting steadily larger. In a relatively brief period of time, briefer in some countries than others, man has changed his way of living from rural to urban. This creates problems such as overcrowding, the journey to work, pollution, and so on, and serves to highlight others such as poverty, which can no longer pass unnoticed in concentrated urban areas. It also makes possible, by the very concentration of numbers, the development of highly specialized services like dentistry. A person specializing in children's dentistry can easily find enough patients and therefore enough income in large towns: he will find neither in a sparsely populated rural area. In these areas, therefore, if dentistry is to come at all, it must be linked with other skills. Taking a British example from another profession, doctors in sparsely populated rural areas are allowed to combine pharmaceutical duties, albeit of a less specialized kind, with their medical duties, this despite the existence of a qualified pharmaceutical profession. *Urbanization is therefore both a concentration of problems whilst at the same time offering opportunities for specialized solutions.* Conversely in many highly urbanized countries the lot of rural people is often in danger of being forgotten as the services provided are inferior, or the solutions sought are urban solutions.

The other factor associated with specialization is the rising standard of living. Even if one could imagine a highly qualified professional group existing in a primitive society, it would have little work as the 'surplus' available for exchange for each family would be insufficient to afford such 'luxuries'. Specialized care is the luxury of the affluent society: specialization alone makes that affluence possible. *The resultant rising standard of living makes what were once 'luxuries' into everyday necessities.* What, however, the increasing standard of living associated with increasing specialization does not ensure is that all share in that rise. The elderly, the young, and the unskilled may miss out, but they share in the desire for these erstwhile luxuries. Increasingly, therefore, the state finds it necessary to intervene to ensure a fairer sharing of this rising standard of living. Here we are now touching on a topic to be taken up again later in this chapter.

Society is changing in other ways too. The overall population is increasing, and within the general population the relative age-structure of society is changing. Both processes are due, at least in part, to improving methods of health care and to rising standards of living. In almost all countries the expectation of life is rising, more and more people are living sixty-five years or more. Increasingly the more developed countries are having to come to terms with a new problem; the problem of the aged, no longer able to make any positive contribution to the productive processes and becoming more and more dependent on their fellows for even the bare necessities of life. More people with handicaps survive previously fatal deficiences. More people are unable to cope, unaided, with the complex requirements of a modern urban society, and more young people are staying on as dependents for longer periods of education and training. *The productive labour force is coming to be a diminishing proportion of the total population as at the same time the burden of caring for its dependents grows.* At the same time this dependency is becoming more and more costly as standards of care improve. In other words, we are slowly building up a new kind of interdependence, where all of us will at various times in our lives be dependent on others for our care and survival.

The rigid social class structure of rural societies is giving way to a new class structure, based to a large extent on the employer/employee division. Traditional elites are being replaced by new managerial elites, those who control large organizations often without actual ownership. A key factor in understanding these elites, and the continuing changes, is the educational system. Education, once a means of maintaining class structures, is more and more becoming a means whereby upward social mobility is being achieved. The able ones climb through the favoured elements of the educational system to the elite positions of the occupational world. At the same time, the general level of education is rising, a fact which may be gradually changing the attitudes of individuals to many things, including medical and dental care.

Societies, then, are changing in many directions. These changes create conditions where improvements in medical and dental services are possible, where the demand for them increases, and where attitudes towards these services are likely to change.

ATTITUDES

Here again the approach must be one of brief summary. As a starting point in the argument, it can be said that in most medical and dental illness situations it is the 'sick' individual, and not the service who takes the initiative. He or she begins by presenting for treatment, and the service responds, although in the case of regular attendance at a dental service, this sequence does not apply in quite the same way. To take the case of the individual patient, we must glance briefly at the concept of the 'iceberg of disease'. This concept presents the natural iceberg, a large proportion of whose bulk floats unseen below the surface of the water, as an analogy for many illness situations in which a sizeable proportion of those persons who are ill remains unnoticed by the formal health services. Recent studies in Britain (Bulman et al., 1968; Gray et al., 1970) have shown the tremendous extent of this underwater proportion of the iceberg of dental disease.

It is, therefore, worth asking the question why this should be so. Some of the factors may be external rather than internal to the individual. For example, he may be unable to afford the prospective monetary cost, which is usually unpredictable before treatment has actually started, he may be unable to gain access to the appropriate practitioner, or he may be totally unaware of his illness, as is often the case with dental disease. These practical factors may, however, be outweighed by more personal and psychological ones. He may be living in a society whose cultural norms throw scorn on the sick, perhaps regarding sickness as an admission of personal wickedness or weakness. He may regard other solutions as more efficacious, such as cure by folk remedies, religious invocation, or consultation with friends or a medical dictionary. He may not regard the doctor or the dentist as providing the services he thinks he needs. He may not be prepared to face the possible consequences of reporting illness, such as time off work, operative techniques, or hospitalization.

Factors like these outlined will vary from person to person, although it is possible to suggest some generalized patterns of difference. Attitudes vary between the social classes, especially towards dental care, they vary by the age of the person concerned, they may vary by the sex of the person, the education he or she has received and by his or her previous experiences of, and images of, a particular service.

To sum up, the equation of forces which decide whether or not the 'patient' seeks treatment may be in part practical, in part the cultural values of his society, and in part his own personal make-up. The patient's personal attributes will in turn be influenced by physiological, psychological, and sociological factors.

In the case of the decision to seek dental treatment, many of the above general points apply. One point, however, needs underlining and a second point needs adding to. The cultural values a society holds towards oral health are clearly important; dental pain is troublesome but rarely crippling or fatal, so that the determination to seek treatment depends considerably on the value attached to oral health. This factor is, perhaps, uniquely reinforced in that the dental patient has to consider seeking examination or treatment when he is not apparently ill. Rather than waiting for pain to signal the need for treatment, he has, ideally to go to the dentist before such warnings appear. This serves to put greater weight on the importance of personal and cultural values in the preliminaries to a dental visit.

There is one final aspect, and the new dimension mentioned in the last paragraph, to attitudes to dental treatment. Unlike almost all forms of medical care, the dentist can offer a replacement for a diseased organ, a replacement which may seem to the patient likely to be equally effective and having no such painful hazards as natural teeth. Attitudes to dentures, to their inevitability at some age, to their cosmetic appearance, and to their efficiency, will affect the patient's behaviour towards the dental services. Ironically, it could be that increasingly efficient and natural looking dentures may, therefore, discourage the proper use of preventive and restorative dental care.

THE ORGANIZATION OF HEALTH CARE SERVICES

As medical care has moved beyond the stage of a one-practitioner care system to services provided by specialist teams, and has therefore become increasingly costly, two things have happened. In the first place, medical care has become increasingly organized, as only then can the effective delivery of proper and complete care be ensured. Secondly, the burden of cost has lead to consumer groups seeking to provide mutual financial protection either through voluntary insurance systems or, in some countries, through state systems. In this sense state systems can be seen as a compulsory extension of mutual voluntary insurance. In this section, the developing role of the state in provision of health care services will be briefly examined.

It is usually possible to trace, in all developed countries, two stages of state intervention. Some countries show a third stage. The first stage is sometimes labelled the 'public health approach'. During the last century, awareness gradually dawned in many countries of the deleterious nature of much of the physical environment. The environment increasingly came to be seen as a direct cause of illness and disease, or at least as a contributory factor in the spread of disease. If the water supply, the housing, and the sewage system could be made effective and healthful, the chances of disease spreading would be lessened. To do this meant regulation and compulsion, something which only the state could ensure. As was soon discovered in Britain, the 'environment' needed ever wider definition: the food which people ate, the existence of people with infectious diseases, pollution of the air, and the effects of noise in more recent times, all were to come to be seen as part of the environment. Britain and other developed countries increasingly responded with legislation to curb these noxious elements of the wider environment.

In time, however, it was discovered that some mortality and morbidity rates, especially those of the newborn, of the young, and of mothers were not materially improved by this approach. In Britain the discoveries at the beginning of this century of the appalling physical condition of many young men led to the state embarking on the next step, a step we might term the 'personal preventive approach'. If the mother and her children could be supervised, protected, and guided, a healthier start to life would ensure in the long run a healthier total population. This attitude has led to the development of maternal and child health services, school medical services, and school meals services. It was, as part of this stage, that the state's direct interest in the provision of dental services grew. It seemed natural to seek to supervise and safeguard the dental health of children and to provide dental health education. In Britain these steps came in the first two decades of this century, in other countries it came later and in others earlier.

The third and final step, when the state moves in to take over from voluntary insurance systems for the direct provision of curative care, came later again and in relatively few countries. In some of these, as for example in Britain under the National Health Service Act of 1946, the dental care of adults as well as children became part of the state medical care system. Now the state was totally involved in environmental protection, personal preventive services and in the curative care of its citizens, or in some cases of its less wealthy citizens.

THE BRITISH NATIONAL HEALTH SERVICE AND DENTISTRY

The final section of this chapter takes a brief general view of the National Health Service in England and Wales; slightly different provisions apply to Scotland and to Northern Ireland. The system provides health care through three main channels: the hospital services, the personal preventive services, and the Executive Council services. The delivery of dental care under these systems is discussed in full detail by Renson in Chapter 7.

For hospital administration the country is divided into regions, in each of which the planning, development and overall control of the hospital services—and most hospitals are now state owned—is the responsibility of a Regional Hospital Board. Below this level, the day-to-day administration of groups of hospitals is entrusted to Hospital Management Committees. The finance for this service is provided from central government monies.

The personal preventive services, together with those associated with the educational system, are the responsibility of the major local authorities within the normal local government system of the country. Regular inspection and treatment of those in the so-called 'priority' classes—children, young people, and pregnant and nursing mothers—is provided in this way, the finance coming both from central and local taxation.

The third element of the National Health Service is that run by a series of local Executive Councils, responsible for the general medical practitioner service, dental services, pharmaceutical, and ophthalmic services. The money for this service, under which the dentist is renumerated on a fee-for-service basis, comes in part from central monies and in part, in the case of the general public, from patient charges.

About four-fifths of the total cost of the services provided under the National Health Service, including dentistry, comes from central government monies, that is from national taxation funds. The Service, despite the charges paid by some patients, and despite the special contribution towards its cost included with the weekly social security contribution, is largely a tax-borne service. This is perhaps inevitable as no preconditions such as age, sex, insurance status, income, or occupation have to be fulfilled before being entitled to health care treatment under the Service.

The cost of the dental services represented about 10 per cent of the total cost of the National Health Service in 1949, but this proportion fell to around 5·5 per cent by 1953 and has remained around that figure since then (Office of Health Economics, 1966). The high early figure chiefly resulted from high pent-up demand for a free service. The subsequent satisfaction of immediate demands, reduction of fees paid to dentists, and the imposition of patients' charges reduced the proportion as did rising expenditure in other parts of the service. Despite the levelling out in the proportional expenditure on dental care, the demand for dental treatment has continued to rise steadily.

The National Health Service, therefore, provides dental services under three separate administrations. Five-sixths of their total costs are borne by the state and one-sixth by the patient. The utilization of the dental services has steadily increased, but despite this increase there are large numbers of adults who do not seek dental treatment at the right time. Britain, like other developed countries, is caught up in the changing nature of society, in its interdependence, and in its increasing specialization: it has come to rely on a state-provided system to meet its health problems. That it has not yet completely succeeded, that many people are still not seeking appropriate dental care, is both a product of manpower difficulties and also of the attitudes and the cultural norms of a society which still does not set a very high price on its values of full dental fitness.

REFERENCES

BULMAN, J. S., RICHARDS, N. D., SLACK, G. L., and WILLCOCKS, A. J. (1968), *Demand and Need for Dental Care; a Socio-dental Study*. London: Oxford University Press and Nuffield Provincial Hospitals Trust.

GRAY, P. G., TODD, J. E., SLACK, G. L., and BULMAN, J. S. (1970), *Adult Dental Health in England and Wales in 1968*. London: H.M.S.O.

OFFICE OF HEALTH ECONOMICS (1966), *The Dental Service*. London: Office of Health Economics.

FURTHER READING

LINDSEY, A. (1962), *Socialized Medicine in England and Wales: The National Health Service 1948–1961*. Chapel Hill, N.C.: University of North Carolina Press.

MARSHALL, T. H. (1965), *Social Policy*. London: Hutchinson.

RICHARDS, N. D., and WILLCOCKS, A. J. (1966), 'The level of dental health: The field for study', in *Nuffield Provincial Hospitals Trust. Problems and Progress in Medical Care*, 2nd Series. London: Oxford University Press.

SUSSER, M. W., and WATSON, W. (1962), *Sociology in Medicine*. London: Oxford University Press.

TITMUSS, R. M. (1958), *Essays on the Welfare State*. London: Allen Unwin.

WILLCOCKS, A. J. (1967), *The Creation of the National Health Service: a Study of Pressure Groups and a Major Social Policy Decision*. London: Routledge & Kegan Paul.

Chapter 2

Prevention in Dental Public Health

William D. McHugh DDSC, FDSRCS
Director, Eastman Dental Center and Associate Dean for Dental Affairs, University of Rochester, NY, USA

Public dental health programmes seek to achieve dental health in a specified population, and so their administration should involve prevention, treatment, and education, and supporting research activities. It is accepted that in any society, a treatment programme without a preventive component can never achieve the long-term objective of dental health for all.

Professor McHugh reviews the currently available mechanisms for preventing the two most prevalent dental diseases, periodontal disease and dental caries. He assesses their efficacy, and their implementation, for the individual patient and for the community as a whole.

The twentieth century has seen a steady increase in the amount of treatment provided by the dental profession in most parts of the world. The rate of increase has been particularly dramatic in the past decade, with improvements in methods of cutting teeth, in analgesia, and in restorative materials, and with greater and more efficient use of ancillary personnel. The effect of this trend has, however, been largely offset by the continued increase in the prevalence of the two major dental diseases: caries and periodontal disease.

Surveys in various parts of the world have shown that, taking the community as a whole, a high proportion of dental disease goes untreated (Hollinshead, 1961; Bulman et al., 1968).

It is apparent that the traditional approach to dental disease, treating disease as it develops, has not been effective and that expansion of treatment facilities would be both difficult and almost prohibitively expensive. Fortunately, preventive methods which are effective and economic have been developed, and these provide an attractive alternative, or rather a supplement to traditional methods. It must be appreciated that the complete prevention of dental disease on a community basis, by any method or combination of methods, is not yet possible. Until it is, the best approach will lie in combining and integrating preventive and therapeutic measures to bring dental diseases under control. Although demonstrated only on a limited basis (Waterman, 1956; Freire, 1964), there is already evidence that such a combination can be very effective.

Certainly, if a dental care programme is ever to reach its long-term goal of dental health for all, it must have a basis in prevention of disease rather than treatment of its consequences. For that reason, methods of prevention will be considered prior to the epidemiology and treatment of dental disease.

PREVENTION OF PERIODONTAL DISEASE

Periodontal disease is primarily due to bacterial products causing breakdown of the periodontal tissues. Methods of prevention can be directed towards eliminating or controlling the bacteria which produce the disease, or to increasing the resistance of the periodontal tissues to these bacterial products.

Dental plaque forming in or close to the gingival sulcus is the primary source of bacterial toxins. Plaque has been shown to consist predominantly of micro-organisms (Socransky et al., 1963). The types and numbers of organisms vary considerably with the age of the plaque (Carlsson and Egelberg, 1965; Theilade et al., 1966; Ritz, 1967), between individuals, between different teeth in the same mouth, and even in different layers of plaque (Ritz, 1967). Efforts to identify a particular type or group of organisms producing periodontal disease have failed. The balance of current evidence suggests that periodontal disease can be produced by a variety of types of organism, that a mixed flora is usually involved, and that the quantity as well as the mere presence of plaque is of major importance.

Methods of preventing periodontal disease are directed at preventing or controlling plaque formation and/or at increasing tissue resistance to disease.

If oral hygiene is defined as 'methods and procedures for the removal of soft deposits from the teeth and surrounding tissues', it can be divided into two types: natural and mechanical.

DETERSIVE FOODS

It has long been assumed that hard or detersive foods have a valuable cleansing action and remove plaque and food debris from the teeth and surrounding tissue. Only recently, however, has this hypothesis been subjected to scientific evaluation. Dogs fed a hard diet consisting of lumps of bovine trachea were found to develop less plaque on the buccal surfaces of their teeth than control animals on a soft diet (Egelberg, 1965). Studies on human subjects who stop toothbrushing have shown, however, that the development of plaque and gingivitis is as rapid in those who eat three large raw carrots, three times a day, as in those who do not follow this regimen (Lindhe and Wicén, 1969). Other studies by Venning (1965) and Bergenholtz et al. (1967) have reached similar conclusions. Thus, the chewing of detersive foods does *not* appear to have any significant plaque-preventing effect in man.

MECHANICAL ORAL HYGIENE

The classical method of cleaning the teeth is by regular use of a toothbrush and toothpaste or other devices such as chewing sticks, wood points, or dental floss. It has been shown that careful toothbrushing can keep the teeth free from plaque and maintain the gingivae in a state of clinical health (Löe et al., 1965; Theilade et al., 1966). Conversely it has been shown that, if normal toothbrushing is discontinued, plaque develops on the teeth within a few hours, and previously healthy gingivae show clinical signs of inflammation within seven to twelve days (Theilade et al., 1966).

Well-motivated patients who have been instructed in effective oral hygiene techniques can keep their mouths almost free from plaque and gingivitis (Lövdal et al., 1961; Lindhe et al., 1966; Lightner et al., 1968; Suomi et al., 1969). There is, however, a considerable amount of evidence that common standards of oral hygiene do not reach this level (McHugh et al., 1964; Bratthall, 1966; Bay, 1967; Ånerud, 1970).

More frequent brushing tends to give better plaque control and improved gingival health (Greene and Vermillion, 1960; McHugh et al., 1964) but there is recent evidence indicating that, as far as maintaining gingival health is concerned, the *efficiency* of toothbrushing may be more important than its frequency since thorough cleaning once every second day will maintain gingival health (Kelner et al., 1973; Lang et al., 1973). The two factors of frequency and efficiency are obviously inter-related, but it seems that the traditional concentration on frequency of brushing should be superseded by equal interests in both frequency and the *care* with which brushing is performed.

One should, however, remember that there is a progressive improvement in gingival health with improvement in plaque control, so that *any* improvement in the efficiency of oral hygiene is of value.

Toothbrushes Although toothbrushes have been in use for many centuries, their general design has not varied much and we still lack concrete information about the relative merits of various types of brush, and the practical significance of variation in hardness, and of bristle or nylon filaments. There is no clear evidence of the superiority of any particular design of toothbrush nor has any difference in cleaning efficiency between nylon and natural bristle brushes been established (Skinner and Takata, 1951; Mooser, 1959; Greene, 1966).

Mechanical toothbrushes driven by electric motors have become widely used in recent years and early studies indicated that they cleaned better than the traditional hand toothbrushes. Subsequent studies lasting over one or two years have shown that, although there is an early advantage, probably related to the 'novelty' of the electrically-driven brush, this is lost within a few months, and thereafter the mechanical brush is not superior to the hand brush in normal use (Ash, 1964; Greene, 1966; McKendrick et al., 1968). The only exception is for those with a physical or mental handicap, for whom the mechanical brush is of great value.

Toothpastes are of significant value as an adjunct to toothbrushing, making the procedure more pleasant and more efficient (Mooser, 1959). The practical effects of variations in abrasiveness and other factors have not been established, and there is a real need for clinical evaluation of such factors. The addition of therapeutic agents to toothpastes has been tried, and, although their value in caries prevention is well-documented and will be described later, none has been shown to have significant value in the prevention or control of periodontal disease.

CHEMICAL PLAQUE CONTROL

Major advances in recent years in our knowledge of the bacterial nature of plaque and of its biochemical components have led to the testing of other methods of plaque control.

Antibacterial agents have been tried over a number of years, although, as Miller (1889) discovered, most antiseptics are too toxic or have such other undesirable effects that they are not satisfactory for this purpose. Mühlemann and his associates carried out clinical tests with a large series of antibacterial agents (Schroeder, 1969). They found that chlorhexidine was the most effective, and recent studies have shown that twice daily rinses with 0·2 per cent chlorhexidine gluconate will prevent plaque formation and the development of gingivitis (Löe and Schiott, 1970).This agent has only been used experimentally for relatively short periods of time, and much more work is necessary to establish its safety and the absence of undesirable side effects before it can be used in clinical practice. It seems, however, that agents of this type have great future value.

Antibiotics have been tested for their effect on the development of plaque. Penicillin and tetracycline have been shown to inhibit plaque formation in animals (Fitzgerald, 1955; Mühlemann et al., 1961; Larson et al., 1963; Keyes, 1966) as do spiramycin and vancomycin (Keyes et al., 1966). Thrice daily rinses of 0·25 per cent vancomycin were not found to have any significant effect on plaque development in human subjects, however (Jensen et al., 1968).

These studies are interesting and are of particular value in studying the effect of selective suppression of different types of plaque micro-organisms. Long-term use of low concentrations of antibiotics tends to induce sensitivity and the development of resistant strains of micro-organisms so that their practical value in preventing plaque formation and gingivitis seems unlikely to be significant.

Enzymes have been tested for their effect on dental plaque, but early results were discouraging (Stewart, 1952; Jensen, 1959; Ennever and Sturzenberger, 1961; Packman et al., 1963; Baumhammers et al., 1968). The discovery by Gibbons and Banghart (1967) that the matrix of dental plaque consists largely of extracellular polysaccharides which are polymers of glucose and fructose gave considerable impetus to work in this area. These extracellular polysaccharides are thought to be important in the cohesion of plaque bacteria and in their adhesion to the tooth surface. It has been shown that the enzyme dextranase will sever the linkages in dextrans which are one type of glucose polymers found in plaque. Feeding this enzyme in food and water to hamsters resulted in a marked reduction in plaque formation and in caries (Fitzgerald et al., 1968). Other work showed, however, that dextranase was not effective in rats which already had an indigenous caries-active flora (Guggenheim et al., 1966) and trials on human subjects have produced disappointing results (Caldwell et al., 1971; Keyes et al., 1971; Lobene, 1971). The lack of clinical effectiveness seems to be due to the high degree of specificity of the enzyme and the variety of dextrans and other glucans found in human dental plaque. Unless some enzyme or combination of enzymes can be found which is effective against all or most of these glucans, clinical plaque control by enzymes will not be practical.

Surface-acting agents which affect the surface tension of the teeth have been tested for their effect on plaque formation. Coating with sulphonated polystyrene (Schaffer et al., 1964) or with silicone (Bowen, 1970) has produced disappointing results. Plaque will form *in vivo* on layers of silicone so that the value of reducing surface tension is questionable.

It is interesting to note in this connexion that water fluoridation tends to reduce both the surface energy of enamel (Glantz, 1969) and its tendency to adsorb proteins (Ericson and Ericsson, 1967). It has not, however, been shown to have any effect on plaque formation.

Increasing Tissue Resistance The resistance of the periodontal tissues to disease varies considerably between individuals and, to a lesser extent, between certain racial and ethnic groups. These differences have not been satisfactorily explained.

Nutrition varies, sometimes dramatically, between developed and less-developed countries, but epidemiological studies comparing the incidence and severity of periodontal disease in adequately nourished and undernourished populations have not found significant differences (Ramfjord, 1961; Russell et al., 1961). The only clear evidence of the significance of general nutrition comes from a study by Pindborg et al.

(1967) in Bangalore, India, of children aged 1–5 years with kwashiorkor: a disease caused by severe protein deficiency. When groups were matched for age and oral hygiene, it was found that the kwashiorkor group had significantly more periodontal disease (PI = 1·52) than the control group (PI = 1·06). Attempts to relate the severity of periodontal disease to deficiency of specific vitamins or other nutritional factors have shown little difference (Russell, 1962).

The only diseases which appear to have a significant direct effect on periodontal disease are diabetes mellitus and cirrhosis of the liver. Studies of 5300 hospitalized patients by Sandler and Stahl (1960) failed to show significant differences in periodontal disease scores between groups with respiratory disease, e.g., tuberculosis, nervous disease, kidney or liver dysfunction, gastro-intestinal tract disease or various other types of disease. Only patients with diabetes mellitus or liver cirrhosis have a greater incidence and severity of periodontitis (Sheridan et al., 1959; Sandler and Stahl, 1960).

Thus, in spite of frequent assumptions to the contrary, general nutritional status, and even the presence of severe chronic disease in other systems of the body, have little, if any, effect on the prevalence of periodontal disease. Equally, it has not been established that supplements of any vitamin or dietary factor are of significant value in increasing the resistance of the periodontal tissues.

Gingival massage has long been advocated as a means of increasing local resistance, and can be produced with a toothbrush, wood sticks, cloth or various special gadgets. It increases the amount of keratinization of the attached gingival epithelium (Robinson and Kitchin, 1948; Stahl et al., 1953; Merzel et al., 1963) and increases the rate of cell turnover in gingival epithelium and connective tissue (Bertolini, 1955; McHugh, 1967). There is, however, no direct evidence that these changes are beneficial. Gingivitis starts with a breach of the epithelium lining the gingival sulcus and this is not keratinized (McHugh, 1964). It is difficult to see how increased keratinization of the attached gingivae will be of significance, since only at a late stage is this area involved in the disease process.

Thus, although massage has been shown to cause specific changes in the gingivae, its value is not established. All of the massaging techniques remove plaque at the same time and it seems likely that therein lies their value.

Immune reactions in the gingivae have long been suspected, and it seemed possible that some means might be found to stimulate them and thus 'immunize' the individual against periodontal disease. Recently, it has been shown, however, that hypersensitivity reactions are involved (Ranney, 1970; Ranney and Zander, 1970; Nisengard and Beutner, 1970). Thus, although immune reactions may initially be favourable to the host, the hypersensitivity induced by repeated challenge with the same bacterial antigen will probably lead to more rapid progress of the disease.

There is much current interest in this field, and, as more becomes understood about immune reactions in the gingivae, it may well be possible to modify these to the benefit of our patients.

PREVENTION OF DENTAL CARIES

Dental caries is a destructive disease of the hard tissues of the teeth and there is good evidence that it is initiated by acids produced by the fermentation of carbohydrate substrates by bacteria in dental plaque. The role of other factors, such as chelation and bacterial enzyme action, is somewhat controversial, but they are probably of little significance in the aetiology of enamel caries.

Dental plaque seems to be essential for the development of caries. It provides the bacteria and the conditions under which they can be supplied with carbohydrate substrates and allowed to ferment them. Plaque also localizes the resultant acid on the tooth surface, preventing its dilution and buffering by the saliva. It contains a great variety of types of micro-organisms, many of which can ferment carbohydrates to produce acid. No specific micro-organism has yet been identified as the 'causative agent' in caries, and, indeed, a number of different micro-organisms have been shown to be capable of producing caries under experimental conditions. On the evidence currently available, it seems that any one of a variety of micro-organisms can cause caries, that mixed cultures are usually associated with the disease, and that streptococci predominate in caries-related plaque.

A number of methods have been shown to be at least partly effective in preventing dental caries. The most effective method, at least on a community basis, is water fluoridation, which will be dealt with in the next chapter. Other methods involve diet, oral hygiene, restorative dentistry, or the topical application of fissure sealants or preventive agents to the teeth. These will now be considered individually.

DIET

There are two components of diet which have a significant relationship to dental caries: its nutritive value and its local action in the mouth.

Nutrition is, of course, of fundamental importance to the general development, growth, and health of the individual. In the early years of this century it was shown that inadequate nutrition during childhood interferes with tooth development, leading to gross or microscopic defects in enamel, either hypoplasia or hypomineralization (Mellanby, 1934). It was assumed that the more perfect a tooth, the more resistant it would be to caries, and great emphasis was, therefore, placed on nutrition. The relative caries-resistance of grossly hypoplastic teeth (Day and Sedwick, 1934; Staz, 1944) and other evidence has shown, however, that 'clinically perfect' teeth are not more caries-resistant than their defective neighbours.

Nutritional influences are greatest during tooth development. Apart from fluoride and possibly other trace elements such as strontium, molybdenum, lithium, boron, and selenium, the only nutritional factor which has been shown to have a direct effect on subsequent susceptibility to caries is vitamin D (Shaw, 1952). Severe protein deficiency causes delay in tooth eruption (Shaw and Griffiths, 1963; Sweeney and Guzman, 1966) and may lead to slightly increased susceptibility to caries.

Studies of caries-free recruits to the US Navy have shown that a high proportion of them come from geographic areas with drinking-water containing relatively high levels of strontium, molybdenum, lithium, and boron, and low levels of selenium (Losee and Adkins, 1969). There is evidence that the method of cooking or preparation of vegetables has a major effect on the consumption of trace elements (Losee and Adkins, 1971). This is potentially a very fruitful field of research which may yield information of considerable practical value in the near future.

Thus, while good nutrition should certainly be encouraged, its significance for caries susceptibility appears limited. Apart from the effects of trace elements, particularly fluorine, the range of nutrition commonly found today seems to bear little relationship to caries.

Local Effect of Diet Although its nutritive value probably has little effect on dental caries, food has a dramatic local effect on the teeth. The classical study of this effect was conducted at the Vipeholm Hospital in Sweden by Gustafsson et al. (1954). Four hundred and thirty-six young adult patients were divided into groups and fed varying diets for a total 5-year period. The major differences between these diets were in the presence, type and amount of carbohydrate eaten between meals. It was found that the control group on the basic Swedish diet, and other groups given supplements of bread or sucrose at meal-times, developed relatively little caries ($<$ 2 DMF teeth) during the 5-year period.

Groups given toffees, chocolate, or caramel *between meals*, however, developed large amounts of new caries. The largest amount of new caries was found in the group eating the greatest amount of sticky toffee; this consisted of 24 large toffees each day! When between-meals eating was discontinued, the caries increment in the following year was much smaller, being of a similar order to that found in the control group.

A complementary study by Lundqvist (1952) attempted to establish the 'oral sugar clearance time' of common foodstuffs and thus to grade their cariogenicity. The foods containing sucrose and with the greatest tendency to stick to the teeth appeared most cariogenic.

Additional evidence linking frequent consumption of carbohydrates with caries has been provided by studies of preschool children (Weiss and Trithart, 1960) and, indirectly, by studies of patients with hereditary fructose intolerance. A review of 11 patients with this rare disease, which makes consumption of sugar potentially fatal, revealed that, although their age at examination ranged from 7 to 41 years, half had no caries and the others very little (Marthaler, 1967).

The other side of the coin has been shown by Bradford and Crabb (1961), who found that the caries prevalence in groups of dentists' children who had *not* had between-meals snacks was considerably lower than that in comparable groups of dentists' children to whom between-meal snacks had been available. This study has additional value in that it shows that some dentists practice restriction of between-meal snacks (i.e., what they preach!) and that the dental health of their children is vastly improved as a result.

Phosphate supplements to the diet have been shown, in recent years, to lead to significant reductions in the incidence of caries in experimental animals (Nizel and Harris, 1964). Human studies have shown variable but encouraging results (Lilienthal et al., 1966) and their continuation will be watched with interest.

ORAL HYGIENE

The belief that 'a clean tooth never decays' has become hallowed by time and constant repetition, but is not supported by clinical studies. The first major scientific study of the relationship of oral hygiene to caries was carried out by Fosdick (1950). University students were taught effective toothbrushing methods and advised to brush within 10 minutes of eating. Those who continued on this regimen were examined at intervals and, after 2 years, were found to have about half as much caries as a control group.

More recent studies were carried out on groups of Swedish children who were initially 9–11 years of age (Koch and Lindhe, 1970). The children were taught how to brush their teeth and brushed under supervision once every school day. After 3 years on this regimen their mouths were markedly cleaner, i.e., their plaque index was lower, than those of children in a control group. In spite of this, there was no significant reduction in dental caries. Even more discouraging is the finding, two years after the supervision ceased, that even the oral hygiene had deteriorated and it and caries prevalence did not differ significantly from that in the other control group.

Epidemiological studies of large groups of children have shown no significant correlation between caries prevalence and the range of oral hygiene commonly found in children (McHugh et al., 1964).

While detersive foodstuffs such as apples, celery, or raw carrots, have long been advocated for their cleansing effect, it has been shown that they are *not* effective plaque-removing agents (Venning, 1965; Bergenholtz et al., 1967; Lindhe and Wicén, 1969). The only scientific study of the effect of detersive foodstuffs on caries incidence was carried out by Slack and Martin (1958) who studied the effect on children of eating pieces of apple after every meal. After 2 years, they found evidence of increased cleanliness and less gingivitis; there was some evidence of reduced caries incidence, but as this was small and the final groups were small, it was of doubtful significance.

On current evidence, it appears that a high standard of oral hygiene with brushing very soon after meals will have a significant anti-caries effect. Large clinical trials and epidemiological studies indicate, however, that it is unrealistic to expect that the necessary standard will be achieved by other than a very small proportion of the population.

TOPICAL APPLICATION OF FLUORIDE COMPOUNDS

Once the correlation between fluorine intake and dental caries experience had been established, it was but a short step to study the effect of applications of fluoride solutions to erupted teeth. Early studies used sodium fluoride, the salt used most commonly in water fluoridation, and showed a worthwhile reduction (Bibby, 1944; Galagan and Knutson, 1947). They involved fairly frequent applications at intervals of 2–6 months and a fairly exacting and time-consuming technique. The results of these and some later studies of topical application of sodium fluoride are summarized in Table 1. This is, by no means, a comprehensive list as the number of such studies is now very large. From the table, however, it is apparent that more recent studies have used 2 per cent NaF applied at 6-monthly intervals. Where the water supply did not contain optimal levels of fluorine, a worthwhile caries reduction was found in almost every case and this averaged $>$20 per cent. Where the water supply did contain an adequate amount of fluorine, the effect was slight and of doubtful significance (Downs and Pelton, 1950; Galagan and Vermillion, 1955).

Research into other fluoride compounds gave encouraging laboratory evidence of their effect on the acid-solubility of enamel and several have been used in clinical trials. Those most widely used have been stannous fluoride and acidulated phosphate-fluoride.

Stannous fluoride was first used as a result of the work of Dr. J. C. Muhler, of Indiana. Table 2 summarizes the results of clinical trials with this agent, and, here again, is only a sample of the more than 50 clinical studies.

In general, 8 per cent SnF_2 has been used, as early studies by Slack (1956) showed that the 2 per cent solution was somewhat less effective. While it may appear, from Table 2, that stannous fluoride is much more effective as an anti-caries agent than sodium fluoride, this may not be true. The studies tend to fall into two distinct groups: those by Muhler and his colleagues in which caries reductions of 50–81 per cent were observed in areas without optimal fluoride and those of other investigators who obtain reductions of 4–26 per cent in similar areas. A similar divergence of data is apparent in studies in areas *with* adequate water fluorine where the Indiana group has obtained reductions of 31–54 per cent compared with reductions of 10–21 per cent observed elsewhere.

TABLE 1

Clinical studies of topical NaF applications

Reference	*Optimal water fluoride*	*Initial age of subjects*	*Percentage of NaF*	*No. of applications*	*Years after initial application*	*Percentage of caries reduction DMFT*	*DMFS*
Bibby (1944)	No	10–12	0·1	3	1	—	46
				6	2	—	28
Galagan and Knutson (1947)	No	7–15	2	2	1	22	14
				4	1	41	34
				6	1	41	28
Davies (1950)	No	9–12	2	4	1	—	58
Downs and Pelton (1950)	Yes	6–18	2	4	1	—	—
Galagan and Vermillion (1955)	Yes	7–16	2	4	1	9	—
Law et al. (1961)	No	7–13	2	4	1	35	35
Torell and Ericsson (1965)	No	10	2	4	2	—	20
Cons et al. (1970)	No	6–11	2	4	3	Not significant	Not significant

TABLE 2

Clinical studies of topical applications of 8 per cent SnF_2

Reference	Optimal water fluoride	Initial age of subjects	No. of applications	Years after initial application	Percentage of caries reduction DMFT	DMFS
Muhler (1960)	Yes	6–17	1	0·5	35	36
			2	1	35	31
Muhler (1960)	Yes	6–17	3	1·5	36	36
			4	2	46	35
			5	2·5	54	50
Mercer and Muhler (1961)	No	6–14	1	1	50	51
			2	1	53	53
Law et al. (1961)	No	7–13	1	1	19	25
Peterson and Williamson (1962)	No	9–13	2	2	26	24
Harris (1963)	No	7–12	1	3	24	—
Mercer and Muhler (1964)	No	5–15	1	1	81	78
				2	68	69
Torell and Ericsson (1965)	No	10	1	2	—	4
Horowitz and Heifetz (1969)	Yes	7–9	1	2	17	10
			2	2	20	12
			3	3	21	21
Cons et al. (1970)	No	6–11	3	3	Not significant	Not significant

TABLE 3

Clinical studies of topical applications of acidulated phosphate–fluoride

Reference	Initial age of subjects	Optimal water fluoride	Agent: Composition	Agent: pH	No. of applications	Years after initial application	Percentage of caries: DMFT	Percentage of caries: DMFS
Wellock and Brudevold (1963)	8–11	No	1·2 per cent (NaF + HF) 0·1m. H_3PO_4	2·8	1 2	1 2	55 67	71 70
Pameijer et al. (1963)	4–10	No	2 per cent NaF 0·15m. $H_3\ PO_4$	3–3·5	4	0·25–1·25	—	51
Wellock et al. (1965)	8–12	No	1·2 per cent (NaF + HF) 0·1m. H_3PO_4	3·5	1 2	1 2	44 44	46 52
Muhler et al. (1965)	6–13	No	8 per cent SnF_2 + 8 per cent NaH_2PO_4	3	2	1	66	67
	6–13	No	3·6 per cent NaF + 1·8 per cent K_2HPO_4	6	2	1	51	51
Averill et al. (1967)	7–11	No	2 per cent NaF + H_3PO_4 + NaH_2PO_4	4·4	4	2	Not significant	Not significant
Cons et al. (1970)	6–11	No	1·2 per cent F(NaF + HF) 0·1m. H_3PO_4	3	3	3	Not significant	Not significant

Analysis of published data offers no ready explanation for these differences between groups of workers. The techniques of application, composition of the solution, and methods of collection and analysis of caries data all appear similar.

It should be noted that a number of studies involved either single applications of stannous fluoride or applications at only yearly intervals, and that, even under these conditions, significant reductions in caries were achieved. Another important point is that, even in areas with adequate fluorine in the drinking-water, applications of 8 per cent stannous fluoride at 6-monthly or yearly intervals do appear to have a slight additional anti-caries effect (Muhler, 1960; Horowitz and Heifetz, 1969).

The use of *acidulated phosphate-fluoride* is based on the fact that the uptake of fluorine is much greater at low *p*H levels. Acidulated fluoride solutions were tried a number of years ago by Roberts et al. (1948) and their use has been greatly stimulated by the work of Dr. Finn Brudevold and his colleagues in Boston. Data from a number of studies with acidulated phosphate–fluoride solutions is summarized in Table 3. Variations in both the composition of the solution and frequency of application should be noted with, again, a wide range of reported reduction in caries incidence. With the exception of the study by Averill et al. (1967), all show fairly high reductions. All of these studies were in areas with drinking-water containing less than the optimal amount of fluorine.

Other fluoride compounds have also been tested in laboratory studies, although experience with their clinical use is still rather limited. The apparent value of potassium fluoride in early studies was not supported by subsequent trials, and other agents, such as lead fluoride, ferric fluoride, stannous chlorofluoride, potassium fluorostannite, sodium silicofluoride, sodium monofluorophosphate, and zirconium fluoride have been found to be either ineffective or less effective than sodium fluoride or stannous fluoride. Stannous hexafluorozirconate has given very promising results in its first clinical trial (Table 4) and the results of further studies will be watched with great interest.

Laboratory studies have shown that titanium fluoride is much more effective in reducing enamel solubility than other agents including NaF, SnF_2, $Sn\,ZrF_6$, ZrF_4 and acidulated phosphate-fluoride (Shrestha, 1970) and clinical trials with this agent are planned. The search for more effective topical agents continues and, almost certainly, improvements will result.

FLUORIDE GELS

One of the problems associated with topical application is keeping the solution in contact with the teeth for sufficient time for adequate amounts of fluorine (and other ions) to be taken up by the enamel. In an effort to overcome this, fluoride gels which adhere to the teeth have been developed. To further simplify the application procedure, these have

TABLE 4

Clinical studies with other fluoride compounds

Reference	*Optimal water fluoride*	*Compound*	*Percentage of fluoride*	*Initial age of subjects*	*No. of applications*	*Years after initial application*	*Percentage of caries reduction*	
							DMFT	*DMFS*
Berggren and Welander (1964)	No	ZrF	0·25	10	5	2	17	—
	No	FeF_3	0·56	10	5	2	33	—
Muhler et al. (1968)	No	$SnZrF_6$	16	5–15	2	1	81	76
	No	$SnZrF_6$	24	5–15	1	1	65	65

TABLE 5

Clinical studies with acidulated phosphate–fluoride gels

Reference	*Optimal water fluoride*	*Initial age of subjects*	*Method of application*	*No. of applications*	*Years after initial application*	*Percentage of caries reduction*	
						DMFT	*DMFS*
Szwejda et al. (1967)	No	7	Foam rubber trays	1	1	Not significant	Not significant
Horowitz (1968)	No	10–11	Cotton-lined wax trays	1	1	12	14
Bryan and Williams (1968)	No	8–12	Wax trays	1	1	45	28
Horowitz (1969)	No	10–11	Cotton-lined wax trays	2	2	12	22
Cons et al. (1970)	No	6–11	Wax trays	3	3	25	18

been used in impression-type trays which the patient can insert, and in some cases treat all teeth in both arches simultaneously. This approach has only had limited use in clinical trials to date and data from these is summarized in Table 5. Only acidulated phosphate–fluorides have been used in this way, and, as can be seen by comparing this data with that in Table 3, the caries reductions have been less than with topically applied aqueous solutions. Nevertheless, any method which simplifies the technique of application or makes self-treatment possible has important implications for cost-effectiveness ratios and community programmes.

FLUORIDE RINSES

Rinsing with fluoride solutions has been tried as a means of treating large groups of children at minimal cost. Most clinical studies utilizing fluoride rinses have been carried out in Scandinavia where the water supplies are, with rare exceptions, deficient in fluorine. Table 6 summarizes some recent studies using fluoride rinses. It will be seen that sodium fluoride in concentrations 0·1 per cent to 0·5 per cent is the most common agent and that the frequency of rinsing varies from daily to once every four months. The advantage of sodium fluoride over stannous fluoride with this method of application is that it is stable and easily prepared. The rinsing was supervised in most studies by dental assistants or schoolteachers. The numbers of subjects varied in the different trials, with the largest being the 40,000 children followed for 5 years by Torell and Ericsson (1967).

While there are the same wide variations between different studies as were found with direct topical application, every study involving rinsing at monthly or 2-weekly intervals with 0·2 per cent or 0·5 per cent NaF resulted in a reduction in caries incidence of at least 20 per cent. In the only study in which children were examined 2 years after cessation of rinsing, however, there was no difference between control and test groups (Koch and Lindhe, 1970).

FLUORIDATED PROPHYLACTIC PASTES

The use of a dental prophylaxis paste containing fluoride was first proposed by Bibby et al. (1946), who found that 2–3 prophylaxes with a paste containing 4 per cent NaF gave reductions in caries incidence of 25–42 per cent. Subsequent studies have utilized stannous fluoride in concentrations of 9–18 per cent, and 6-monthly prophylaxes with this paste have given caries reductions of 30–42 per cent (Bixler and Muhler, 1964; Gish and Muhler, 1965). Yearly application of pastes containing acidulated phosphate–fluoride or a SnF_2 zirconium silicate abrasive prophylaxis system have been reported to give reductions of 14–17 per cent in non-fluoride areas, and, surprisingly, reductions of 6–19 per cent in areas with optimal water fluoridation (Peterson et al., 1969).

TABLE 6

Clinical studies with fluoride rinses

Reference	*Agent*	*Fluoride concentration (percentage)*	*Frequency of rinsing*	*Initial age of subjects*	*Years after initial application*	*Percentage of caries reduction*	
						DMFT	*DMFS*
Torell and Siberg (1962)	NaF	0·2	Monthly	8–9	1	—	21
Berggren and Welander (1964)	NaF	0·5	Five times in 2 years	10	2	19	—
	ZrF_4	0·25	Five times in 2 years	10	2	17	—
	FeF_3	0·56	Five times in 2 years	10	2	33	—
Forsman (1965)	NaF	0·2	Twice monthly	10–12	1	—	50
					2	—	80
Torell and Ericsson (1967)	NaF	0·2	Twice monthly	6–15	5	—	51
Ollinen (1966)	NaF	0·5	Monthly	—	$3\frac{1}{2}$	—	64
Kasakura (1966)	NaF	0·1	Daily	10–11	2	60	92
Horowitz (1968 and 1969)	NaF + PO_4(*p*H 3)	0·6	Five times per year	11–14	2	8	8
	NaF + PO_4(*p*H 3)	0·6	Five times per year	11–14	2	+9	2
	NaF + PO_4(*p*H 3)	1·2	Five times per year	11–14	2	9	5
Koch (1967)	NaF	0·5	Twice monthly for 3 years	10	3	—	25
					5	—	—

TABLE 7

Clinical studies of the application of fluoride solutions by toothbrushing

Reference	*Agent*	*Fluoride concentration (percentage)*	*Frequency of brushing*	*Initial age of subjects*	*Years after initial application*	*Percentage of caries reduction*	
						DMFT	*DMFS*
Goaz et al. (1963)	Na_2PO_3F	6	Daily	7–14	1	—	42
Berggren and Welander (1964)	NaF	0·5	Five times in 2 years	10	2	19	—
	ZrF_4	0·25	Five times in 2 years	10	2	17	—
	FeF_3	0·56	Five times in 2 years	10	2	33	—
Hundstadbraaten (1966)	NaF	1	Four times per year	7–13	3	—	43
Conchie et al. (1969)	NaF + PO_4 (*p*H 3)	1·2	Nine times in 2 years	12–13	1	18	17
					2	23	24
					3	24	25

TOOTHBRUSHING WITH FLUORIDE SOLUTIONS

In an attempt to increase the effectiveness of fluoride rinses, some workers have had children brush with the solution rather than merely rinse with it. The results of some of these studies are summarized in Table 7.

A wide variation between the results of different trials is once again apparent. This may be partly due to variations in the type or concentration of fluoride solution used, or in the frequency of brushing. All studies, however, do show a reduction in caries incidence of 17 per cent or better. In the study of Berggren and Welander (1964) it was found that, whichever of the three fluoride solutions was used, brushing twice a year did not result in a significant reduction in caries incidence, whereas brushing five times a year did.

TOOTHPASTES

Toothpastes are valuable adjuncts to oral hygiene as they make brushing more pleasant and more effective. Attempts have been made at various times to add 'therapeutic' agents to toothpastes with the object of interfering with the oral flora, limiting plaque formation, or making the teeth more resistant to caries.

Chlorophyll was one of the earliest of these agents, and is still present in some toothpastes today. Although *in vitro* tests showed that chlorophyll-containing toothpaste limits bacterial growth, clinical trials have not shown any anti-caries effect.

Ammoniated toothpastes, usually containing urea, were produced in an attempt to control acid production in plaque. A number of clinical trials were carried out, but these produced either a small reduction in caries, or inconclusive results. Ammoniated pastes have largely been superseded by more effective agents.

Antibiotic toothpastes, containing penicillin, or topical antibiotics such as tyrothricin, have been tried. Their use is based on the premise that if acidogenic bacteria are destroyed, caries will be controlled. Although early clinical studies showed that penicillin-containing pastes do result in reduction in caries incidence, toothpastes containing antibiotics are no longer used because of the dangers of inducing hypersensitivity and resistant strains of micro-organisms.

Anti-enzyme pastes have also been tried. They are thought to interfere with the enzyme systems of bacteria, and thus, with their growth and function. Their effectiveness has not been evaluated in clinical trials.

Fluoride dentifrices of varying composition have been in use since 1945 and have been shown to be of real value as anti-caries agents.

Early studies with pastes containing NaF failed to show any cariostatic effect (Bibby, 1945; Winkler et al., 1953) but it is now believed

TABLE 8

Clinical trials with fluoride-containing toothpastes

Reference	*Dentifrice*	*Brushing supervision*	*Initial age of subjects*	*Percentage of caries reduction DMFS*
Jordan and Peterson (1959)	$SnF_2 + Ca_2P_2O_7$	No	8–11	12 (not significant)
Jordan and Peterson (1959)	$SnF_2 + Ca_2P_2O_7$	Once daily	7–8	21
Peffley and Muhler (1960)	$SnF_2 + Ca_2P_2O_7$	Three times daily for 5 months	10–19	57
Kyes et al. (1961)	$SnF_2 + Ca_2P_2O_7$	No	17–24	14 (not significant)
Muhler (1962)	$SnF_2 + Ca_2P_2O_7$	No	6–18	21
Henriques (1964)	SnF_2 + insoluble metaphosphate	No	5–17	17
Slack and Martin (1964)	SnF_2 + insoluble metaphosphate	No	11–13	0
Brudevold and Chilton (1966)	SnF_2 + insoluble metaphosphate	No	8–17	24
Slack, Berman, Martin, and Young (1967)	SnF_2 + insoluble metaphosphate	No	11–12	27–29
Naylor and Emslie (1967)	Monofluorophosphate	No	11–12	15–30
	SnF_2 + insoluble metaphosphate	No	11–12	12–22
Slack, Berman, Martin, and Hardie (1967)	$SnF_2 + Ca_2P_2O_7$	No	11–12	17–36
James and Anderson (1967)	$SnF_2 + Ca_2P_2O_7$	No	11–12	15–49
Jackson and Sutcliffe (1967)	$SnF_2 + Ca_2P_2O_7$	No	11–12	0–50
Thomas and Jamison (1968)	Monofluorophosphate	Twice daily for 2 years	9–15	34
Fanning et al. (1968)	Monofluorophosphate	No	12–14	20
Møller et al. (1968)	Monofluorophosphate	Daily for $2\frac{1}{2}$ years	10–12	19
Mergele (1968)	Monofluorophosphate	No	9–19	20
Koch and Lindhe (1970)	NaF	Once per school day	9–11	53

that this was due to a reaction between the fluoride and the calcium carbonate or calcium orthophosphate abrasive in the toothpaste, which resulted in an insoluble compound so that the fluoride was not available to act on the teeth.

Later trials with a stannous fluoride/calcium pyrophosphate toothpaste gave promising results (Muhler et al., 1955) which have largely been borne out in subsequent studies. A number of more recent studies are summarized in Table 8.

Most studies show that a reduction in caries of around 20 per cent resulted from the unsupervised use of a fluoride-containing toothpaste. Supervised brushing, which is presumably more regular and more efficient, seems to cause a slightly greater caries reduction.

A dentifrice containing amine fluoride has produced caries reductions of 28–32 per cent in a 7-year trial of unsupervised brushing (Marthaler, 1968). In view of this favourable result, and the supporting laboratory data, it is surprising that this system has not had wider trials which certainly seem justified.

In evaluating the results of these and other clinical trials it should be realized that, because of the wide range of caries incidence between different subjects in a group, differences between test and control groups of up to about 10 per cent are usually not significant unless the groups are very large. Examples of this can be seen in Table 8 where reductions of 12 per cent (Jordan and Peterson, 1959) and 14 per cent (Kyes et al. 1961) are not statistically significant. Between-group differences are significant, however, in most trials, and it seems clear that fluoride-containing dentifrices have a significant anti-caries effect.

While there are differences in overall caries incidence between test and control groups in these studies, analyses of caries incidence in specific types or surfaces of teeth have shown that there is considerable variation in relative effectiveness. It is clearly established that the effect is greatest on erupting teeth (Slack et al., 1967; James and Anderson, 1967; Naylor and Emslie, 1967) and on the proximal surfaces of both anterior (Jackson and Sutcliffe, 1967) and posterior teeth (James and Anderson, 1967; Slack et al., 1967).

The development of a brown stain on teeth brushed with stannous fluoride dentifrice has proved to be a minor disadvantage. This is a very superficial staining of the pellicle on the enamel surface and can be removed by occasional brushing with a more abrasive paste. No such stain develops with the monofluorophosphate pastes.

FISSURE SEALANTS

Pits and fissures are usually the first parts of the teeth to be attacked by caries, and the occlusal is the most caries-susceptible of all tooth surfaces. An agent which would prevent caries developing in fissures would, thus, be of particular value. The concept of sealing the fissures of newly erupted teeth with adhesive resins was introduced some years ago, primarily by Dr. M. G. Buonocore, of Rochester, New York. The first material to be subjected to clinical trial consisted of a methyl-2-cyanoacrylate with a powder filler. The technique of application involved the prior 'conditioning' of the enamel surface by treating it for 45 seconds with 50 per cent phosphoric acid. This pretreatment has been found to increase the penetration of the resin into the enamel surface, and thus greatly improve bonding.

In an early study, the cyanoacrylate was applied every six months to caries-free molars and premolars. The sealant was retained on 71–80 per cent of the teeth, and after one year there was an 86 per cent reduction in caries in the treated compared with the control teeth (Cueto and Buonocore, 1967). Another study using the same material applied on only one occasion showed complete retention of the sealant in only 32 per cent of treated teeth after one year with an 84 per cent reduction in occlusal caries (Ripa and Cole, 1970). A more recent report of a study using a single application of a modification of this material reported almost complete loss of the sealant within six months and no difference in caries incidence between treated and control teeth (Parkhouse and Winter, 1971).

A more recent development has been the use of a bisphenol A-glycidyl methacrylate reaction product with benzoin methyl ether as a catalyst to make the curing process sensitive to ultraviolet light (Buonocore, 1970). This material is painted on the teeth in liquid form and polymerized in situ by the application of ultraviolet light. Early results are most encouraging as, after 2 years, there was 87 per cent retention in permanent and 50 per cent in deciduous teeth, and caries reductions of 99 per cent and 87 per cent respectively (Buonocore, 1971a). A preliminary report from a larger study in Montana noted that 90 per cent of the treated teeth had retained all sealant for nine months (McCune and Cvar, 1971).

Other fissure sealant agents such as polyurethane and zinc polycarboxylate have been proposed, but no clinical trials of their use have yet been reported. Laboratory tests of polycarboxylate cements have shown excellent bonding to enamel (Smith, 1967). A clinical trial of this material is currently in progress in Maracaibo, Venezuela (McCune and Cvar, 1971).

The use of fissure sealants holds considerable promise as a method of controlling fissure caries, although much further work is needed before the precise value and potential of this approach can be established. Laboratory studies indicate that sealant penetrates into 'conditioned' white-spot caries lesions and this makes them considerably more resistant to acid dissolution (Buonocore, 1971b), and also that, when caries is sealed into a tooth for one month the count of viable organisms in the lesion drops dramatically (Handelman et al., 1972).

A study of the large-scale application of fissure sealants by dental hygienists to schoolchildren is in progress in Rochester, New York, and should give some indication of the value of this approach on a community basis.

THE APPLICATION OF PREVENTIVE MEASURES

Earlier sections of this chapter have reviewed the now numerous methods available for the prevention of periodontal disease and dental caries. These have to a large extent revolutionized dental practice since complete control of dental disease is now possible by combinations of preventive and therapeutic measures. The ideal balance between prevention and treatment has not been clearly demonstrated and will probably vary with individual circumstances. Preventive methods are generally much more humane and probably also more economic than restorative treatment of developed lesions. However, there may not always be an economic advantage if the preventive treatment involves a large amount of chairside time and produces only small reductions in the incidence of disease. Dr. Charles W. Gish, of the Indiana State Board of Health, has estimated that for every $100,000 spent, water fluoridation will prevent 620,000 cavities, self-application of fluorides 230,000 cavities, professional application of fluorides 80,000 cavities, and that about 60,000 cavities could be restored for this sum.

The data given in the preceding sections have shown that many different preventive methods are available, but that the relative value of each, and the degree to which they complement each other, are not clearly established. An attempt will now be made to outline the way in which these methods should be applied to the individual patient and to the community.

FOR THE INDIVIDUAL

Providing adequate information to the patient, and, if appropriate, to his parents, is an essential part of any programme of preventive dentistry. This subject is dealt with by Davis in Chapter 12 and is mentioned here only to emphasize its importance. Motivation is a most important part of education for it has been clearly shown that merely knowing that something should be done is not sufficient in itself to cause a person to do it.

Motivation can probably be best developed on a person-to-person basis, and depends to a large extent on the clinician's enthusiasm and sincerity.

Water fluoridation is, beyond question, the most effective, simplest, and cheapest means of preventing caries, and is dealt with in detail by Burt in the following chapter. Where adequate amounts of fluorine cannot be made available in drinking-water, children with developing teeth (i.e., from birth to approximately 12½ years of age) should be given fluoride tablets. These usually consist of 2·2 mg. of NaF providing 1 mg. of fluorine. In areas with less than 0·1 p.p.m. fluorine, a half tablet should be taken daily up to 2 years of age, and a whole tablet daily thereafter.

Diet counselling is an important part of any preventive programme. Unless there are clinical signs suggestive of inadequate nutrition, or the individual comes from a background where this might be suspected, analysis of food intake and general nutrition is probably not justified.

The essential feature of any dental diet counsel is advice on restriction of between-meal eating. The dangers of indiscriminate consumption of snacks should be explained and the patient advised to eat adequately nutritious meals with enough protein so that he does not feel hungry until the next meal is due. For those who find that complete elimination of between-meal eating is too difficult, non-cariogenic items such as nuts, fresh or dried fruit, popcorn, or sugarless chewing gum should be recommended.

It may be necessary to limit carbohydrate intake in patients with rampant caries, and, in such cases, serial lactobacillus counts can be useful in monitoring the change.

Oral hygiene is important for gingival health, although as mentioned earlier it is of very limited value as a caries preventive measure unless a very high standard is achieved. Disclosing tablets are useful in demonstrating plaque and in enabling the patient to monitor his own efforts. The most important aspect of teaching oral hygiene is regular follow-up and supervision. It is relatively easy to engender enthusiasm for toothbrushing, but this will soon evaporate unless there is regular follow-up and the patient is continually reminded and encouraged.

Fluoride toothpastes have been clearly shown to be of value, and should be routinely recommended to all patients. Although a case can be made for recommending them only to children, but not to adults in whom caries incidence is usually low, there seems no point in limiting their use in this way since they have a side-benefit in combating sensitivity of exposed cervical dentine and are as pleasant and as efficient as non-fluoride dentifrices.

Prophylaxis should be carried out at an early stage in the treatment of every patient. It has several important advantages. The feeling of freshness and well-being which results is valuable in encouraging patients to maintain cleanliness, and the removal of calculus is essential for improvement in gingival health.

Fluoride-containing prophylaxis pastes have been shown to be effective in reducing caries incidence. They are as efficient for cleaning and polishing as other such pastes and should therefore entirely supersede their use in dental practice.

Topical fluoride should be applied to every child patient and to adults who have a high incidence of caries. No particular fluoride compound, method, or frequency of application has yet been demonstrated to be clearly superior to all others. A number of studies have been carried out to compare the effectiveness of different preparations. In some, NaF solutions have been found to be more effective than SnF_2 (Nevitt et al., 1958; Torell and Ericsson, 1965; Averill et al., 1967) while, in others, the reverse has been found (McLaren and Brown, 1955; McDonald and Muhler, 1957; Gish and Howell, 1962). A comparison of stannous fluoride with acidulated phosphate–fluoride solutions failed to demonstrate any difference (or any significant effect) although the acidulated phosphate–fluoride gel did prove superior (Cons et al., 1970). In the face of this conflicting and inconclusive evidence, selection of topical fluoride must remain a matter of personal choice.

Frequency of application is probably important and a maximum of 6 months between treatments seems desirable. This should not cause any hardship since fluoride treatments can readily be integrated with routine recall visits.

Where the water supply contains adequate amounts of fluorine, topical application of fluoride solution or gel is not so important, although there is evidence that an additional reduction in caries incidence can be achieved (McDonald and Muhler, 1957).

Fissure sealants should be applied to newly erupted teeth when the whole of the occlusal surface becomes visible in the mouth, or as soon as possible thereafter. Some effective products have been developed to date; continuing clinical trials will help decide which ones will be the most effective.

Dental hygienists and possibly other types of auxiliaries can apply all of the preventive measures outlined so far. This reduces the cost of application and increases the availability of the measures. The concept of the 'dental team' has become well established and the team approach to preventive dentistry and indeed to modern dental practice, has so many advantages that it is very difficult to think of circumstances in which it should not be used. Hygienists and other ancillaries are further discussed by Elderton in Chapter 9.

Restorative dentistry of high quality is important in preventing the extension or recurrence of both caries and periodontal disease, and the novelty and ease of application of other preventive measures should not be allowed to obscure its great importance.

Even by applying all currently known preventive measures, we cannot expect complete prevention of dental disease in most patients. The stage has been reached, however, at which preventive measures can so reduce the amount of disease that the remainder can be completely controlled by therapeutic measures. The two 'approaches' are complementary to one another and should be carefully integrated and incorporated into every modern dental practice.

TO THE COMMUNITY

Community measures are those which are applicable to large sections of the population on a large-group or mass basis. Water fluoridation is the best and most effective example of such a measure, and should form the 'cornerstone' of any community dental health programme.

While children are usually an accessible and receptive population, it is difficult to reach substantial numbers of adults with dental community preventive programmes, unless these are focused on special groups such as employees in a particular office, store, or factory. Dental disease starts and tends to progress most rapidly in children, however, so that they are the most important and susceptible segment of the population and the principal focus of almost every community dental programme. In addition to water fluoridation, the following measures are suitable for such programmes.

Topical Fluoride Application Although topical fluorides probably have some additional effects, their use on a community basis is hardly justified if the water supply contains optimal fluoride levels. The only exception to this generalization is the use of fluoride toothpastes. Where the water supply is deficient in fluorine, the topical application of fluoride solution or gel is a valuable procedure which should form part of every programme. The methods of application which have been used are:

1. Topical application by ancillary personnel (such as dental hygienists).
2. Supervised rinsing or brushing with a fluoride solution.
3. Supervised application of fluoride gels in rubber or wax trays.

The relative effectiveness of these methods has been reviewed earlier in this chapter. In most studies, topical application by dental personnel (usually hygienists) has been carried out at yearly intervals (Tables 1, 2, and 3). Significant reductions in caries have been reported in all except two recent studies (Averill et al., 1967; Cons et al., 1970). None of the fluoride solutions has been clearly shown to be more effective than the others, although the average reported reduction in caries is higher with stannous fluoride and acidulated phosphate–fluoride than with sodium fluoride. Also, the early studies with the highest reductions reported for sodium fluoride involved very frequent application. The choice would thus appear to lie between stannous fluoride and acidulated phosphate–fluoride.

Acidulated phosphate–fluoride in gel form has been applied in trays of rubber or wax. In most studies, this has been preceded by a prophylaxis and has been carried out on an individual rather than a group basis. The results should thus be compared with those obtained from application of solutions, compared to which they appear to be inferior (Table 5). This method could, however, be applied on a group basis if the prophylaxis was omitted and the trays loaded with the gel and used by the children under supervision of a dental ancillary. Clinical studies of this approach seem desirable, while further studies of its utilization on an individual basis do not.

Supervised rinsing or brushing with fluoride solutions has been tried as a convenient method of topically applying fluorides to groups of children. The technique of rinsing is simple and can be applied to groups of 20–40 children in a total of 10–15 minutes. It is usually supervised by a specially trained dental assistant, although schoolteachers supervise the procedure in some areas. Sodium fluoride has been used in most studies because of its ease of preparation and the stability of the solution. It appears that its effectiveness is directly proportional to the frequency of application with reductions of 20 per cent or less from monthly rinsing (Table 6) ranging up to 92 per cent for daily rinsing (Kasakura, 1966).

Supervised toothbrushing with fluoride solution involves a similar approach, although it requires more complicated equipment and facilities (toothbrushes, sinks, etc.) and cannot thus be carried out in school classrooms. Its effectiveness seems to vary with frequency of use (Table 7) but it does not appear to offer any advantages over rinsing.

The choice of 'community' method for topical fluoride therapy thus appears to lie between frequent rinsing and topical application by auxiliary personnel at yearly intervals. Both methods show a similar range of effectiveness in reported studies (Tables 2, 3, and 6) although the choice should not be based entirely on clinical efficacy.

Economic factors are important for this and any other community health measure. Data on the cost-effectiveness of the various techniques and frequency of application is needed before a logical choice can be made. It may be found, for instance, that each application of a particular solution by ancillary personnel costs $5, and that yearly application gives a 30 per cent caries reduction while 6-monthly application gives a 40 per cent reduction. A decision would then have to be made as to whether the additional 10 per cent reduction justified doubling the cost of the programme from $5 to $10 per child per annum.

It has been shown that when caries is reduced by preventive measures to a very low level, the unit cost of treating the lesions that do occur increases considerably (Freire, 1964).

Ideally, all future reports of clinical trials of preventive measures should include data on the cost of each method (including the cost of personnel, equipment and materials) as well as on its effectiveness.

Fluoride toothpastes can be used on a community basis and their promotion has largely been left to the manufacturers. Since they have been clearly shown to be of value, especially in children (Table 7), they should form part of every dental health programme, and their use should be actively encouraged by dentists.

Oral hygiene is currently the only effective means of preventing and controlling periodontal disease. It has been shown that, by teaching effective methods of cleaning, oral hygiene can be dramatically improved in both adults (Lövdal et al., 1961) and in children (Koch and Lindhe, 1965). These studies involved a degree of supervision by regular recall examination or supervision of brushing and, when this is discontinued, deterioration to pre-existent levels takes place (Koch and Lindhe,

1970). The depressing fact is that, although effective toothbrushing is a simple, easy, and very inexpensive method of controlling periodontal disease, its practice on a community basis cannot be readily engendered by any means known at present. Oral hygiene education is the 'cornerstone' of most dental health campaigns, yet even the most vigorous campaigns have produced only short-term improvements, with subsequent deterioration to pre-existent levels of oral hygiene (Rowntree, 1959; Goose, 1960; Finlayson and Pearson, 1967; Koch and Lindhe, 1970).

Since it appears that significant improvements in oral hygiene and plaque control can only be achieved on an individual patient–clinician basis, community programmes should take account of this fact. The value of dental hygienists in providing personal dental health education and the importance of regular prophylaxis are well established. Hygienists provide an appropriate and relatively inexpensive means of providing these services. Thus community programmes should include provision for dental hygienists to carry out regular prophylaxis, preferably at 6-monthly intervals. Continuing education in personal oral hygiene procedures should, of course, be incorporated into this programme.

Where such a programme can be instituted, application of topical fluorides can be incorporated into it with minimal trouble and expense. The child is seen every six months by a dental hygienist and the following done:

1. Oral hygiene is checked, and any necessary steps taken to effect an improvement.
2. The teeth are scaled, if necessary, and polished with a fluoridated prophylactic paste.
3. A topical solution of either stannous fluoride or acidulated phosphate–fluoride is applied to the teeth.
4. The child's mouth is examined and arrangements made to treat any lesions of teeth or soft tissues.

Community programmes integrating preventive and therapeutic measures are in progress in various parts of the USA (Waterman, 1956, Jordan et al., 1959), in Brazil (Freire, 1964), and in Britain (McKendrick, 1970), and are proving very successful. There is limited evidence that they are less expensive as well as more effective than any other approach to community dental health, and as more such evidence is forthcoming, this will surely prove to be the pattern for tomorrow.

REFERENCES

Ånerud, A. (1970), 'The effect of preventive measures upon oral hygiene and periodontal health', Thesis, University of Oslo.

Ash, M. M. (1964), 'A review of the problems and results of studies on manual and power toothbrushes', *J. Periodont.*, **35,** 202.

AVERILL, H. M., AVERILL, J. E., and RITZ, A. G. (1967), 'A 2-year comparison of three topical fluoride agents', *J. Am. dent. Ass.*, **74,** 996.

BAUMHAMMERS, A., LANDAY, M. A., and PINKUS, D. T. (1968), 'Dental calculus inhibition in rats through pancreatin applications', *Archs oral Biol.*, **13,** 353.

BAY, I. (1967), 'Undersögelse över plaqueforekomsten og gingivans tilstånd hos skolebarn i ålderen 11–13 år', Thesis, University of Copenhagen.

BERGENHOLTZ, A., HUGOSON, A., and SOHLBERG, F. (1967), 'Den plaqueavlägsnande formogan hos några munhygeiniska hjälpmedel', *Svensk Tandläk. Tidskr.*, **60,** 447.

BERGGREN, H., and WELANDER, E. (1960), 'Supervised tooth brushing with a sodium fluoride solution in 5,000 Swedish school children', *Acta odont. scand.*, **18,** 209.

— — — — (1964), 'The caries-inhibiting effect of sodium, ferric and zirconium fluorides', *Ibid.*, **22,** 401.

BERTOLINI, A. (1955), 'Experimental research on the effects of mechanical gingival massage', *Parodontologie*, **9,** 144.

BIBBY, B. G. (1944), 'Use of fluorine in the prevention of dental caries. II. Effects of sodium fluoride applications', *J. Am. dent. Ass.*, **31,** 317.

— — (1945), 'Test of the effect of fluoride-containing dentifrices on dental caries', *J. dent. Res.*, **24,** 297.

— —, ZANDER, H. A., MCKELLEGET, M., and LABUNSKY, B. (1946), 'Preliminary reports on the effect on dental caries of the use of sodium fluoride in a prophylactic cleaning mixture and in a mouthwash', *Ibid.*, **25,** 207.

BIXLER, D., and MUHLER, J. C. (1964), 'Combined use of three agents containing stannous fluoride: a prophylactic paste, a solution and a dentifrice', *J. Am. dent. Ass.*, **68,** 792.

BOWEN, W. H. (1970), 'The prevention or control of dental plaque', in *Dental Plaque* (ed. MCHUGH, W. D.). Edinburgh: Livingstone.

BRADFORD, E. W., and CRABB, H. S. M. (1961), 'Carbohydrate restriction and caries incidence', *Br. dent. J.*, **111,** 273.

BRATTHALL, D. (1966), 'Effektan på plaqueutbredningen hos skolbarn efter engångsupplysning med audiovisuell teknikk', *Sver. TandläkFörb. Tidn.*, **58,** 176.

BRUDEVOLD, F., and CHILTON, N. W. (1966), 'Comparative study of a fluoride dentifrice containing soluble phosphate and a calcium-free abrasive: second year report', *J. Am. dent. Ass.*, **72,** 889.

— — and DEPAOLA, P. F. (1966), 'Studies on topically applied acidulated phosphate fluoride at Forsyth Dental Center', *Dent. Clin. N. Am.*, July, 299.

BRYAN, E. T., and WILLIAMS, J. E. (1968), 'The cariostatic effectiveness of a phosphate-fluoride gel administered annually to school children', *J. publ. Hlth Dent.*, **28,** 182.

BULMAN, J. S., RICHARDS, N. D., SLACK, G. L., and WILLCOCKS, A. J. (1968), *Demand and Need for Dental Care*. London: Oxford University Press.

BUONOCORE, M. G. (1970), 'Adhesive sealing of pits and fissures for caries prevention with use of ultraviolet light', *J. Am. dent. Ass.*, **80,** 324.

— — (1971a), 'Caries prevention in pits and fissures sealed with an adhesive resin polymerized by ultraviolet light: a two-year study of a single adhesive application', *Ibid.*, **82,** 1090.

— — (1971b), personal communication.

CALDWELL, R. C., SANDHAM, H. J., MANN, W. V., FINN, S. B., and FORMICOLA, A. J. (1971), 'The effect of a dextranase mouthwash on dental plaque in young adults and children', *J. Am. dent. Ass.*, **82,** 124.

CARLSSON, J., and EGELBERG, J. (1965), 'Effect of diet on early plaque formation in man', *Odont. Revy*, **15,** 23.

CONCHIE, J. M., MCCOMBIE, F., and HOLE, L. W. (1969), 'Three years of supervised brushing with a fluoride-phosphate solution', *J. publ. Hlth Dent.*, **29,** 11.

CONS, N. C., JANERICH, D. T., and SENNING, R. S. (1970), 'Albany topical fluoride study', *J. Am. dent. Ass.*, **80,** 777.

CUETO, E. I., and BUONOCORE, M. G. (1967), 'Sealing of pits and fissures with an adhesive resin: its use in caries prevention', *J. Am. dent. Ass.*, **75,** 121.
DAVIES, G. N. (1950), 'Dental caries control and the dental practitioner', *N. Z. dent. J.*, **46,** 25.
DAY, C. D. M., and SEDWICK, H. J. (1934), 'The fat-soluble vitamins and dental caries in children', *J. Nutr.*, **8,** 309.
DOWNS, R. A., and PELTON, W. J. (1950), 'The effect of topically applied fluorides on dental caries experience in children residing in fluoride areas', *J. Colo. St. dent. Ass.*, **29,** 7.
EGELBERG, J. (1965), 'Local effect of diet on plaque formation and development of gingivitis in dogs. I. Effect of hard and soft diets', *Odont. Revy*, **16,** 31.
ENNEVER, J., and STURZENBERGER, O. P. (1961), 'Inhibition of dental calculus formation by use of an enzyme chewing gum', *J. Periodont.*, **32,** 54.
ERICSON, T., and ERICSSON, Y. (1967), 'Effect of partial fluorine substitution on the phosphate exchange and protein adsorption of hydroxylapatite', *Helv. odont. Acta*, **11,** 10.
FANNING, E. A., GOTJAMANOS, T., and VOWLES, N. J. (1968), 'The use of fluoride dentifrices in the control of dental caries: methodology and results of a clinical trial', *Aust. dent. J.*, **13,** 201.
FINLAYSON, D. A., and PEARSON, J. C. G. (1967), 'Dundee dental health campaign: a study of its value six years later', *Br. dent. J.*, **123,** 535.
FITZGERALD, R. J. (1955), 'Influence of antibiotics on experimental rat caries', *Am. Ass. adv. Sci.*, 187.
— —, KEYES, P. H., STOUDT, T. H., and SPINNELL, D. M. (1968), 'The effects of a dextranase preparation on plaque and caries in hamsters: a preliminary report', *J. Am. dent. Ass.*, **76,** 301.
FORSMAN, B. (1965), 'Effekten av munskölningar med natriumfluoridlösning vid skolor i Växjö', *Sver. TandläkFörb. Tidn.*, **57,** 705.
FOSDICK, L. S. (1950), 'Reduction of the incidence of dental caries. I. Immediate toothbrushing with a neutral dentifrice', *J. Am. dent. Ass.*, **40,** 133.
FREIRE, P. S. (1964), 'Planning and conducting an incremental dental program', *Ibid.*, **68,** 199.
GALAGAN, D. J., and KNUTSON, J. W. (1947), 'Effect of topically applied sodium fluoride on dental caries experience. V. Report of findings with two, four and six applications of sodium fluoride and lead fluoride', *Publ. Hlth Rep.*, **62,** 1477.
— — and VERMILLION, J. R. (1955), 'Effect of topical fluoride on teeth matured on fluoride-bearing water', *Ibid.*, **70,** 1114.
GIBBONS, R. J., and BANGHART, S. B. (1967), 'Synthesis of extracellular dextran by cariogenic bacteria and its presence in human dental plaque', *Archs oral Biol.*, **12,** 11.
GISH, G. W., and HOWELL, C. L. (1962), 'A new approach to the topical application of fluorides for the reduction of dental caries in children; results at the end of five years', *J. Dent. Child.*, **29,** 65.
——, ——, and MUHLER, J. C. (1965), 'Effect on dental caries in children in a natural fluoride area of combined use of three agents containing stannous fluoride: a prophylactic paste, a solution and a dentifrice', *J. Am. dent. Ass.*, **70,** 914.
GLANTZ, P.-O. (1969), 'On wettability and adhesiveness. A study of enamel, dentine, some restorative materials and dental plaque', *Odont. Revy*, **20,** supplement 17.
GOAZ, P. W., MCELWAINE, L. P., BISSEL, H. A., and WHITE, W. E. (1963), 'Effect of daily applications of sodium monofluorophosphate solutions on caries rate in children', *J. dent. Res.*, **42,** 965.
GOOSE, D. H. (1960), 'Oral hygiene campaign in Wellingborough', *Dent. Practnr dent. Rec.*, **10,** 258.
GREENE, J. C. (1966), 'Oral health care for the prevention and control of periodontal disease—Review of literature', in *World Workshop in Periodontics* (ed. RAMFJORD, S. P., KERR, D. A., and ASH, M. M.), University of Michigan.

GREENE, J. C., and VERMILLION, J. R. (1960), 'Oral hygiene index; a method for classifying oral hygiene status', *J. Am. dent. Ass.*, **61,** 172.

GUGGENHEIM, B., KÖNIG, K. G., HERZOG, E., and MÜHLEMANN, H. R. (1966), 'The cariogenicity of different dietary carbohydrates tested on rats in relative gnotobiosis with a streptococcus-producing extracellular polysaccharide', *Helv. odont. Acta*, **10,** 101.

GUSTAFSSON, B. E., QUENSEL, C.-E., LANKE, L. S., LUNDQVIST, C., GRAHNEN, H., BONOW, B. E., and KRASSE, B. (1954), 'The Vipeholm dental caries study', *Acta odont. scand.*, **11,** 195.

HANDELMAN, S. L., BUONOCORE, M. G., and HESECK, D. J. (1972), 'A preliminary report on the effect of fissure sealant on bacteria in dental caries', *J. prosth. Dent.*, **27,** 390.

HARRIS, R. (1963), 'Observations on the effect of eight per cent stannous fluoride on dental caries in children', *Aust. dent. J.*, **8,** 335.

HENRIQUES, J. (1964), 'Council on Dental Therapeutics evaluation of CUE toothpaste', *J. Am. dent. Ass.*, **69,** 197.

HOLLINSHEAD, B. S. (ed.) (1961), *The Survey of Dentistry*. Washington, D.C.: American Council of Education.

HOROWITZ, H. S. (1968), 'The effect on dental caries of topically applied acidulated phosphate-fluoride: results after one year', *J. oral Ther.*, **4,** 286.

—— (1969), 'Effect on dental caries of topically applied phosphate-fluoride: results after two years', *J. Am. dent. Ass.*, **78,** 568.

—— and HEIFETZ, S. B. (1969), 'Evaluation of topical applications of stannous fluoride to teeth of children born and reared in a fluoridated community: final report', *J. Dent. Child.*, **36,** 355.

HUNDSTADBRAATEN, K. (1966), 'Effect on dental caries in children of supervised toothbrushing with a sodium fluoride; results after three years', *Norske Tandlægeforen. Tid.*, **76,** 164.

JACKSON, D., and SUTCLIFFE, P. (1967), 'Clinical testing of a stannous fluoride-calcium pyrophosphate dentifrice in Yorkshire school children', *Br. dent. J.*, **123,** 40.

JAMES, P. M. C., and ANDERSON, R. J. (1967), 'Clinical testing of a stannous fluoride-calcium pyrophosphate dentifrice in Buckinghamshire school children', *Ibid.*, **123,** 33.

JENSEN, S. B. (1959), 'Use of dehydrated pancreas in oral hygiene', *J. Am. dent. Ass.*, **59,** 923.

——, LÖE, H., SCHIÖTT, C. R., and THEILADE, E. (1968), 'Experimental gingivitis in man. IV. Vancomycin induced changes in bacterial plaque composition as related to development of gingival inflammation', *J. periodont. Res.*, **3,** 284.

JORDAN, W. A., and PETERSON, J. K. (1959), 'Caries inhibiting value of a dentifrice containing stannous fluoride: final report of a two-year study', *J. Am. dent. Ass.*, **58,** 42.

——, SNYDER, J. R., PETERSON, J. K., and JOHNSON, R. A. (1959), 'Askov Dental Demonstration: A.D.A. ten-year study of a community dental health program. 1948–1958. Final Report', *N.W. Dent.*, **38,** 445.

KASAKURA, T. (1966), 'Dental observation on school feeding. Part 3. Effect on dental caries prevention by oral rinsing with sodium fluoride solution after school meals', *Odontology*, **54,** 22.

KELNER, R. M., WOHL, B. R., and DEASY, M. J. (1973), 'Gingival inflammation as related to frequency of plaque removal', *J. dent. Res.*, **52,** Special General Session Issue. Abstract 154.

KEYES, P. H. (1966), 'Evaluation of two topical application methods used to assess the anti-dental caries potential of drugs in hamsters', *J. oral Ther. Pharm.* **2,** 285.

——, HICKS, M. A., GOLDMAN, B. M., MCCABE, R. M., and FITZGERALD, R. J. (1971), 'Dispersion of dextranous bacterial plaques on human teeth with dextranase', *J. Am. dent. Ass.*, **82,** 136.

KEYES, P. H., ROWBERRY, S. A., ENGLANDER, H. R., and FITZGERALD, R. J. (1966), 'Bio assays of medicaments for the control of dento-bacterial plaque, dental caries and periodontal lesions in Syrian hamsters', *J. oral Ther. Pharm.*, **3,** 157.

KOCH, G. (1967), 'Effect of sodium fluoride in dentifrice and mouthwash on incidence of dental caries in school children', *Odont. Revy*, **18,** supplement 12.

— — and LINDHE, J. (1965), 'The effect of supervised oral hygiene on the gingiva of children. The effect of toothbrushing', *Ibid.*, **16,** 327.

— — — — (1970), 'The state of the gingivae and the caries-increment in school children during and after withdrawal of various prophylactic measures', in *Dental Plaque* (ed. MCHUGH, W. D.). Edinburgh: Livingstone.

KYES, F. M., OVERTON, N. F., and MCKEAN, J. W. (1961), 'Clinical trials of caries-inhibitory dentifrice', *J. Am. dent. Ass.*, **63,** 189.

LANG, N. P., CUMMING, B. R., and LÖE, H. (1973), 'Toothbrushing frequency as it relates to plaque development and gingival health', *J. Periodont.*, **44,** 396.

LARSON, R. H., ZIPKIN, I., and FITZGERALD, R. J. (1963), 'Effect of dehydroacetic acid and tetracycline on caries activity and its transmission in the rat', *J. dent. Res.*, **42,** 95.

LAW, F. E., JEFFREYS, M. H., and SHEARY, H. C. (1961), 'Topical applications of fluoride solutions in dental caries control', *Publ. Hlth Rep.*, **76,** 287.

LIGHTNER, L. M., O'LEARY, T. J., JIVIDEN, G. J., CRUMP, P. P., and DRAKE, R. B. (1968), 'Preventive periodontic treatment procedures: results after one year', *J. Am. dent. Ass.*, **76,** 1043.

LILIENTHAL, B., BUSH, E., BUCKMASTER, M., GREGORY, G., GAGOLSKI, J., SMYTHE, B. M., CURTIN, J. H., and NAPPER, D. H. (1966), 'The cariostatic effect of carbohydrate phosphates in the diet', *Aust. dent. J.*, **11,** 388.

— —(1967), 'The effect of supervised oral hygiene on the gingivae of children. Lack of prolonged effect of supervision', *J. periodont. Res.*, **2,** 215.

LINDHE, J., KOCH, G., and MANSSON, U. (1966), 'The effect of supervised oral hygiene on the gingiva of children', *Ibid.*, **1,** 268.

— —, and WICÉN, P.-O. (1969), 'The effects on the gingivae of chewing fibrous foods', *Ibid.*, **4,** 193.

LOBENE, R. R. (1971), 'A clinical study of the effect of dextranase on human dental plaque', *J. Am. dent. Ass.*, **82,** 132.

LÖE, H. (1970), 'A review of the prevention and control of plaque', in *Dental Plaque* (ed. MCHUGH, W. D.). Edinburgh: Livingstone.

— —, and SCHIOTT, C. R. (1970), 'The effect of suppression of the oral microflora upon the development of dental plaque and gingivitis', *Ibid.*

— —, THEILADE, E., and JENSEN, S. B. (1965), 'Experimental gingivitis in man', *J. Periodont.*, **36,** 177.

LOSEE, F. L., and ADKINS, B. L. (1969), 'A study of the mineral environment of caries-resistant navy recruits', *Caries Res.*, **3,** 23.

— —, — — (1971), 'Trace elements related to dental caries and other diseases', in *Environmental Geochemistry in Health and Disease* (ed. CANNON, H. L., and HOPPS, H. C.). Boulder, Colorado: Geological Society of America Inc.

LÖVDAL, A., ARNÖ, A., SCHEI, O., and WAERHAUG, J. (1961), 'Combined effect of subgingival scaling and controlled oral hygiene on the incidence of gingivitis', *Acta odont. scand.*, **19,** 537.

LUNDQVIST, C. (1952), 'Oral sugar clearance', *Odont. Revy*, **3,** supplement 1.

MCCUNE, R. J., and CVAR, J. F. (1971), 'Pit and fissure sealants: preliminary results', *Int. Ass. dent. Res. Abstr.*, No. 745.

MCDONALD, R. E., and MUHLER, J. C. (1957), 'The superiority of topical application of stannous fluoride on primary teeth', *J. Dent. Child.*, **24,** 84.

MCHUGH, W. D. (1964), 'The keratinization of gingival epithelium', *J. Periodont.*, **35,** 338.

— — (1966), 'Dentistry and the community', *Br. dent. J.*, **121,** 428.

— — (1967), 'Effect of brushing on cell-turnover in the gingivae of the monkey', *J. dent. Res.*, **46,** 1269.

McHugh, W. D., McEwen, J. D., and Hitchin, A. D. (1964), 'Dental disease and related factors in 13-year-old children in Dundee', *Ibid.*, **117**, 246.

McKendrick, A. J. W. (1970), 'Control of dental caries by the school dental service', *Ibid.*, **128**, 185.

— —, Barbenel, L. M. H., and McHugh, W. D. (1968), 'A two-year comparison of hand and electric toothbrushes', *J. periodont. Res.*, **3**, 224.

McLaren, H. R., and Brown, H. K. (1955), 'A study of the use of topically applied stannous fluoride solution in prevention of dental caries', *Can. J. Publ. Hlth*, **46**, 387

Marthaler, T. M. (1967), 'Epidemiological and clinical dental findings in relation to intake of carbohydrates', *Caries Res.*, **1**, 222.

— —, (1968), 'Caries inhibition after seven years of unsupervised use of an amine fluoride dentifrice', *Br. dent. J.*, **124**, 510.

Mellanby, M. (1934), *Diet and the Teeth. Part III. The Effect of Diet on Dental Structure and Disease in Man.* London: H.M.S.O.

Mercer, V. H., and Muhler, J. C. (1961), 'Comparison of a single application of stannous fluoride with a single application of sodium fluoride or two applications of stannous fluoride', *J. Dent. Child.*, **28**, 84.

— —, — — (1964), 'The effect of a 30-second topical SnF_2 treatment on dental caries reductions in children', *J. oral Ther.*, **1**, 141.

Mergele, M. E. (1968), 'Report II. An unsupervised brushing study on subjects residing in a community with fluoride in the water', *Bull. Acad. Med. New Jersey*, **14**, 251.

Merzel, J., Viegas, A. R., and Munhoz, C. O. G. (1963), 'Contribution to the study of keratinization in human gingiva. Brushing action', *J. Periodont.*, **34**, 127.

Miller, W. D. (1889), *The Micro-organisms of the Human Mouth.* Philadelphia: S. S. White Co.

Møller, I. J., Holst, J. J., and Sorensen, E. (1968), 'Caries reducing effect of a sodium monofluorophosphate dentifrice', *Br. dent. J.*, **124**, 209.

Mooser, M. (1959), 'Abrasive action of toothbrushes with natural and synthetic bristles, and of toothpaste', *Parodontologie*, **13**, 131.

Mühlemann, H. R., Meyer, R. W., König, K. G., and Marthaler, T. M. (1961), 'Cariostatic effect of some antibacterial compounds in animal experimentation', *Helv. odont. acta*, **5**, 18.

Muhler, J. C. (1960), 'The anticariogenic effectiveness of a single application of stannous fluoride in children residing in an optimal fluoride area. II. Results at the end of 30 months', *J. Am. dent. Ass.*, **61**, 431.

— — (1962), 'Effect of a stannous fluoride dentifrice on caries reduction in children during a three-year study period', *Ibid.*, **64**, 216.

— — Bixler, D., and Stookey, G. K. (1968), 'The clinical effectiveness of stannous hexafluorozirconate as an anticariogenic agent', *Ibid.*, **76**, 558.

— — Radike, A. W., Nebergall, W. H., and Day, H. G. (1955), 'Comparison between the anticariogenic effects of dentifrices containing stannous fluoride and sodium fluoride', *Ibid.*, **51**, 556.

— — Stookey, G. K., and Bixler, D. (1965), 'Evaluation of the anticariogenic effect of mixtures of stannous fluoride and soluble phosphates', *J. Dent. Child.*, **32**, 154.

Naylor, M. N., and Emslie, R. D. (1967), 'Clinical testing of stannous fluoride and sodium monofluorophosphate dentifrices in London school children', *Br. dent. J.*, **123**, 17.

Nevitt, G. A., Witter, D. H., and Bowman, W. D. (1958), 'Topical applications of sodium fluoride and stannous fluoride', *Publ. Hlth Rep.*, **73**, 847.

Nisengard, R. J., and Beutner, E. H. (1970), 'Relation of immediate hypersensitivity to periodontitis in animals and man', *J. Periodont.*, **41**, 223.

Nizel, A. E. (1967), *The Science of Nutrition and its Application in Clinical Dentistry.* 2nd ed. Philadelphia: Saunders.

NIZEL, A. E., and HARRIS, R. S. (1964), 'The effects of phosphates on experimental dental caries: a literature review', *J. dent. Res.*, **43,** 1123.

OLLINEN, P. (1966), 'Munsköljning eller borstning med olika fluoridlösningar', *Sver. TandläkFörb. Tidn.*, **58,** 913.

PACKMAN, E. W., ABBOT, D. D., SALISBURY, G. B., and HARRISON, J. W. E. (1963), 'Effect of enzyme chewing gums upon oral hygiene', *J. Periodont.*, **34,** 255.

PAMEIJER, J. H. N., BRUDEVOLD, F., and HUNT, E. E. (1963), 'A study of acidulated fluoride solutions. III. The cariostatic effect of repeated topical sodium fluoride applications with and without phosphate: a pilot study', *Archs oral Biol.*, **8,** 183.

PARKHOUSE, R. C., and WINTER, G. B. (1971), 'A fissure sealant containing methyl-2-cyanoacrylate as a caries preventive agent. A clinical evaluation', *Br. dent. J.*, **130,** 16.

PEFFLEY, G. E., and MUHLER, J. C. (1960), 'Effect of a commercial stannous fluoride dentifrice under controlled brushing habits on dental caries incidence in children: preliminary report', *J. dent. Res.*, **39,** 871.

PETERSON, J. K., HOROWITZ, H. S., JORDAN, W. A., and PUGNIER, V. A. (1969), 'Effectiveness of an acidulated phosphate fluoride-pumice prophylactic paste: a two-year report', *Ibid.*, **48,** 346.

— — and WILLIAMSON, L. (1962), 'Effectiveness of topical application of eight per cent stannous fluoride', *Publ. Hlth Rep.*, **77,** 39.

PINDBORG, J. J., BHAT, M., and ROED-PETERSEN, B. (1967), 'Oral changes in South Indian Children with severe protein deficiency', *J. Periodont.*, **38,** 218.

RAMFJORD, S. P. (1961), 'The periodontal status of boys 11 to 17 years old in Bombay, India', *Ibid.*, **32,** 237.

RANNEY, R. R. (1970), 'Specific antibody in gingiva and submandibular nodes of monkeys with allergic periodontal disease', *J. periodont. Res.*, **5,** 1.

— — and ZANDER, H. A. (1970), 'Allergic periodontal disease in sensitized squirrel monkeys', *J. Periodont.*, **41,** 12.

RIPA, L. W., and COLE, W. W. (1970), 'Occlusal sealing and caries prevention: results 12 months after a single application of adhesive resin', *J. dent. Res.*, **49,** 171.

RITZ, H. L. (1967), 'Microbial population shifts in developing human dental plaque', *Archs oral Biol.*, **12,** 1561.

ROBERTS, J. F., BIBBY, B. G., and WELLOCK, W. D. (1948), 'The effect of an acidulated fluoride mouthwash on dental caries', *J. dent. Res.*, **27,** 497.

ROBINSON, H. B. G., and KITCHIN, P. C. (1948), 'The effect of massage with a toothbrush on keratinization of the gingivae', *Oral Surg.*, **1,** 1042.

ROWNTREE, F. S. D. (1959), 'Dental health education. An experiment at Braintree', *Br. dent. J.*, **107,** 238.

RUSSELL, A. L. (1962), 'Periodontal disease in well- and malnourished populations', *Archs envir. Hlth*, **5,** 132.

— — CONSOLAZIO, C. F., and WHITE, C. L. (1961), 'Periodontal disease and nutrition in Eskimo scouts of the Alaska National Guard', *J. dent. Res.*, **40,** 604.

SANDLER, H. C., and STAHL, S. S. (1960), 'Prevalence of periodontal disease in a hospitalized population', *Ibid.*, **39,** 439.

SCHAFFER, E. M., SCHINDLER, C. W., and MCHUGH, R. B. (1964), 'The effects of two ion-exchange resins on the inhibition of calculus-like deposits in vitro', *J. Periodont.*, **35,** 296.

SCHROEDER, H. E. (1969), *Formation and Inhibition of Dental Calculus*. Hans Hüber.

SHAW, J. H. (1952), 'Nutrition and dental caries', in *Survey of the Literature on Dental Caries* (ed. TOVERUD, G.). Washington D.C.: National Academy of Science.

— — and GRIFFITHS, D. (1963), 'Dental abnormalities in rats attributable to protein deficiency during reproduction', *J. Nutrit.*, **80,** 123.

SHERIDAN, R. C., CHERASKIN, E., FLYNN, F. H., and HUTTO, A. C. (1959), 'Epidemiology of diabetes mellitus: II. A study of 100 dental patients', *J. Periodont.*, **30,** 298.

SHRESTHA, B. M. (1970), 'In vitro chemical effect of different fluoride and non-fluoride compounds on enamel solubility', M. S. Thesis, University of Rochester, New York, U.S.A.

SKINNER, E. W., and TAKATA, G. K. (1951), 'Abrasions of tooth surfaces by nylon and natural bristle toothbrushes', *J. dent. Res.*, **30,** 522 (abstract).
SLACK, G. L. (1956), 'The effect of topical application of stannous fluoride on the incidence of dental caries in 6-year-old children', *Br. dent. J.*, **101,** 7.
—— BERMAN, D. S., MARTIN, W. J., and HARDIE, J. M. (1967), 'Clinical testing of a stannous fluoride-calcium pyrophosphate dentifrice in Essex schoolgirls', *Ibid.*, **123,** 27.
—— —— —— and YOUNG, J. (1967), 'Clinical testing of a stannous fluoride-insoluble metaphosphate dentifrice in Kent schoolgirls', *Ibid.*, **123,** 9.
—— and MARTIN, W. J. (1958), 'Apples and dental health', *Ibid.*, **105,** 366.
—— —— (1964), 'Use of a dentifrice containing stannous fluoride in the control of dental caries', *Ibid.*, **117,** 275.
SMITH, D. C. (1967), 'A new dental cement', *Ibid.*, **123,** 540.
SOCRANSKY, S. S., GIBBONS, R. J., DALE, A. C., BORTNICK, L., ROSENTHAL, E., and MACDONALD, J. B. (1963), 'Microbiota of the gingival crevice area of man. I. Total microscopic and viable counts of specific organisms', *Archs oral Biol.*, **8,** 275.
STAHL, S. S., WACHTEL, N., DECASTRO, C., and PELLETIER, G. (1953), 'The effect of toothbrushing on the keratinization of the gingiva', *J. Periodont.*, **24,** 20.
STAZ, J. (1944), 'Hypoplastic teeth and dental caries', *J. dent. Res.*, **23,** 220.
STEWART, G. G. (1952), 'Mucinase—a possible means of reducing calculus formation', *Ibid.*, **23,** 85.
SUOMI, J. D., GREENE, J. C., VERMILLION, J. R., CHANG, J. J., and LEATHERWOOD, E. C. (1969), 'The effect of controlled oral hygiene procedures on the progression of periodontal disease in adults: Results after two years', *Ibid.*, **40,** 416.
SWEENEY, E. A., and GUZMAN, M. (1966), 'Oral conditions in children from three highland villages in Guatemala', *Archs oral Biol.*, **11,** 687.
SZWEJDA, L. F., TOSSY, C. V., and BELOW, D. M. (1967), 'Fluorides in community programs: results from a fluoride gel applied topically', *J. Publ. Hlth Dent.*, **27,** 192.
THEILADE, E., WRIGHT, W. H., JENSEN, S. B., and LÖE, H. (1966), 'Experimental gingivitis in man. II. A longitudinal clinical and bacteriological investigation', *J. periodont. Res.*, **1,** 1.
THOMAS, A. E., and JAMISON, H. C. (1968), 'Effect of a combination of two cariostatic agents on caries in children: two year clinical study of supervised brushing in children's homes', *Bull. Acad. Med. New Jersey*, **14,** 241.
TORELL, P., and ERICSSON, Y. (1965), 'Two-year clinical tests with different methods of local caries-preventive fluorine application in Swedish school children', *Acta odont. scand.*, **23,** 287.
—— —— (1967), 'The value in caries prevention of methods for applying fluorides topically to the teeth', *Int. dent. J.*, **17,** 564.
—— and SIBERG, A. (1962), 'Mouthwash with sodium fluoride and potassium fluoride', *Odont. Revy*, **13,** 62.
VENNING, P. (1965), personal communication.
WATERMAN, G. E. (1956), 'Richmond-Woonsocket studies on dental care services for school children', *J. Am. dent. Ass.*, **52,** 676.
WEISS, R. L., and TRITHART, A. H. (1960), 'Between-meal eating habits and dental caries experience in pre-school children', *Am. J. Publ. Hlth*, **50,** 1097.
WELLOCK, W. D., and BRUDEVOLD, F. (1963), 'A study of acidulated fluoride solutions. II. The caries inhibiting effect of single annual topical applications of an acidic fluoride and phosphate solution; a two-year experience', *Archs oral Biol.*, **8,** 179.
——, MAITLAND, A., and BRUDEVOLD, F. (1965), 'Caries increments, tooth discoloration and state of oral hygiene in children given single annual applications of acid phosphate-fluoride and stannous fluoride', *Ibid.*, **10,** 453.
WINKLER, K. C., BACKER-DIRKS, O., and VAN AMERONGEN, J. (1953), 'Reproducible method for caries evaluation. Test in a therapeutic experiment with a fluorinated dentifrice', *Br. dent. J.*, **95,** 119.

Chapter 3

Fluoridation of Public Water Supplies

Brian A. Burt PHD, BDSC, MPH, FRACDS
Lecturer, Community Dentistry Unit,
The London Hospital Medical College Dental School

In the previous chapter, Professor McHugh pointed out that fluoridation of water supplies is the most effective method of reducing the prevalence of dental caries on a community level. It is also the most controversial. It is unique as the only preventive measure which does not require individual involvement, and so merits special consideration.

In this chapter, Dr. Burt looks at the background to fluoridation, weighs up its advantages for a community, and then considers some of the social and political problems in implementing fluoridation.

In the year 1908, a young Philadelphia dentist named Frederick McKay travelled west and began dental practice in the town of Colorado Springs. Today, some 129 million people around the world are drinking water which contains minute quantities of fluoride ion (World Health Organization, 1969). The link between these two statements is one of the most fascinating stories in public health. It is a story which has established fluoridation of water supplies as the major contribution which dental science has made towards public health; for it is now accepted that this simple and inexpensive measure can substantially reduce the prevalence of dental caries in a population (World Health Organization, 1969).

DEFINITION

Fluoridation may be defined as the upward adjustment of the concentration of fluoride ion in a public water supply in such a way that the concentration of fluoride ion in the water may be consistently maintained at one part per million (p.p.m.) by weight. Some communities, where the climate is hot, maintain the fluoride concentration at slightly less than 1·0 p.p.m. This is to compensate for the greater quantities of water consumed in a hot climate (Galagan et al., 1957).

There are some communities where the public water supply has a natural concentration of fluoride which is higher than is desirable. If this concentration is considerably more than 1·0 p.p.m. it is usually deemed advisable to remove the excess fluoride to bring the concentration down to 1·0 p.p.m. This downward adjustment of fluoride concentration is called de-fluoridation.

THE BACKGROUND TO FLUORIDATION

When Frederick McKay began dental practice in Colorado Springs in 1908, he soon noticed a feature of dental enamel among local residents which he had not previously encountered elsewhere. This condition was known simply as Colorado Brown Stain, and exhibited itself as a stain of varying intensity in many individuals, ranging from fine pale lacy markings to a pronounced dark-brown mottling which could be quite ugly. It was common among long-term residents of the area and the local people who were accustomed to the condition attached little importance to it. McKay became interested in the condition, and with some help from his dental society he began to investigate it seriously.

His investigations showed that the stain was prevalent in the area around Colorado Springs, and in a number of other districts in the general vicinity as well. His methodical investigations led him to the conclusion that the causative agent was to be found in the drinking water of the communities concerned, and that it was a substance absorbed during the formative years of the dentition (McClure, 1962). McKay also observed that in areas where the mottled enamel condition was found, the prevalence of dental caries appeared lower than would be expected (McKay, 1928).

These observations, which time has shown to be correct, were made by McKay before the causative agent had been identified as fluoride. This discovery only came in 1931, following the development of new methods of spectrographic analysis (Russell, 1969).

It was known that under certain conditions fluoride was a protoplasmic poison, so the discovery of fluoride as the causative agent in mottled enamel was a matter of sufficient concern to attract the attention of the US Public Health Service. H. Trendley Dean was the dentist from that agency who continued the investigations, and his studies through the 1930s and the early 1940s remain as classics of epidemiology.

Dean began by devising an index of mottled enamel. This index, still used today, was based on six grades of severity of the condition, ranging from the mildest discernible form of fine, lacy markings through to the severe pitting and brown staining seen in the worst form of mottling (Dean, 1934). Armed with this index, he was then able to make comparisons of relative severity of the condition among different communities, and in time he documented mottled enamel over much of the United States (Dean, 1936). At the same time as he quantified the prevalence of mottled enamel, Dean would also assess the concentration of fluoride in each community's water supply. The emergent pattern enabled him to conclude that where the fluoride concentration exceeded 1·0 p.p.m., undesirable mottling began to be seen in about 10 per cent of the population. Dean then referred to the concentration of 1·0 p.p.m. as the 'minimal threshold of endemic fluorosis' (Dean et al., 1939). It also became apparent from these studies that large numbers of people had been drinking water containing moderate amounts of fluoride all their lives without apparent ill-effects, other than the mottled enamel.

In 1938 and 1939, several studies by Dean in South Dakota, Colorado and Wisconsin added support to McKay's earlier observation that there was a link between fluorosis, as mottled enamel came to be called, and allow prevalence of caries. Later in 1939, to pursue the fluoride-caries association, Dean examined 885 children aged 12–14 in four cities in Illinois. Two of these cities (467 children) had water supplies where fluoride was naturally present at 1·7–1·8 p.p.m., the other two (418 children) had water containing fluoride at the negligible concentration of 0·2 p.p.m. The children in the higher-fluoride cities had about half the amount of caries seen in the children in the low-fluoride cities (Dean et al., 1939).

Although the evidence was mounting that fluoride was associated with low caries prevalence, it was still necessary to examine the effect of fluoride at lower concentrations, as concentrations of 1·7 p.p.m. and higher caused undesirable fluorosis among some of the population. Dean therefore embarked on what has become known as his '21 cities' study, in which he examined 7257 children aged 12–14 in 21 cities, in which the natural fluoride concentrations in the drinking water varied from 0 to 2·6 p.p.m. This investigation showed that caries prevalence tended to fall sharply as the fluoride concentration rose from 0 to 1·0 p.p.m., and that the caries prevalence declined at a much less dramatic rate as the fluoride concentration rose higher (Dean et al., 1941; Dean et al., 1942). As Dean had previously identified 1·0 p.p.m. as the threshold level beyond which endemic fluorosis became unacceptable, an hypothesis was now able to be formulated. This hypothesis stated that where fluoride was present in drinking water at 1·0 p.p.m., a significant reduction in dental caries would be found without undesirable fluorosis in a population. Previously unpublished data from Dean's studies is described by Young and Striffler (1969).

Once it became established that the experiment could be conducted safely, the hypothesis was ready to be tested and the first artificial fluoridation projects began. In 1945 and 1946, four cities began to add fluoride at 1·0 p.p.m. to their water supplies, the beginning of long-term studies in which they were to be compared with similar neighbouring communities whose water contained negligible fluoride. The four cities were Grand Rapids in Michigan, Newburgh in New York State, Evanston in Illinois, and Brantford in Ontario, Canada. The results from all four were remarkably similar, namely that the addition of fluoride to bring its concentration to 1·0 p.p.m. in drinking water reduced the prevalence of new caries by about one-half, and that this could be done cheaply and safely. These studies, and the host of others which followed in many parts of the world, did indeed prove the hypothesis which Dean had evolved from McKay's early observations. The proof is such that the results of fluoridating a water supply can now be predicted with complete confidence.

WHERE IS FLUORIDATION NEEDED?

Any population which has a public water supply and a moderate-to-high prevalence of dental caries needs fluoridation. A high prevalence of dental caries is found in Western Europe, North and South America, and Australasia (Dunning, 1970). Caries is less prevalent in Asia and Africa, though prevalence does seem to be increasing in many areas where it had not been a public health problem previously (Russell, 1963; Russell et al., 1965; World Health Organization, 1971).

Attempts have been made to associate the prevalence of caries with a number of demographic variables in different regions of the earth (Dunning, 1970). The most consistent association on a global basis comes with diet, in particular with consumption of sugars (Russell, 1969). As many so-called 'developing' countries are tending to adopt the dietary patterns associated with Western European culture, the prevalence of caries in these areas is likely to increase in the future.

In Western countries, the high prevalence of dental caries makes fluoridation practically a universal necessity. In the United States, the National Health Examination Survey (Kelly et al., 1967) showed that persons aged 18–20 had an average of 13·4 DMF (decayed, missing, or filled) teeth, that number representing the total number of teeth which had been affected by caries at some time. (The DMF Index is described in detail by James and Beal in Chapter 5.) In Britain, persons aged 20–24 in a provincial town had been shown to average 14·9 DMF teeth (Bulman et al., 1968), while in Australia a group of 20-year-old army recruits were found to have 19·4 DMF teeth each (Dale, 1969). Beck (1968) in New Zealand, assessed the mean DMF of 20-year-olds in Palmerston North at 19·95. Prevalence rates of this order have not been recorded in Africa and Asia, but that is not to say that they could not be approached in the future if social and cultural change continue to affect dietary patterns there. Anticipating this trend, a number of Asian countries are implementing fluoridation at the present time (World Health Organization, 1969).

There may be communities where caries prevalence is low, and where it is unlikely to rise. Fluoridation may not be necessary in these cases, nor would it be in those communities where the drinking water already contains fluoride which is present naturally at or near the optimal concentration. It would certainly not be necessary, in fact it would be undesirable, in those parts of the world where endemic fluorosis is seen.

Fluoridation requires an efficient public water supply. A certain sophistication in water distribution equipment is necessary to control the precise degree of fluoride concentration in the mains supply. If the public water supply does not reach a reasonable number of persons, or if water from some other source such as wells or individual rain-water tanks is used for drinking and cooking purposes, then fluoridation may not be indicated.

WHY IS FLUORIDATION NEEDED AS A PUBLIC HEALTH MEASURE?

No country believes that it has enough dentists. Even Norway and Sweden with dentist-to-population ratios in the order of 1: 1200 (Federation Dentaire Internationale, 1970) are actively expanding their dental services. In Britain, a dental survey in two towns showed that the adult population examined required twice as many dentists as were available, working full-time for a year, simply to treat the backlog of existing disease (Bulman et al., 1968). In the Australian State of Queensland, Davies et al. (1969) showed that existing dental services were capable of providing less than half the treatment required for dental caries in schoolchildren alone. New Zealand, with its scheme of school dental nurses, probably has come closer to treating all existing dental caries in its schoolchildren than any other country (Beck, 1968), but even there this ultimate goal of dental health for all schoolchildren is only likely to be reached now that the number of fluoridation projects is spreading (Walsh, 1970).

These statements make even clearer what was already apparent, namely that the problem of dental caries will never be met solely by means of treatment of existing disease. Mass educative efforts by dental health educators to change dietary habits have not been proved successful. Fluoridation, where it can be implemented, is left as the most feasible way to substantially reduce the prevalence of caries. As will be discussed later, the economic advantages of preventing caries as opposed to treating it are impressive. More difficult to measure, but a factor to be considered nevertheless, is the savings in work time lost through toothache and other manifestations of caries.

Finally, the savings in human suffering and misery brought on by the sequelae of caries, and the savings in the mental and physical trauma which dental treatment brings to many cannot be measured, but they must be one of fluoridation's greatest intangible benefits.

CURRENT WORLD SITUATION IN FLUORIDATION

The World Health Organization in 1969 estimated that the number of persons drinking fluoridated water was 129 million, this figure being compiled from information received from governments, WHO's own Regional Offices, and the Federation Dentaire Internationale (World Health Organization, 1969). Bernhardt (1970) made the conservative estimate of 110 million people drinking fluoridated water in 32 countries. These countries covered all geographic regions of the earth and included all political persuasions.

The majority of people receiving fluoridated water are in the United States. The first controlled fluoridation projects began in the USA in 1945 and now nearly 4000 communities are fluoridated there (World Health Organization, 1969). These communities include the major cities of New York, which is the world's largest single fluoridation project, Chicago, Philadelphia, Cleveland, San Francisco, Washington DC, Baltimore, and Detroit. The USSR has fluoridation in 24 communities, including Leningrad, serving a total of 13 million people (Bernhardt, 1970). New Zealand now has two-thirds of its public water supplies fluoridated (Walsh, 1970), and Australia has 4 million people, one-third of its total population, receiving fluoridated water (Barnard, 1969). In Canada, 6·6 million people receive fluoridated water, also about one-third of its total population (Goldstein, 1970).

Fluoridation is making steady progress in Latin America. Paraguay and Puerto Rico both have nearly 100 per cent of piped water supplies fluoridated, and in Panama fluoridation reaches 72 per cent of the population receiving piped water. Brazil has fluoridation in 86 communities. Systematic national programmes are being developed in Colombia (5 communities, a total of 1·15 million people, now fluoridated), Chile (86 communities), and Surinam (World Health Organization, 1970a).

The Irish Republic is still the only nation to have a mandatory fluoridation law for the whole country, and progress towards fluoridation of all water supplies is proceeding steadily (*British Dental Journal*, 1971a). Progress in Europe generally, however, has been slow. Czechoslovakia has 10 per cent of its population receiving fluoridated water, and in Poland, Warsaw is fluoridated (Bernhardt, 1970). Five per cent of Britain's population receive fluoridated water (*British Dental Journal*, 1971b), including the nation's second largest city, Birmingham. Forrest (1967) stated that the subject was also under study in the Netherlands, Belgium, Finland, Democratic German Republic, and Switzerland.

In Asia, fluoridation is established in Malaysia, where six projects reach 3 million people, in Singapore and in Hong Kong (World Health

Organization, 1969). There is an unconfirmed report from China that Canton is fluoridated (Bernhardt, 1970).

THE SAFETY OF FLUORIDE INGESTION

The identification of fluoride as the causative agent in mottled enamel in 1931 created a great deal of concern. Studies into the possible injurious effects of fluoride ingestion began soon after, and studies into the physiology of fluoride absorption continue today.

Before artificial fluoridation could commence, it was necessary to establish the safety of adding fluoride to a public water supply at a concentration of around 1·0 p.p.m. It was already seen that fluoride could cause mottled enamel in certain circumstances, and in 1937 Roholm published his works on industrial fluoride intoxication.

The initial effects on the physiological effects of fluoride were carried out by epidemiological and clinical research in areas where fluoride was naturally present in the water. Some of these studies have been described already in the earlier part of this chapter, others are listed and reproduced by McClure (1962). These studies show that at the recommended concentration, fluoride had no deleterious effects on the human organism. Physiological effects were included as subjects for study in the early artificial fluoridation projects, and the previous findings were confirmed. Briefly, it has been found that fluoride has an affinity for the calcified tissues, and hence deposition of fluoride does occur in the bones and teeth. Storage in the soft tissues appears negligible (Ericsson, 1967).

The whole subject of fluoride physiology has been reviewed by the World Health Organization in its monograph *Fluorides and Human Health* (1970b). This publication treats all aspects of the subject in exhaustive detail and it should be a standard text for all dental public health workers. The weight of evidence it presents shows conclusively that ingestion of fluoride at recommended dosage is safe.

DENTAL BENEFITS OF FLUORIDATION

The studies of Dean and others up to 1943 had shown that fluoride was associated with a lower prevalence of caries and that there was a sound basis for hypothesizing that the introduction of fluoride into a water supply would result in a lower communal prevalence of caries. All the studies up to this stage were retrospective in nature, that is, they looked at communities and situations where fluoride was already present in the water. While the weight of circumstantial evidence to support the hypothesis was impressive, it could not be proven until prospective studies were undertaken. In other words, the hypothesis could not be considered to be substantiated until it could be tested and the results shown to be predictable.

It is worth considering for a moment what conditions must be met before a hypothesis can be considered substantiated to the extent that it becomes accepted as scientific fact. Let us suppose that we want to know if an action X causes an event Y, or in other words, we wish to test the hypothesis that X causes Y. To do so, we would need to show that:

1. An association existed between X and Y.
2. Action X preceded Y in time.
3. That no outside variable or chance factors were affecting the outcome.

Applied to fluoridation, it was known by 1943 that a strong association existed between the presence of a certain concentration of fluoride in a water supply and a low prevalence of caries. Dean's studies had shown this association. It was not definitely known whether the second condition was fulfilled, that is whether the presence of fluoride preceded the lower prevalence of caries. The main unknown factor, however, was the third one, that is, could it be that the association between the two factors was completely spurious, and that some other factor, so far unknown and unconsidered, could be responsible for the lowered prevalence of caries? Hence the need for prospective study projects.

These projects needed to be carefully designed. Condition (1), the association of the two factors, was already known. Condition (2), the time factor, could be met by introducing fluoride to a community's water supply and then studying the effects. Condition (3), the chance factors, is always the most difficult part of any biological study. Here it was met by the use of a control community, a town as similar as possible in all respects to the community under study in terms of population, race, age-structure, socio-economic status, and way of life. This use of a 'control group', a standard procedure in biological experiments, made it possible to say the two communities were identical in all respects except for the variable under study. Any chance factors which might occur, such as changes in communal affluence or dietary habits, were likely to affect both communities equally, so that any differences later observed in caries prevalence between the two communities could be attributed solely to the presence of the fluoride in the water supply of the study community. The use of control groups in clinical trials is described in more detail by James and Beal in Chapter 5.

In January 1945, the town of Grand Rapids, Michigan, began adding fluoride to its water supply so as to bring the fluoride concentration to 1·0 p.p.m. (Knutson, 1954). The town of Muskegon, 30 or so miles away, was the control community. In May of the same year, Newburgh, a town in the Hudson valley in New York, began fluoridating as part of a controlled comparative study with Kingston, 25 miles away. These projects were soon followed by Evanston (study) and Oak Park (control), two suburban Chicago communities, and then, in Ontario, Canada, by Brantford (study) and Sarnia (control), with Stratford (naturally fluoridated) also being included in the latter study.

Within a few years dental benefits were noted in Grand Rapids (Dean et al., 1950) and by the seventh year of the study these benefits had become more pronounced (Arnold et al., 1953). By the tenth year of fluoridation, the mean DMF of 9-year-olds in Grand Rapids, which was 3·90 when the project began, had dropped to 1·97. By contrast the DMF for 9-year-olds in Muskegon, 3·81 at the commencement of the study, had dropped to only 3·16 (Arnold et al., 1956). Muskegon was lost to the study as a true control community when it began fluoridating in 1951.

By the fifteenth year of fluoridation in Grand Rapids, results were clearcut. The mean DMF for 15-year-old children in that year (1959) was 6·22, compared with 12·48 for the same age-group in 1944, a reduction of 50·2 per cent in caries prevalence (Arnold et al., 1962).

Similar results were obtained from the Newburgh–Kingston study, where after ten years of fluoridation 10–12-year-old children in Newburgh had 53 per cent less caries than their counterparts in Kingston (Hilleboe et al., 1956). The Evanston study was assessed in a special issue of the *Journal of the American Dental Association* in January 1967; the results from it were closely comparable to Grand Rapids and Newburgh. It should be noted that all of these studies looked at questions of general health effects of artificial fluoridation, but no deleterious effects were discovered in any of them. Russell (1962) noted a slight increase in the mildest forms of fluorosis in Grand Rapids children after 17 years of fluoridation, but these mildest forms are not observable except by a trained examiner. Russell found that unaesthetic enamel opacities due to other causes were notably reduced by fluoridation and Diefenbach et al. (1965) also found that fluoridation generally improves the appearance of teeth.

The fourth of the initial studies, that in Brantford, Ontario, also provided results that were remarkably similar to the other three (Hutton et al., 1956). This close replication of results, by different examiners in different conditions, was in itself strong evidence in favour of fluoridation's efficacy. Since these initial four studies fluoridation has continued to find acceptance in North America so that in 1969 there were 3827 communities in USA and 459 in Canada with fluoridated water (World Health Organization, 1969). Many of these projects have published findings to show the dental benefits of fluoridation, the results generally follow the pattern of the earlier studies.

Studies have been conducted in other parts of the world as well, where governments wish to assess the degree to which the North American experiences can be replicated in the different cultural pattern of their own countries. In Britain, an 11-year study conducted by the Ministry of Health (now the Department of Health and Social Security), concluded by saying that fluoridation is 'a highly effective way of reducing dental decay and is completely safe' (Department of Health and Social Security, 1969). British results are similar to those found elsewhere in the world.

In New Zealand, 10 years of fluoridation in Hastings produced reductions in mean DMF of 10-year-old children from 5·48 before fluoridation began in 1954 to 2·46 in 1964, a reduction of 55 per cent (Ludwig, 1965). The number of caries-immune 5-year-olds had increased from 4 per cent in 1954 to 27 per cent in 1964.

Studies into the effects of fluoridation in the Netherlands, German Democratic Republic (Backer-Dirks, 1969), Australia (Martin, 1969), Brazil, Chile, Colombia, Czechoslovakia, Finland, Ireland, Japan, Puerto Rico, Switzerland, and USSR (World Health Organization, 1969), have shown in every instance a pronounced reduction in the prevalence of dental caries.

The most dramatic reductions in prevalence of caries with fluoridation have been found among those who have drunk the fluoridated water all their lives. But all the major studies also show that some reduction occurs when fluoridated water is ingested for only part of the period of tooth calcification. Thus, a 4-year-old child who moves from a non-fluoridated to a fluoridated area can be expected to show benefits, especially in those teeth which are still calcifying. Fluoridation also reduces caries in the primary dentition (Ast and Fitzgerald, 1962; Tank and Storvick, 1964) and the beneficial effects have been shown to be lifelong, rather than merely to delay the onset of caries (Russell and Elvove, 1951; Englander and Wallace, 1962; Murray, 1971). The study by Russell and Elvove was carried out in Colorado Springs; it is worth recalling here that one of Frederick McKay's original clinical impressions there was the presence of teeth in adults among whom he expected to find a greater degree of tooth loss.

The question of whether fluoridation affects the developing teeth in the foetus has been studied and views have tended to be conflicting. Some authorities (Blayney and Hill, 1964; Martin, 1969) hold to the view that a beneficial effect is seen when a pregnant mother-to-be drinks fluoridated water, others (Horowitz and Heifetz, 1967; Backer-Dirks, 1967) do not.

Research has also shown that smooth surfaces of teeth benefit more than do pit and fissure surfaces. Results from the Hastings project in New Zealand showed that in 12-year-olds, after 10 years of fluoridation, reduction in caries on buccal and lingual smooth surfaces was 89 per cent, on proximal surfaces 58 per cent, and on occlusal surfaces 40 per cent (Ludwig, 1965). In the Tiel–Culemborg study in the Netherlands, Backer-Dirks (1969) reported comparable figures. In England, comparing the naturally fluoridated community of Hartlepool with nearby fluoride-free York, Murray (1969) found that 15-year-olds in Hartlepool had a mean DMF of 4·96 compared to the York children's 8·95. But the number of carious approximal surfaces of molars was eleven times greater in York than in Hartlepool.

Perhaps the most telling indication of fluoride's efficacy has come from two communities where fluoridation has been instituted and then stopped some years later as a result of political pressures. These communities are Kilmarnock, Scotland (Department of Health and Social

Security, 1969), and Antigo, Wisconsin, USA (Lemke et al., 1970). In both cases caries prevalence dropped after fluoridation began, only to begin rising back towards its previous levels again after fluoridation stopped. Antigo took a further step by recommencing to fluoridate, so caries prevalence can be expected to drop again there.

The dental benefits of fluoridation in a community can be summarized by saying that a 50–60 per cent reduction in caries prevalence is observed when children receive fluoridated water during the total period of tooth calcification. Both dentitions are affected and the benefits last throughout adult life. The protective effects of fluoride are more pronounced in the smooth surfaces of the teeth than they are in pit and fissure surfaces.

PUBLIC HEALTH BENEFITS OF FLUORIDATION

It is accepted that fluoridation will substantially reduce the prevalence of dental caries in a community. Questions then arise on what the costs of implementing the measure are and what are the savings to the community in economic terms. Dental practitioners will want to know how their practices will be affected. A public health administrator may also want to know what the effects would be on the treatment requirements of his community and hence on the manpower needed for his programme.

Costs of installing the necessary equipment to fluoridate a water supply will naturally vary a great deal from country to country, and will also depend on type of equipment, size of community to be served, nature of the water treatment plant, and type of fluoride material used (Ingram, 1961). Running costs vary with the same factors. A brief examination of these costs from a number of countries shows, however, that they are reasonable when compared to the results obtained.

Maier puts the overall cost of fluoridation in the USA in 1957 at \$1·23 per million gallons of water treated, an average of 7·9 cents per person per year (Maier, 1963). In Canada the current cost of installing the equipment was between \$2000 and \$5000, and running costs were between 8 cents and 12 cents per person per year (Goldstein, 1970). Barnard (1969) states that in Sydney, Australia, a city of some $2\frac{1}{2}$ million people, fluoridation costs 6 cents per person per year, while annual costs in Latin America have been assessed as between 5 cents and 12 cents (American) per person per year (World Health Organization, 1970a). Puerto Rico's annual expenditure on fluoridation for 1·5 million people is \$140,000 (American), Brazil's \$45,000 for 86 communities (World Health Organization, 1970a).

Records from the Water Department at Watford, England, show that the most modern equipment at The Grove plant cost £2849 to install. This plant uses sodium silicofluoride. Two older sets of equipment cost £1163 (using sodium fluoride) and £1116 (using hydrofluosilicic acid). Combined costs for all of Watford is £1·53 per million gallons of water treated, and 2½p per person, per year.

Considering the financial saving in the costs of dental treatment, Ast et al. (1970) studied the time and cost factors involved in bringing regular dental care to children in fluoridated and non-fluoridated communities. They found that with children receiving initial care at ages 5 and 6 there were twice as many primary tooth extractions per child from the non-fluoridated community than from the fluoridated. Bearing out the findings that fluoridation has its greatest effect on smooth surfaces of teeth, Ast and his group found that in the non-fluoridated community, 75 per cent of the average number of restorations per child were multi-surface type compared to 55 per cent in the fluoridated community. This finding should mean that considerable time would be saved in a public health programme where children from a fluoridated area are being treated.

Ast's study also showed that the number and types of treatment services required in the incremental care programmes were reduced for children from the fluoridated area. In cash terms, initial care for 6-year-olds from the fluoridated community averaged $16·93, compared to $40·78 for children from the non-fluoridated area (1966 fees from New York). Looking at the USA as a whole, *Time* magazine considers that universal fluoridation there would save patients $700 million per year (*Time*, 1970). An editorial in the *Journal of the American Dental Association* (1969) stated that the economic benefits of fluoridation are the major reason for its support among both labour and management groups.

Douglas and Coppersmith (1965, 1966) have looked at the effect of fluoridation on dental practice, and concluded that the type of dentistry carried out does indeed change, but that dentists are not suffering financially and that many appear to be getting more satisfaction out of their work. Apart from the reduced prevalence of caries, a study shows that the prevalence of malocclusion is reduced in a fluoridated area, mainly because of the reduction in premature tooth loss (Ast et al., 1962). Another study, however, does not substantiate this view (Hill et al., 1959).

An illustration of fluoridation's ability to reduce manpower requirements comes from New Zealand. It has been found there that a school dental nurse, who previously was responsible for the dental care of 450 children per year, could care for 690 children after 10 years of fluoridation (Denby and Hollis, 1966).

To summarize, this weight of evidence indicates that fluoridation can have immense public health benefits. It is relatively inexpensive to install and cheap to run, and it would appear that the initial costs are soon offset by savings in the costs of public treatment services. The nature of private dental practice can change where fluoridation has been instituted for some time, but practitioners appear not to suffer financially, and may even enjoy their work more.

FLUORIDATION IN THE COMMUNITY

FLUORIDATION AS A POLITICAL AND LEGAL ISSUE

Fluoridation hardly needs further scientific studies to demonstrate its efficacy. There are few engineering problems, costs are not high, and the measure has been shown to be safe. Why, then, is fluoridation not more widespread?

The answer is that fluoridation is now no longer simply a health issue, it is a political one. Dentists and other health science personnel who promote fluoridation are as a rule not trained to operate in politics, and may even find the necessity to do so odious. Druiff (1967) puts it succinctly when he says that the problems of fluoridation promotion are no longer associated with health considerations but rather are problems of human and public relations. Knutson (1969) states bluntly that fluoridation is a political issue, and that its widespread adoption requires a study of the political system.

There are several reasons why fluoridation must be treated as a political issue. They are:

1. Fluoridation affects health, and most societies now regard access to health care as a fundamental human right. This attitude forces all aspects of health care, including fluoridation, to be regarded as political issues.

2. The decision to implement fluoridation must ultimately come from public authorities, who are usually responsive to political pressures.

3. The public debate on whether or not to fluoridate heard in many parts of the world must have political repercussions.

The form that the political issue takes will vary from country to country. With the infinite variety of political systems in the world, any promoter of fluoridation is advised to know his own political system well, to be aware of its subtleties, and to know which agencies, boards, councils, ministries, authorities, commissions, and influential individuals are involved in the decision-making.

In the USA, the decision to fluoridate has most often been one made by the local community, and a public referendum is a common method of deciding any community decision in that country. There have been over 900 referenda on fluoridation in the USA, and it is interesting to note that in two-thirds of these referenda fluoridation has lost Knutson, 1969). Knutson believes that the political inexperience of the measure's proponents was responsible for many of these failures. Many communities which have begun fluoridation have had legal suits brought against them by citizens in an effort to stop the measure. Some of these suits have been successful, though it should be noted that no American court has ever struck down fluoridation on the grounds that it is harmful (Bergen, 1970). Successful lawsuits to stop fluoridation have usually been fought on the issues of personal liberty and religious beliefs, and the legal and political aspects of these issues, *vis-à-vis* fluoridation, have been reviewed by Strong (1968). He provides reasons why the legality of fluoridation is usually upheld in American courts, especially in more recent years. There have been occasions where a favourable decision by a state court has been challenged in the Supreme Court of the United States, but on all occasions the Supreme Court has upheld the states' decisions (Butler, 1962; Roemer, 1965). At the present time, there are seven states of the USA which have mandatory fluoridation laws in operation (Editorial, 1969), but there are others, such as Massachusetts and Utah, where the political and social climate makes promotion of fluoridation difficult.

McNeil (1957), traces the growth of opposition to fluoridation. His account of the referendum at Stevens Point, Wisconsin, in 1950 describes how fluoridation can quickly become inflated into a major political issue in a community. Referenda are regarded as best avoided if possible, because of the little time available for the public education campaign required in addition to the political organization, all in the face of opposition which can be vociferous. Ontario, Canada, has a law which states that a referendum on fluoridation can be held if requested by only 10 per cent of the citizens of a community (Goldstein, 1970). The adoption of a law like this makes it difficult to implement fluoridation, because as soon as a favourable decision is taken, opponents can readily force a further referendum. The town of Hamilton, Ontario, for example, has had three referenda (Goldstein, 1970).

In Britain, the decision to fluoridate is taken at Local Authority level. Referenda are not commonly held in Britain, though one on fluoridation was held in Bolton, Lancashire, in 1968 and fluoridation was defeated. Although central governments have supported fluoridation, and even gone as far as indemnifying local authorities against the costs of litigation brought against them (Editorial, 1965), mandatory legislation is unlikely to be forthcoming in the near future. In the present British political climate such a move would be unpopular, so the final decision must be made by local authorities. As councillors in one authority have already been unseated as a result of accepting fluoridation (*Lancet*, 1958), it is understandable that many other councils are unwilling to make positive decisions. But even when a Local Health Authority, or a group of them supplied by one water undertaking, has decided in favour of fluoridation, the water undertaking supplying the area is not always obliged to act (Department of the Environment, 1971). Administrative relationships between these bodies is complicated, as illustrated by the fact that in late 1971 there were 97 of the 186 Local Health Authorities in England favouring fluoridation, but only 14 of the 171 water undertakings in England actually fluoridating (Department of Health and Social Security, 1971). The conservative policy of the British Waterworks Association (British Waterworks Association, 1971) and the absence of a court ruling on the legality of fluoridation has added to the stalemate position that fluoridation is in in Britain, although a writ was once issued and then withdrawn before it came to court (Oral Hygiene Service, 1967).

Countries with political and legal systems based on the British model, however, have had a number of notable court cases and public hearings concerning fluoridation. Eire, still the only country in the world to have nationwide mandatory fluoridation, saw the longest court case in its history when the 1960 Eire Health (Fluoridation of Water Supplies) Act was challenged by a Dublin housewife and the case brought to the Eire High Court. The court ruled that fluoridation was constitutional and did not accept that it could be classed as mass medication. The Supreme Court of Ireland upheld this judgment in 1964 (Department of Health, Dublin, 1963, 1964). In New Zealand, the Court of Appeal refused an order seeking to restrain the Lower Hutt Corporation from fluoridating. This judgment was appealed by the plaintiffs, but the Judicial Committee of the Privy Council upheld the Court of Appeal's decision in *Attorney-General of New Zealand vs. Lower Hutt City Corporation* (1964), A.C. 1469. In Tasmania, Australia, a Royal Commission sat for over a year before reporting in favour of fluoridation (Crisp, 1968). In the light of these decisions in Eire, New Zealand, and Australia, it would seem that if a court case were brought against fluoridation in Britain it would be unlikely to succeed.

Czechoslovakia is proceeding steadily with fluoridation now that the Water Fluoridation Commission has succeeded in ensuring that fluoridation equipment is included in the designs of new waterworks (Jiraskova et al., 1969). In Sweden, opposition to fluoridation has been strong, a predictable situation in view of that country's commitment to personal liberties. The field-trial at Norrköping was blocked by legal action brought on by opponents of fluoridation and an unsuccessful attempt to repeal enabling legislation had been made in the Swedish Parliament in 1968. A second attempt in November 1971 succeeded by a narrow majority in a vote that closely followed party lines (Burt and Petterson, 1972). The future of fluoridation in Sweden remains uncertain.

Fluoridation is supported by a large number of professional organizations around the world, the most notable endorsement coming in 1969 when the World Health Assembly adopted fluoridation as official policy of the World Health Organization (World Health Organization, 1969).

The evidence shows that where fluoridation has advanced most it has been treated as a political and legal issue. Certainly, in any nation or smaller community where it is being promoted, all the evidence of efficacy, safety, and economic benefits must be collected and used. But it must never be forgotten that the ultimate decision must be made by a public authority which may have no particular feeling on the issue, but which may react in response to its own political needs and goals. Knowledge of political realities in any governmental system is a basic need if fluoridation is to be implemented.

PUBLIC ATTITUDES TO FLUORIDATION

Fluoridation is established as a safe, effective, and practical public health measure, but as political decision-makers usually act on it only when their public so demands, public attitudes to fluoridation must be reasonably positive if the measure is to be promoted. In a sociological appraisal of fluoridation, Motz (1971) stated that social scientists have been attracted to the issue by the community conflict which it frequently sparks off. The assessment of a public attitude has emerged as a difficult and complex problem.

Why is fluoridation opposed by some people, often with a degree of vehemence that borders on the hysterical? Those promoting fluoridation have frequently been surprised by the seeming irrationalities of opponents and they become frustrated when they see non-scientific arguments influencing decision-makers at least as much as their own apparently lucid and objective case in favour of fluoridation. The basic error of many people trained in scientific thinking is the bland assumption that all persons think in rational terms and are therefore able to be convinced by a scientific argument. This assumption is quite false, and the problem that then arises for anyone promoting fluoridation is that he or she is often ill-equipped for dealing with the conflicts aroused by the issue in the community. When attitudes other than complete approval are based on honest doubts, or where they have some rational foundation, they can be identified and perhaps modified to some extent. But where opposition stems from irrational opinions or unconscious anxieties, or is based on cultural viewpoints different from those held by the promoter, then the problem is far greater.

There have been many attempts to categorize the antifluoridationist, the rationale being that if this can be done then individual and group opposition to fluoridation can be predicted and steps taken to counter it when promotional efforts are made. Unfortunately, social science research by its very nature is considerably more diffuse than physical or even biological science. The vagaries of human nature, and the infinite range of complex factors which contribute to human beliefs and behaviour, have resulted in a picture of the antifluoridationist which is confused and even contradictory.

A number of studies in the USA have concentrated on the attitudes of persons who vote against fluoridation at referenda in that country. Some of these studies concluded that the antifluoridationist felt a sense of deprivation, or of powerlessness, an alienation from the forces which direct society, and a grudge against the people whom they see to be directing these forces. In this 'anti-establishment' view, opposition to fluoridation is seen by alienated persons as a means of expressing their general discontent with society at large, rather than being more directly concerned with the merits of the measure itself. This hypothesis was suggested in several similar forms by Simmel (1961), Horton and Thompson (1962), and McDill and Ridley (1962). Green (1961) expressed a similar conclusion from his interviews with leading antifluoridationists in Massachusetts, he suggested that government and big business were perceived as agents responsible for a loss of personal freedom. 'Alienation' has become a fashionable word and hence is in danger of losing its precise meaning, but here it means the process by which the complications, the value scales, the pace and the pressures of life in competitive western society act as forces which produce conscious or unconscious effects in an individual. The individual reacts, consciously or unconsciously, against these social forces in a variety of ways. As alienation has been suggested as the root cause for much of the social unrest in the USA, it is likely that where social divisions are present there will be numbers of people who will use the fluoridation issue to express their vague and even unconscious desires to articulate discontent. O'Shea and Kegeles (1963) stated that some persons opposed fluoridation because they considered it undemocratic and Cohen (1966) discusses the 'anti-scientific' attitude held by some people, an attitude which could combine with alienation to promote a deep feeling of frustration.

How many antifluoridationists are there in the USA? Podshadley (1966) describes results of a nationwide survey which indicated that only 4 per cent were actively opposed to fluoridation. A similar figure for persons strongly opposed was found in a 1968 survey (O'Shea and Cohen, 1969), while the same survey showed that 11 per cent held varying degrees of opposition to fluoridation and 77 per cent considered fluoridation desirable.

It has been suggested that the antifluoridationist is more likely to be an older, childless person of lower than median income and education, but Shaw (1969) described a referendum which failed in a young, high-income, and high-education community. Shaw found, as did Metzner (1957), that some opposition came from those who were merely doubtful or uncommitted. The conclusion that opposition to fluoridation can be based on complex motives and that caution is needed in interpreting sociological data was reached by Hirabayashi and Hirabayashi (1964) and Hahn (1965). As relatively few people appear to be actively opposed to fluoridation, it appears that more knowledge is needed concerning the motives of the doubtful, uncommitted, or merely uninterested person who is moved to oppose it.

The prevailing image of the profluoridationist in the USA is of the younger married person with small children, and having above-median income and education (Mausner and Mausner, 1955; Kegeles, 1962; Cohen, 1966). But even this image is confused by Gamson (1961) finding support for fluoridation in all socio-economic groups, and Hahn's (1965) citing of an investigation in California where greater opposition to fluoridation was found among non-manual groups than among manual workers. Linn (1969) reviewed public attitudes towards fluoridation and concluded that opposition stems from multiple causes and that the only single factor to emerge with any consistency was alienation. Linn stated that the evidence showed that persons who expressed dissatisfaction with their social or political world, or who otherwise took a stand not generally valued by middle-class society, tended more than others to oppose fluoridation.

In Britain, the extent of ignorance and apathy concerning fluoridation appears greater. Bulman et al. (1968) found that in Salisbury 65 per cent of adults interviewed had either not heard of fluoridation or had no opinion on it, and that the corresponding figure in Darlington was 52 per cent. This latter figure is of interest considering that fluoridation was a political issue in the town shortly before the survey and had received considerable publicity. This study confirmed the result of many American studies in finding that favourable attitudes towards fluoridation were associated with younger age-groups, and to a lesser extent with higher social class. Dickson (1968) in Manchester also concluded that ignorance and apathy about fluoridation were widespread. In a study in a working-class area of Inner London, Burt (1971) found that only 44 per cent of persons interviewed reported that they had heard of fluoridation, and only 75 per cent of this group had even a general idea of what fluoridation was, and fewer still had any specific feelings about the subject.

In the Anglo-Saxon nations, there is some reason for believing that the more extreme arguments against fluoridation are winning few new adherents. Certainly in Britain, the strongest argument against fluoridation that has emerged is the 'civil liberties' argument, which essentially says that no-one should be compelled to ingest any specific substance against their will. This view is put forward by Douglas of Barloch (1969), and more lucidly by Joll (1966). While it is not difficult to produce counter-arguments against it, the civil-liberties argument goes outside the realm of science and becomes more of a philosophical discussion. The current social climate of Britain certainly favours acceptance of this argument by many persons, and it is well in evidence in other countries as well.

The attitudes towards fluoridation in developing countries have received little study, perhaps in many cases there are no discernible attitudes, or if there are they may not affect political decisions. Where they do matter, public attitudes and their subsequent effects upon the political process have more bearing upon whether fluoridation is implemented or not than does the direct results of scientific research. It then becomes necessary to consider how public attitudes may be shaped to help produce favourable decisions from political leaders.

THE ROLE OF THE DENTIST IN PROMOTING FLUORIDATION

In most communities which have implemented fluoridation, dentists have played an important role in having the measure adopted. The nature of this role, however, will vary with the community.

Where the society is largely illiterate, or for some other reason takes little part in influencing the decision-making process, public education may not be a major priority. The case for fluoridation could be made by dentists directly to the political leadership, stressing the economic and community health benefits that will result. Careful action by the dental profession in such societies could eliminate the acrimonious debate which surrounds the issue in so-called 'developed' nations. In the 'developed' nations, dentists have to undertake more of a public education role. In these cases it is first of all necessary for dentists themselves to know the subject well, for Podshadley (1966) has described a study which showed that a dentist's attitude towards fluoridation is positively correlated with the knowledge of the subject which he possesses. Some dentists are known to be even opposed to fluoridation, mostly for reasons of personal prestige, in the opinion of Galagan (1959).

Douglas (1962) stated that many persons who voted in favour of fluoridation had first heard about the measure from their dentists, and Sturgeon (1958), in Canada, considered that a successful referendum in Thorold, Ontario, was largely due to the efforts of the profession. Knutson (1969) agrees that dentists see their own role as educational in fluoridation campaigns, but urges a stronger political role in pushing the issue. Martin (1969) describes how the profession in Australia adopted both an educative and a political role. This approach has met with some moderate successes; in New South Wales some 72 per cent of the population on piped water now receive fluoride (Barnard, 1969), and Western Australia has mandatory fluoridation.

The fluoridation law in Connecticut, USA, came about after a well-organized campaign, which was primarily led by lay persons (Hirakis and Foote, 1967). Dentists, however, had a vital though unpublicized educative role in this campaign. Earlier, Metzner (1956) had advocated this quiet role for dentists, as too-obvious involvement could lead to public suspicion of the profession's motives in supporting a cause which could appear to reduce the need for its services. Discussing the publicity efforts during a community's fluoridation campaign, Bishop (1962) outlined a number of educative roles for the dental profession.

It would appear that dentistry must take an active educative role in communities where fluoridation is needed. Both private practitioners and public health dentists can educate their patients and influential groups and individuals in the community. Where the profession as a whole organizes a community-wide campaign to reach key groups and individuals in the community, the measure must have a good chance of success.

SUMMARY

A considerable weight of evidence, collected over a number of years, shows that the addition of fluoride to a public water supply so as to bring the total concentration of fluoride ion up to 1 part per million will substantially reduce the prevalence of new tooth decay. This procedure can be safely carried out with fairly simple equipment at water treatment and distribution plants, and can be easily supervised by ordinary waterworks personnel. Both the capital cost of the equipment and the running costs are not high.

The physiology and metabolism of fluoride ingestion have been studied for many years, no deleterious effects on human or animal health have been found when fluoride is taken in the recommended dosage. The savings in costs of dental treatment, both to the individual paying his dental bills and to the community operating a public treatment programme, are substantial.

Opposition to fluoridation is found, but the measure has been accepted as a correct public health action in different countries with different legal systems. Reasons for this opposition are complex, and a better knowledge of human behaviour is required before they can be totally countered. Dentists have an important educative role to play wherever fluoridation is being considered.

The World Health Organization, together with numerous national medical, dental, and allied health organizations, completely and actively endorse fluoridation. Wherever it is implemented, fluoridation has shown itself to be a significant factor in improving the public health of the community.

REFERENCES

ARNOLD, F. A., jun., DEAN, H. T., and KNUTSON, J. W. (1953), 'Effects of fluoridated public water supplies on dental caries prevalence. Results of the seventh year of study at Grand Rapids and Muskegon, Michigan', *Publ. Hlth Rep.*, **68,** 141.

——————— (1956), 'Effect of fluoridated public water supplies on dental caries prevalence. Tenth year of the Grand Rapids–Muskegon study', *Ibid.*, **71,** 652.

—— LIKINS, R. C., RUSSELL, A. L., and SCOTT, D. B. (1962), 'Fifteenth year of the Grand Rapids fluoridation study', *J. Am. dent. Ass.*, **65,** 780.

AST, D. B., ALLAWAY, N., and DRAKER, H. L. (1962), 'The prevalence of malocclusion, related to dental caries and lost first permanent molars, in a fluoridated city and a fluoride-deficient city', *Am. J. Orthodont.*, **48,** 106.

——, CONS, N. C., POLLARD, S. T., jun., and GARFINKEL, J. (1970), 'Time and cost factors to provide regular, periodic dental care for children in a fluoridated and non-fluoridated area: Final report', *J. Am. dent. Ass.*, **80,** 770.

—— and FITZGERALD, B. (1962), 'Effectiveness of water fluoridation', *J. Am. dent. Ass.*, **65,** 581.

BACKER-DIRKS, O. (1967), 'The relation between the fluoridation of water and dental caries experience', *Int. dent. J.*, **17,** 582.

—— (1969), 'The effectiveness of fluoridation in Europe', in *International Symposium on Fluoridation and Preventive Dentistry*. New York: American Dental Association and Federation Dentaire Internationale.

BARNARD, P. D. (1969), 'Communities fluoridated in Australia, 1968', *Aust. dent. J.*, **14,** 392.

BECK, D. J. (1968), *Dental Health Status of the New Zealand Population in Late Adolescence and Young Adulthood.* Special Report Series No. 29. Wellington, NZ National Health Statistics Centre, Department of Health.

Bergen, R. P. (1970), 'Legal status of fluoridation', *J. Am. med. Ass.*, **211,** 555.
Bernhardt, M. E. (1970), 'Fluoridation international', *J. Am. dent. Ass.*, **80,** 731.
Bishop, E. M. (1962), 'Publicity during a fluoridation campaign', *Ibid.* **65,** 663.
Blayney, J. R., and Hill, I. N. (1964), 'Evanston dental caries study XXIV. Prenatal fluorides—value of waterborne fluorides during pregnancy', *Ibid.*, **69,** 291.
British Dental Journal (1971a), 'Fluoridation of water supplies in Ireland', **130,** 97.
— — — (1971b), 'Parliamentary news', **130,** 412.
British Waterworks Association (1971), personal communication.
Bulman, J. S., Richards, N. D., Slack, G. L., and Willcocks, A. G. (1968), *Demand and Need for Dental Care; a Socio-dental Study*. London: Oxford University Press and Nuffield Provincial Hospital Trust.
Burt, B. A. (1971), unpublished data.
— —, and Petterson, E. O. (1972), 'Fluoridation: Developments in Sweden', *Br. dent. J.*, **133,** 57.
Butler, H. W. (1962), 'Legal aspects of fluoridating community water supplies', *J. Am. dent. Ass.*, **65,** 653.
Cohen, L. (1966), 'A sociologist looks at fluoridation', *Ore. St. dent. J.*, **35,** 26.
Crisp, M. P. (1968), *Report of the Royal Commissioner into the Fluoridation of Public Water Supplies*. Hobart, Tasmania: Government Printing Office.
Dale, J. W. (1969), 'Prevalence of dental caries and periodontal disease in military personnel', *Aust. dent. J.*, **14,** 30.
Davies, G. N., Kroger, B. J., and Homan, B. T. (1969), 'Dental survey of children in country districts of Queensland', *Ibid.*, **14,** 153.
Dean, H. T. (1934), 'Classification of mottled enamel diagnosis', *J. Am. dent. Ass.*, **21,** 1421.
— — (1936), 'Chronic endemic dental fluorosis (mottled enamel)', *J. Am. med. Ass.*, **107,** 1269.
— — Jay, P., Arnold, F. A., jun., and Elvove, E. (1939), 'Domestic water and dental caries, including certain epidemiological aspects of *L. acidophilus*', *Publ. Hlth Rep.*, **54,** 862.
— — — — — — — — (1941), 'Domestic water and dental caries. II. A study of 2,832 white children, aged 12–14 years, of 8 suburban Chicago communities, including *Lactobacillus acidophilus* studies of 1,761 children', *Ibid.*, **56,** 761.
— — — — — — (1942), 'Domestic water and dental caries. V. Additional studies of the relation of fluoride domestic waters to dental caries experience in 4,425 white children, aged 12–14 years, of 13 cities in 4 states', *Ibid.*, **57,** 1155.
— — — —, Jay, P., and Knutson, J. W. (1950), 'Studies on mass control of dental caries through fluoridation of the public water supply', *Ibid.*, **65,** 1403.
Denby, G. C., and Hollis, M. J. (1966), 'The effect of fluoridation on a dental public health programme', *N.Z. dent. J.*, **62,** 32.
Department of the Environment (1971), personal communication.
Department of Health and Social Security, Scottish Office, Welsh Office, and Ministry of Housing and Local Government (1969). *The Fluoridation Studies in the United Kingdom and the Results Achieved After Eleven Years*. London: HMSO.
— — — — (1971), personal communication.
Department of Health, Dublin (1963), *Gladys Ryan vs. Attorney-General for Ireland*. Judgment in the High Court, Ireland, delivered by Mr. Justice Kenny, 31 July, 1963.
— — — — (1964). *Gladys Ryan vs. Attorney-General for Ireland*. Judgment of the Supreme Court, Ireland, delivered by Chief Justice O'Dalaigh on appeal from Mr. Justice Kenny, 3 July, 1964.
Dickson, S. (1968), 'Attitudes to fluoridation in a North-West industrial area', *Br. J. Sociol.*, **18,** 231.

DIEFENBACH, V. L., NEVITT, G. A., and FRANKEL, J. M. (1965), 'Fluoridation and the appearance of teeth', *J. Am. dent. Ass.*, **71**, 1129.

DOUGLAS, B. L. (1962), 'Dentistry and the fluoridation issue: The dentist in the social and political arena', *N.Y. St. dent. J.*, **28**, 347.

—— and COPPERSMITH, S. (1965), 'The impact of water fluoridation on dental practice', *Ibid.*, **31**, 439.

———— (1966), 'The impact of water fluoridation on the practice of dentistry for children', *J. Dent. Child.*, **33**, 128.

DOUGLAS OF BARLOCH (1969), 'Medical, dental, political and moral aspects of fluoridation of water supplies', *Pakist. dent. Rev.*, **19**, 107.

DRUIFF, D. P. (1967), 'The public reaction to fluoridation', *J. dent. Ass. S. Afr.*, **22**, 243.

DUNNING, J. M. (1970), *Principles of Dental Public Health*, 2nd ed. Cambridge, Mass.: Harvard University Press.

EDITORIAL (1965), 'Fluoridation: An urgent public health measure', *Br. dent. J.*, **119**, 283.

— (1969), 'How new trends in health care generate support for fluoridation', *J. Am. dent. Ass.*, **78**, 901.

ENGLANDER, H. R., and WALLACE, D. A. (1962), 'Effects of naturally fluoridated water on dental caries in adults', *Publ. Hlth Rep.*, **77**, 887.

ERICSSON, Y. (1967), 'Medical aspects of fluoridation. A review', *Br. dent. J.*, **123**, 276.

FEDERATION DENTAIRE INTERNATIONALE (1970), *Basic Facts Sheets.*

FORREST, J. (1967), 'The effectiveness of fluoridation in Europe. A review', *Br. dent. J.*, **123**, 269.

GALAGAN, D. J. (1959), 'Nature of the fluoridation controversy in the United States', *Aust. dent. J.*, **4**, 149.

——, VERMILLION, J. R., NEVITT, G. A., STADT, Z. M., and DART, R. E. (1957), 'Climate and fluid intake', *Publ. Hlth Rep.*, **72**, 484.

GAMSON, W. A. (1961), 'Public information in a fluoridation referendum', *Hlth Educ. J.*, **19**, 47.

GOLDSTEIN, P. (1970), 'Fluoridation, Canada, 1970', *J. Can. dent. Ass.*, **36**, 206.

GREEN, A. L. (1961), 'The ideology of anti-fluoridation leaders', *J. Soc. Issues*, **17**, 33.

HAHN, H. D. (1965), *Fluoridation and Patterns in Community Politics.* Ann Arbor: University of Michigan, mimeograph.

HILL, I. N., BLAYNEY, J. R., and WOLF, W. (1959), 'The Evanston dental caries study. XIX: Prevalence of malocclusion of children in a fluoridated and control area', *J. dent. Res.*, **38**, 782.

HILLEBOE, H. E., SCHLESINGER, E. R., CHASE, H. C., CANTWELL, K. T., AST, D. B., SMITH, D. J., WACHS, B., OVERTON, D. E., and HODGE, H. C. (1956), 'Newburgh–Kingston caries–fluorine study: final report', *J. Am. dent. Ass.*, **52**, 290.

HIRABAYASHI, E. S., and HIRABAYASHI, G. K. (1964), 'Sociological aspects of fluoridation', *J. Can. dent. Ass.*, **30**, 11.

HIRAKIS, S., and FOOTE, F. M. (1967), 'Statewide fluoridation: How it was done in Connecticut', *J. Am. dent. Ass.*, **75**, 174.

HOROWITZ, H. S., and HEIFETZ, S. B. (1967), 'Effects of prenatal exposure to fluoridation on dental caries', *Publ. Hlth Rep.*, **82**, 297.

HORTON, J. E., and THOMPSON, W. E. (1962), 'Powerlessness and political negativism: A study of defeated local referendums', *Am. J. Sociol.*, **67**, 485.

HUTTON, W. L., LINSCOTT, B. W., and WILLIAMS, D. D. (1956), 'Final report of local studies on water fluoridation in Brantford', *Can. J. Publ. Hlth*, **47**, 89.

INGRAM, W. T. (1961), 'Water fluoridation is feasible', *Post-grad. Med.*, n.v., 108.

JOLL, A. E. (1966), 'The politics of fluoridation', *Br. dent. J.*, **121**, 154.

JIRASKOVA, M., et al. (1969), 'Water fluoridation in Czechoslovakia', *Czech. Stomat.*, **3**, 129.

JOURNAL OF THE AMERICAN DENTAL ASSOCIATION (1967), 'Special issue: Fluorine and dental caries', **74.**

KEGELES, S. S. (1962), 'Contributions of the social sciences to fluoridation', *J. Am. dent. Ass.*, **65,** 667.

KELLY, J. E., VAN KIRK, L. E., and GORST, C. C. (1967), *Decayed, Missing and Filled Teeth in Adults, United States, 1960–1962.* Washington, D.C.: Dept. of Health Education and Welfare, Public Health Service, National Center for Health Statistics, Series 11, Number 23, Government Printing Office.

KNUTSON, J. W. (1954), 'An evaluation of the Grand Rapids water fluoridation project', *J. Mich. St. med. Soc.*, **53,** 1001.

—— (1969), 'Water fluoridation after 25 years', in *International Symposium on Fluoridation and Preventive Dentistry.* New York: American Dental Association and Federation Dentaire Internationale.

LANCET (1958), 'Fluoridation', **2,** 592.

LEMKE, C. W., DOHERTY, J. M., and ARRA, M. C. (1970), 'Controlled fluoridation: The dental effects of discontinuation in Antigo, Wisconsin', *J. Am. dent. Ass.*, **80,** 782.

LINN, E. L. (1969), 'An appraisal of sociological research on the public's attitudes towards fluoridation', *J. Publ. Hlth Dent.*, **29,** 36.

LUDWIG, T. G. (1965), 'The Hastings fluoridation project, V: Dental effects between 1954 and 1964', *N.Z. dent. J.*, **61,** 175.

MCCLURE, F. J. (ed.) (1962), *Fluoride Drinking Waters.* Bethesda: US Department of Health, Education and Welfare, National Institute of Dental Research.

MCDILL, E. L., and RIDLEY, J. C. (1962), 'Status, anomia, political alienation and political participation', *Am. J. Sociol.*, **68,** 205.

MCKAY, F. S. (1928), 'The relation of mottled enamel to caries', *J. Am. dent. Ass.*, **15,** 1429.

MCNEIL, D. R. (1957), *The Fight for Fluoridation.* London: Oxford University Press.

MAIER, F. J. (1963), *A Manual of Water Fluoridation Practice.* New York: McGraw-Hill.

MARTIN, N. D. (1969), 'Introducing fluoridation to a continent', in *International Symposium on Fluoridation and Preventive Dentistry.* New York: American Dental Association and Federation Dentaire Internationale.

MAUSNER, B., and MAUSNER, J. (1955), 'A study of the antiscientific attitude', *Scient. Am.*, **192,** 35.

METZNER, C. (1956), 'Referenda for fluoridation', *Am. Ass. Publ. Hlth dent. Bull.*, **16,** 2.

—— (1957), *Some Possible Reasons Why Public and Professional Acceptance of Water Fluoridation has been Slow.* Geneva: WHO. Mimeograph.

MOTZ, A. B. (1971), 'The fluoridation issue as studied by social scientists', in *The Social Sciences and Dentistry* (ed. RICHARDS, N. D., and COHEN, L. K.). The Hague: Sijthoff and Federation Dentaire Internationale.

MURRAY, J. (1969), 'Caries experience of 15-year-old children from fluoride and non-fluoride communities', *Ibid.*, **127,** 128.

—— (1971), 'Adult dental health in fluoride and non-fluoride areas', *Br. dent. J.*, **131,** 391.

ORAL HYGIENE SERVICE (1967), *A Symposium on the Role of Fluoride in Preventive Dentistry.* London: Oral Hygiene Service.

O'SHEA, R. M., and COHEN, L. (1969), 'The social sciences and dentistry; public opinion on fluoridation, 1968', *J. Publ. Hlth Dent.*, **29,** 57.

——, and KEGELES, S. S. (1963), 'An analysis of antifluoridation letters', *J. Hlth Human Behav.*, **4,** 135.

PODSHADLEY, D. (1966), *Removing Social Blocks to Fluoridation.* San Francisco: US Public Health Service. Mimeograph.

ROEMER, R. (1965), 'Water fluoridation: Public health responsibility and the democratic process', *Am. J. Publ. Hlth*, **55,** 1337.

ROHOLM, K. (1937), *Fluorine Intoxication. A Clinical-Hygienic Study with a Review of the Literature and some Experimental Investigations.* London: Lewis.

RUSSELL, A. L. (1962), 'Dental fluorosis in Grand Rapids during the seventeenth year of fluoridation', *J. Am. dent. Ass.*, **65,** 608.

—— (1963), 'International nutrition surveys: A summary of preliminary dental findings', *J. dent. Res.*, **42,** 233.

—— (1969), 'Epidemiology and the rational bases of dental public health and dental practice', in *The Dentist, his Practice, and his Community*, 2nd ed. (YOUNG, W. O., and STRIFFLER, D. F.). Philadelphia: Saunders.

——, and ELVOVE, E. (1951), 'Domestic water and dental caries. VII. A study of the fluoride–caries relationship in an adult population', *Publ. Hlth Rep.*, **66,** 1389.

——, LEATHERWOOD, E. C., LE VAN HIEN, and VAN REEN, R. (1965), 'Dental caries and nutrition in South Vietnam', *J. dent. Res.*, **44,** 102.

SHAW, C. T. (1969), 'Characteristics of supporters and rejectors of a fluoridation referendum and a guide for other community programs', *J. Am. dent. Ass.*, **78,** 339.

SIMMEL, A. (1961), 'A signpost for research on fluoridation projects; the concept of relative deprivation', *J. soc. Issues*, **17,** 26.

STRONG, G. A. (1968), 'Liberty, religion, and fluoridation', *J. Am. dent. Ass.*, **76,** 1398.

STURGEON, L. W. (1958), 'A plebiscite on continuing fluoridation in Thorold, Ontario', *Can. J. Publ. Hlth*, **49,** 425.

TANK, G., and STORVICK, C. A. (1964), 'Caries experience of children one to six years old in two Oregon communities (Corvallis and Albany). I. Effect of fluoride on caries experience and eruption of teeth', *J. Am. dent. Ass.*, **69,** 749.

TIME (1970), 'Fluorides revisited', Issue of Mar. 2nd.

WALSH, J. (1970), 'The changing face of dentistry in New Zealand', *N.Z. dent. J.*, **66,** 214.

WORLD HEALTH ORGANIZATION (1969), 'Fluoridation and dental health', *WHO Chron.*, **23,** 505.

——— (1970a), 'Program of fluoridation of water supplies', *Proceedings of the 21st Meeting of the Regional Committee of WHO for the Americas.* Typescript.

——— (1970b), 'Fluorides and human health', *Monograph Series No. 59.* Geneva: WHO.

——— (1971), personal communication.

YOUNG, W. O., and STRIFFLER, D. F. (1969), *The Dentist, his Practice and his Community*, 2nd ed. Philadelphia: Saunders.

Chapter 4

Dental Health Services in Europe: The Regional Role of the World Health Organization

Jarmil Kostlan MD, DS, FDSRCS (ENG)
Regional Officer for Dental Health, Regional Office for Europe of the World Health Organization, Copenhagen

We have seen how dental services have developed in society, and then the mechanisms for preventing dental disease were reviewed. Dr. Kostlan begins the section on care services with a brief look at the World Health Organization, followed by a broad review of the various systems of dental care operating in WHO's European Region. Dr. Kostlan discusses the various types of private practitioner services, dental health insurance schemes, and national dental services which characterize the delivery of dental care in the region.

THE WORLD HEALTH ORGANIZATION

The World Health Organization was founded in 1948 as a specialized agency of the United Nations. It is a governmental organization, supported by its member states. It helps the member countries to strengthen their national health service systems and to train health personnel. It also supplies them with information, surveys international standards and health control measures, and assists member states in numerous other ways as well. Its Headquarters are in Geneva and six Regional Offices have been established around the world.

Problems of dental health have been followed by the World Health Organization since 1950. Special Dental Health Officers have been appointed at Headquarters and in the American and European Regional Offices. The Dental Health Unit at WHO Headquarters follows

TABLE 1

Survey of main systems of delivery of dental care in the European Region of WHO around 1970

Country	Population per dentist	Dental care based primarily on: Private practice	Social Security: DHI	Social Security: NDS	Benefit offered by Social Security to: Major part of population	Minor part of population	Service delivered by DPH care to: Major part of children	Minor part of children
Monaco	800	×				Limited	Ref.	
Sweden	1,250	×			—	—	S/C	
Norway	1,270	×			—	—	S/C	
Denmark	1,500		×		Cons.		S/C	
Germany	2,000		×		Cons.			Ref.
Finland	2,050	×			—	—	S/C	
Austria	2,150		×		Cons.			Ref.
Iceland	2,200	×			—	—		LT
Greece	2,200	×				Cons.		Em.
Switzerland	2,200	×			—	—	S/C	Ref.
France	2,300		×		Cons.		—	—
Poland	2,300			×	Cons.		S/C	
Bulgaria	2,400			×	Cons.		S/C	
Czechoslovakia	2,600			×	Cons.		S/C	
USSR	2,600			×	Cons.		S/C	
Luxembourg	3,200		×		Cons.		Ref.	LT
Italy	3,400	×			Limited			LT
Belgium	3,450		×		Cons.		—	—
UK*	3,500			×	Cons.		Ref.	LT
Hungary	3,800			×	Cons.		LT	
Netherlands	3,900		×		Cons.		LT	
Ireland	4,300		×		Cons.		Ref.	LT
Yugoslavia	5,000			×	Cons.		LT	
Romania	5,500			×	Cons.		LT	S/C
Spain	10,300	×			Limited		—	Em.
Malta	12,000	×			—	—		Em.
Turkey	14,500	×				Cons.	—	—
Albania	17,000			×	Cons.	—		LT
Portugal	19,000	×			—	—	—	—
Algeria	60,000	×			—	—	—	—
M[illegible]	80,[illegible]							

crucial problems of dental health on a world-wide basis, surveys epidemiological and planning methods, and organizes research in dental health.

The programme in dental health of the European Region is based mainly on international activities related to dental education, prevention of dental disease, and organization of dental services. Particular attention is being paid to the analysis of the delivery of the dental care services and to their rational management. The following outline of dental health services in Europe shows several problems relating to management of services in this Region.

DENTAL SERVICES IN THE EUROPEAN REGION

The European Region of the World Health Organization has 31 member countries. It extends beyond the geographical boundaries of the European continent and includes Algeria, Morocco, and the whole territories of both Turkey and the USSR. Every country in the Region has particular features in its economy, political history, and cultural traditions. Thus, it is hardly surprising that in Europe many different programmes of dental care exist next to each other.

Table 1 illustrates the overall situation from several points of view. The sequence of countries in the table corresponds to their ratio of dentists per head of population. Among the first ten, there are five Nordic countries, three central European ones, and two from the Mediterranean area. This corresponds to the general decrease in density of dental manpower from north to south. The scarcity of manpower in the southern Mediterranean strip of the region reflects the low priority of dental care in developing countries. The Nordic peak, however, corresponds not only to advanced economy but also to the highest European prevalence of dental caries, for it seems that in Norway and Sweden its prevalence may be twice as high as in central Europe or in the United Kingdom.

Notes to Table 1

Column 1	Countries arranged according to the density of dentists
Column 2	Approximate dentist-to-population ratios, mostly corresponding to dentists in active practice in 1969
Column 3	Private practice with full fee paid directly by patients
Column 4	Dental health insurance (DHI)
Column 5	National dental service (NDS)
Columns 6 and 7	The columns show what proportion of the population is eligible for the benefit indicated below (Cons. = considerable)
Columns 8 and 9	The columns show what proportion of children receives service indicated below S/C = Systematic and comprehensive dental treatment LT = Limited treatment Em. = Emergency treatment Ref. = Referral

* UK has a General Dental Service in addition to its local authority and hospital services. See Chapter 7.

In Table 1, columns 3–5 show prevailing systems of the delivery of dental care. In about one-half of the countries of the Region, the majority of the population is treated by private dental practitioners and pays directly a fee for service. Most of these countries are located in the Mediterranean and the Nordic areas.

On the other hand, schemes of social security in dental care exist in two-thirds of all countries and play a leading role in 16 of them (columns 6–7). They are represented by dental health insurance (DHI) in 13 countries and by national dental services (NDS) in 8. The former prevails in central Europe, the latter in the eastern part of the Region. Dental health insurance is a system by which a patient becomes eligible for care by payment of a regular contribution, whether this payment is voluntary or compulsory. Payment can be to a state-operated or to a private organization. Care is usually received in facilities operated by dentists who are private practitioners in the sense that they are not salaried employees of the state. The patients' contributions usually do not cover the whole costs of treatment, so some patients' charges at the time of treatment are common.

National dental services refer to a system where state-employed dentists provide care in state-operated facilities. Many items of care are provided free of charge, but some items require a payment by the patient to the clinic.

Social security, which makes dental services more easily accessible to broad layers of the population, represents the first of two general trends in European dental care. The second trend aims to establish priority care for certain groups of population, mostly children, and has materialized in numerous systems of dental public health services (DPHS). These exist in 24 countries of the Region and in 16 of them they provide care for the majority of children (columns 8–9). They can be found in almost the whole of the well-developed part of the Region. The organization of dental public health services is discussed by Burt in Chapter 6.

From the geographical point of view, systems of delivery of the dental care in the Region form a complex pattern. Eastern Europe is the only homogeneous area. It is a domain of national dental health services, covering the whole population, and combining, to a degree dependent on their economical resources, broad accessibility of basic dental care with priority service for children.

A similar basic pattern exists in the United Kingdom, services in that country are described fully by Renson in Chapter 7. Some of the central European countries also have relatively strong programmes in both social security and public dental care. This is the case in Denmark, Luxembourg, and the Netherlands. Ireland could also be grouped in this category.

Other central European countries adopted broad schemes of dental health insurance but have remained far behind the previous group as far as the dental public care is concerned. This is the case in Germany and Austria, and particularly in Belgium and France.

The opposite pattern: insignificant schemes of dental health insurance but well-supported dental public care, is characteristic of the major part of the Nordic area (Norway, Sweden, and Finland) as well as Switzerland.

In most of the Mediterranean countries dental care programmes are still developing and both the dental health insurance and priority dental care for children are either non-existent or remain considerably limited in eligibility and scope of the benefits offered. The pattern of future development of dental care services in this area is not yet clear.

SPECIFIC EXAMPLES OF DENTAL CARE SERVICES

In Czechoslovakia, as in most eastern European countries, access to health care is granted to every citizen as a right. Dental care is a part of the integrated health care system and is financed from the national budget. Overall planning and co-ordination is with the republican Ministries of Health, whereas the operation of dental services is a matter of co-operation between regional, district, and municipal health administrations. Nearly the whole population is eligible for care, which is performed in public dental clinics free of charge except for limited charges for inlays and fixed prostheses paid to the clinic. Children and priority groups of adults are exempted from payment of charges. Specialist treatment is available in district dental centres or in regional dental hospitals. All the dental health personnel are employed by the health administration and receive fixed salaries. One practising dentist cares, on an average, for an area with about 3000 inhabitants, the choice of dentist by patient being limited in practice to a dentist working either near the patient's home or near his place of work. Private dental practice is very limited, probably accounting for less than one per cent of the total volume of dental care.

Priority dental care for children and selected groups of adults is organized as a sub-system of the general dental service and is delivered in school dental surgeries or public dental clinics. The children are systematically examined and treated comprehensively. Practically all school children and about one-quarter of preschool children and adolescents are treated regularly once a year.

Other countries of Eastern Europe exhibit the same fundamental patterns of organization, though some variations do exist. Services in the USSR are similar to those in Czechoslovakia, and in Bulgaria a higher proportion of preschool children receive treatment. In Hungary, some 20 per cent of total dental care is delivered through private practice, and in Romania there is a smaller proportion of children receiving systematic care than in the other countries. Yugoslavia has a decentralized administration of dental services and dentists there are paid on an item-of-service basis. Financing in Yugoslavia is through the state social security system.

The central European schemes of dental care based on health insurance are exemplified by the Federal Republic of Germany. The German dental health insurance scheme has been established for more than half a century. At present, the insurance is compulsory for most of the citizens, depending on their income level. It is financed by contributions from both employees and employers, and is administered by numerous private insurance companies. The service is delivered in private dental surgeries, nearly all dentists having contracts with the insurance companies. The dentists treat patients on the basis of a scale of fees per item of service, which is reviewed periodically on the national level by representatives of the insurance companies and the dental association. The government's only concern is with the legal basis for these arrangements. Over 95 per cent of the population is eligible for care under this system. The benefits are the same for insured persons and for their dependents, and vary little from one insurance company to another. Surgical and conservative treatment is free of charge to the patient whereas the cost of prosthetic and orthodontic treatment is partly subsidized and partly paid for by the patient. Even though only 3 per cent of patients receive care on a purely private basis, the average dentist receives up to half his income from patient payments. The subsidy has been increasing steadily. It has risen six times during the last 20 years, and for prosthetic treatment alone by 50 per cent over a 10-year period. The dental service is available in all regions of the country.

In other countries of this area the proportion of the insured population is about the same, though in the Netherlands it drops to only 70 per cent. The benefits offered, however, are somewhat lower. In Austria only acrylic dentures are partly subsidized. In France and Denmark the benefits cover 75 per cent and 66 per cent respectively of the total expenses, but prosthetic treatment must be paid for in full. On the other hand, in France the whole approved orthodontic treatment is free of charge. In many of these countries some dental treatment is provided in the dental clinics organized by the Sick Funds.

In contrast to the insurance scheme, the dental public health service in Germany developed only in three of the nine federal states. It is organized by municipalities and partly supported by the respective states. It covers, in general, regular inspection of schoolchildren and their referral for treatment to private dental practitioners, when the treatment itself is covered by the DHI. Each of the salaried public health dentists inspects yearly up to 20,000 children. In Hessen, routine data are collected systematically for evaluation of their care. Practically all children have received regular check-ups, 60 per cent of them have been treated completely, and 20 per cent have received partial treatment.

The Austrian system is similar in extent and scope, though some of the Viennese children are treated in municipal clinics. In Luxembourg, the proportion of children both inspected and treated is higher. In Denmark, half of the schoolchildren are treated systematically and comprehensively in school clinics. In the Netherlands, the dental public health service is organized in most places through both the local municipality and the Sick Funds, and over 60 per cent of schoolchildren receive a more or less complete treatment.

The 'nordic' pattern of dental care is represented by the Norwegian and Swedish systems, which are rather similar to each other. In these countries the role of dental insurance is negligible. The whole population is eligible to receive care through the dental public service system, but up till now the public service has been organized primarily for dental care of schoolchildren, and its facilities and manpower are still insufficient to be able to cope with the treatment of the remaining part of the population. Consequently, 75 per cent of all adult patients and most of the preschool children depend on private treatment for which they pay the full fee. The dental insurance covers only 2 per cent of total expenses for dental care. Over 70 per cent of dentists work purely on this private basis. As for the public dental care, the initiative, organization, and main financial responsibility is either with the municipalities or with the counties. The national governments participate, as a rule, by covering part of the salaries. Some 27 per cent of the dentists work for the dental public service and receive either a fixed salary or fee per item of service. The service is delivered in school or community dental clinics. Fifty-five per cent of the working time is devoted to children and 45 per cent to adults. Schoolchildren aged 6–16 years in Sweden, and 6–17 years in Norway, are treated free of charge. Preschool children and adolescents receive the service at a reduced charge, whereas adults pay full fixed fees, which are lower than those prevailing in private practice. About 10–20 per cent of the adults are treated through the DPHS. Their interest in this treatment is much higher and long waiting lists for adults exist in most public clinics. In Norway 80 per cent of schoolchildren, and 75 per cent in Sweden, are treated systematically and comprehensively. Dental services in Norway are described in more detail by Burt in Chapter 6.

As far as Finland is concerned, the dental public services work under a set of general conditions which is similar to that in Norway and Sweden. It is centred on elementary school children, on an age-priority basis, the first priority is for those aged 7–10 years and the second priority for those from 11–14 years. All children in the first group and half in the second are examined by school dentists and 85 per cent of those inspected are treated regularly and comprehensively.

In the Mediterranean area there is a variable organizational pattern for dental services. The number of dentists varies tremendously not only among countries, but also within individual countries; the density of dental manpower in the urban areas is up to 150 times higher than in the rural areas. In the developing countries problems of general health have a high priority and only limited resources can be allocated to dental care. The usual pattern consists of a private practice service, sometimes with very limited assistance from DHI in cities, and a loose network of public dental health facilities in rural areas. The latter are usually situated in hospitals or community health centres, and they provide, free of charge, simple emergency treatment for broad layers of the indigent population. Some of these features can be found even in those countries of this area which are relatively rich in manpower. Even in those with limited manpower, such as Algeria and Turkey, there are strong trends to expand and organize dental care, but the design of the future services remains to be seen. Collection of data to be used in organizing dental services has started already in Malta and Spain.

CONCLUSION

Different areas of the European Region face different problems in the development of dental health care. In the southern area the main task may be the analysis of conditions determining future development of dental services. The central and northern areas might profit from an evaluation of different programmes and comparisons of their effectiveness, whereas countries with national health services may be interested in the efficiency and economy of preventive measures, in the use of dental auxiliaries, and in system analysis which would improve the co-ordination within their programmes. It seems that these diverse problems can be related to one common denominator, namely to the need for further research in the advancement of dental public health.

Chapter 5

Dental Epidemiology and Survey Procedures

P. M. C. James MDS (LOND.), LDSRCS, DPD (ST AND.)
John Humphreys Professor of Dental Health, University of Birmingham
J. F. Beal LDSRCS, BDS (LOND.), PHD (BIRM.)
Lecturer in Dental Health, University of Birmingham

To be delivered effectively, dental services must be carefully planned, operated, and evaluated. Epidemiology is the basic measuring device employed in all three steps, and should always be considered as an integral part of the administration of the service.

Professor James and Dr. Beal outline the way in which epidemiology has developed historically, and take us past many landmarks in dental epidemiology. This is followed by a step-by-step description of how a study should be organized, then a detailed study of examination methods, diagnostic criteria, and indices. Later chapters will apply the application of epidemiology to various aspects of dental service administration.

INTRODUCTION

The word 'epidemiology' is derived from the Greek *epi*—upon, *demos*—the people, and *logos*—discourse or science. The scope of this branch of science was originally confined to the origins, development, and distribution of communicable disease or epidemic infections, but nowadays it has a wider and more literal meaning. It can be defined as 'the orderly study of diseases and other conditions in human populations where the group rather than the individual is the unit of interest'. Groups may vary in size from the family or the school to the country, continent, or the world, and the observations may involve not only clinical diagnosis but a number of special investigations such as those concerned with microbiology, genetics, or haematology. Numerous other factors may be considered, including environment, social status, and even religion.

The objects of epidemiology are two-fold: the investigation of disease and other conditions in populations to ascertain the public health needs, and to conduct research into the factors that may influence the occurrence of the disease or conditions with a view to their ultimate prevention or control. The activities of the epidemiologist are aptly expressed by Englander (1962):

> He collects and tabulates data, searches for causes, and tests hypotheses in the field. He attempts to correlate morbidity and mortality rates with appropriate agent, host and environmental factors in order to detect relative risks among and within populations.

There are two basic types of epidemiology. The first, known as *descriptive epidemiology*, is concerned with the observation and reporting of the distribution of a disease or condition in a population or populations. Later, hypotheses may be formulated to explain those observations and studies of the second type, *analytical epidemiology*, are designed to test these hypotheses. In this type of investigation the epidemiologist seeks to discover factors and mechanisms associated with the distribution and prevention of the disease.

HISTORY

The history of epidemiology cannot be separated from that of medicine, especially up to the nineteenth century. Man's belief about the cause of epidemics has undergone radical change through the ages. It was originally believed that disease was the result of demons or divine judgment by a wrathful god or gods; later this was refined to an acceptance that illness was part of God's plan for man. With the development of ancient Greece came the advent of rational theory and it was then thought that infections were caused by miasma or effluvium, a putrid matter in the atmosphere associated with dead bodies and filthy living conditions. Not until after the work of Louis Pasteur (1822–95) and Robert Koch (1843–1910) was this philosophy refuted and the germ-theory accepted.

The founder of logical thought in medicine and the first known epidemiologist was Hippocrates of Cos (460–375 BC). Hippocrates believed, in an age when hardly any exact data or observation existed, that the world was ordered and that this order could be understood by the intellect of man. After his death, the Greeks returned to their priest healers and, with a few exceptions, scientific method was lost to medicine for five hundred years. It was revived by Claudius Galen (130–200 AD), a Greek who lived in Rome for much of his life. Galen wrote that 'reason alone discovers some things, experience alone discovers some, but to find others requires both experience and reason'.

By about the mid-thirteenth century, the first medical schools in Europe were founded and scientific reasoning was resurrected, especially in the field of anatomy where dissections were carried out on executed criminals. Some time was still to elapse, however, before the first glimmerings of epidemiological science started to emerge. An important development took place in the seventeenth century. Like Hippocrates, Thomas Sydenham (1624–89), a London physician, stressed the importance of careful clinical observation. Unlike Hippocrates, who wrote the histories of sick persons, Sydenham wrote the history of disease and thus became the founder of epidemiology as we know it today.

John Snow (1813–58), one of the greatest of all epidemiologists, carried out the classic study on cholera recorded in his treatise *On the Mode of Communication of Cholera* (Snow, 1855). He pointed out that sailors were attacked by cholera only when visiting ports where the disease already existed. He cited several instances of infected individuals going to a new locality and initiating a fresh chain of infection, suggesting that the disease was transmitted to those having physical contact with the soiled clothes of a diseased person, and that infection could also occur after the drinking of water contaminated by an adjacent sewer. The central part of the work is his description of the cholera epidemic in Soho, London, in 1854, during which over 500 deaths occurred within a period of 10 days. Marking the location of each death on a map he found a distribution with a dense central point thinning towards the periphery (*Fig*. 1). At this central point, situated in Broad Street, was a pump from which the local inhabitants obtained their water.

He followed this up by the investigation of a number of individual cases. For example, one man had come to London from Brighton to visit his brother, only to find that he had recently died. After a quick meal, with which he drank some of the pump water, he left and went on to Pentonville. The next evening he was taken ill with cholera and he died the following night. Another much-quoted example was that of an old woman living in Hampstead, who liked the water from the Broad Street pump and had a bottle of it taken to her each day. Her niece from Islington visited her and drank some of the water before returning home. They both contracted cholera and died; no other cases of the disease were reported in either Hampstead or Islington. At Snow's insistence the handle of the Broad Street pump was removed and immediately the epidemic subsided. Snow's work demonstrates the train of logical inference that leads to important public health developments.

Similar reasoning was employed by William Budd (1811–80) a contemporary of Snow, who did for typhoid fever what Snow had done for cholera. There are many other examples of this type of epidemiological work.

This century has seen numerous important epidemiological studies, only a brief mention of two will be made. The first was by McAlistair Gregg in 1941, drawing attention to the association between rubella in early pregnancy and the unusually frequent occurrence of congenital cataract in the infant. This was followed by further epidemiological surveys and also studies in embryology and virology which clearly demonstrated a causal relationship.

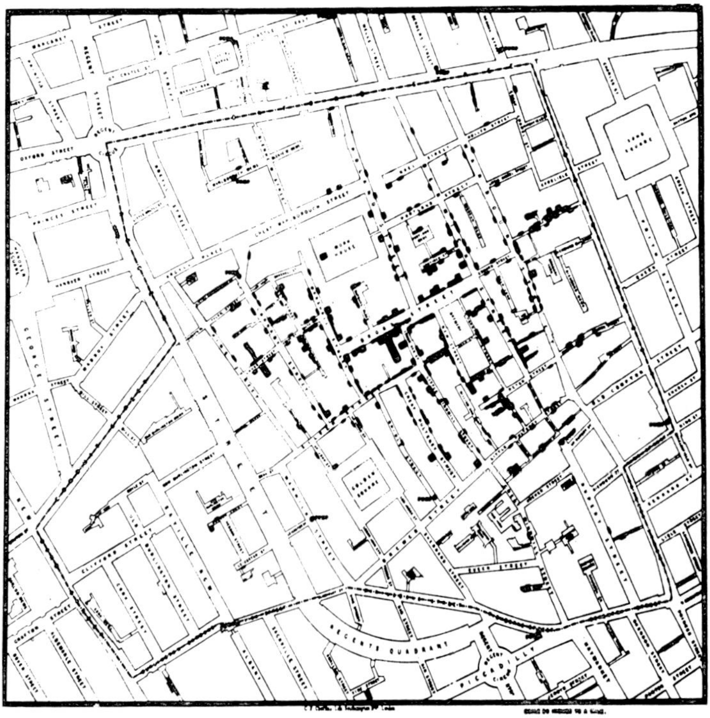

Fig. 1. John Snow's map of the Soho area in London, showing the distribution of deaths from cholera in the epidemic of 1854.

The second is a group of studies conducted by R. Doll and A. Bradford Hill (1950, 1964) into the association between smoking and carcinoma of the lung. In the initial enquiries patients with established carcinoma of the lungs were questioned about their smoking habits and the findings compared with those from a control group which was similarly interrogated. Following this, further studies were carried out by recording the smoking habits of 40,000 doctors and subsequently relating their cause of death, as recorded on their death certificates, with these habits. These investigations demonstrated the relationship between smoking and lung cancer.

DENTAL EPIDEMIOLOGY

Early work was limited to the descriptive type of study based on the clinical examination of individuals. This can be illustrated by two examples from the *Books of Epidemics* by Hippocrates, quoted by Guerini (1967): 'The third upper tooth is found to be decayed more frequently than all the others' and 'among those individuals whose heads are long shaped, some have thick necks, strong members and bones; others have strongly arched palates, their teeth are disposed irregularly, crowding one on the other . . .' Organized epidemiological research

390 LONGEVITY, &c. OF GREENWICH PENSIONERS.

Age.	Names of pensioners upwards of 80 years of age.	How long in the King's service.	Whether they lived in cold or warm climates	If ever married.	If in the habit of drinking freely.	If in the habit of using tobacco freely.	The state of their organs, and mental faculties.	The state of their teeth
86	George Forbes	18 years	Warm	20 years	Freely	Snuffs freely	Very dim-sighted. Hearing bad	Bad teeth
85	Richard Oldston	32 years	Cold	60 years	Moderate	Never used tobacco	Middling eye sight. Hard of hearing	Bad teeth
81	Peter Eager	14 years	Warm	50 years	Very little	Chews freely	Rather dim-sighted. Otherwise good	Very bad teeth
82	Edward Collins	36 years	Cold	40 years	Very freely	Chews freely	Very dim-sighted. Otherwise good	Middling teeth
82	George Diffiny	20 years	Both	30 years	Freely	Chews freely	Very dim sighted. Otherwise good	Middling teeth
83	William Wright	50 years	Warm	24 years	Freely	Smokes freely	Very hard of hearing	Middling teeth
92	Edward Skinner	25 years	Cold	43 years	Moderate	Chews freely	Very hard of hearing	Bad teeth
98	Daniel M'Neal	37 years	Cold	22 years	Moderate	Chews freely	Ditto, and blind of one eye	Middling good teeth
82	Jeffery Moore	16 years	Cold	22 years	Very little	Never used any	Dim-sighted. Very infirm	Bad teeth
87	Nathaniel Chapman	15 years	Warm	2 years	Moderate	Snuffs freely	Dim sighted. Very infirm	Not a tooth left
81	Robert Hannaway	21 years	Mostly warm	49 years	Moderate	Snuffs freely	Very deaf. Otherwise very good	Front teeth pretty good
102	John Moore	31 years	Mostly cold	60 years	Pretty freely	Chews freely	Rather dim-sighted. 4 new teeth—3 lost	Bad teeth
91	Daniel Coughlan	30 years	Mostly warm	40 years	Moderate	Snuffs freely	Very good	Good teeth
89	John Hutchins	22 years	Mostly warm	45 years	Moderate	Chews freely	Sight bad	Not a tooth left
95	John Jackson	19 years	Mostly cold	50 years	Freely	Smokes freely	Very short of breath	Not a tooth left
83	John Blackwell	16 years	Both	60 years	Freely	Snuffs freely	Very infirm	Not a tooth left
90	John M'Pearson	22 years	Mostly warm	22 years	Freely	Smokes freely	Very good	Not a tooth left
94	Thomas Lansdown	14 years	Mostly warm	22 years	Freely	Chews freely	Very dim sighted	Middling good teeth
80	James Archer	12 years	Mostly warm	14 years	Freely	Chews freely	Very good	Not a tooth left
85	Adam Malcum	14 years	Mostly warm	19 years	Moderate	Chews freely	Dim sighted and palsy	Not a tooth left
84	Thomas Vaughan	14 years	Mostly warm	34 years	Freely	Chews freely	Quite blind. Otherwise good	Not a tooth left
80	John Carbery	14 years	Mostly warm	14 years	Freely	Chews freely	Dim-sighted	Not a tooth left
81	Isaac Rutter	21 years	Mostly warm	40 years	Freely	Smokes freely	Very dim-sighted. Otherwise good	Bad teeth
81	James Patch	8 years	Moderate	30 years	Freely	Chews freely	Very infirm. Very dim-sighted	Bad teeth

Fig. 2. Tabulated findings from Greenwich pensioners, reported by Sinclair in 1803.

appeared to be completely lacking until the end of the eighteenth and the beginning of the nineteenth centuries.

One of the first field studies of the teeth in Britain was reported in the *Naval Chronicle* of 1803. Sir John Sinclair had collected details of the health habits and dental state of 96 old men, all aged over 80 years, from Dr. Robert Robertson, physician to Greenwich Hospital, where all the subjects were spending their remaining years as ex-service pensioners (Sinclair, 1803). It is interesting to note that 21 were edentulous, 9 had 'very bad' teeth, 48 'bad' teeth, 11 'middling' teeth, 2 'middling good' teeth, and 5 'good' teeth. *Fig.* 2 shows one page of the tabulated findings. Unfortunately the criteria for diagnosis were not defined.

THE

TEETH A TEST OF AGE,

CONSIDERED WITH REFERENCE

TO THE

FACTORY CHILDREN.

ADDRESSED TO THE

MEMBERS OF BOTH HOUSES OF PARLIAMENT.

BY EDWIN SAUNDERS,

FELLOW OF THE MEDICO-BOTANICAL SOCIETY;
AUTHOR OF
"FIVE MINUTES' ADVICE ON THE CARE OF THE TEETH," ETC.

LONDON:
H. RENSHAW, 356, STRAND.
M DCCC XXXVII.

Fig. 3. Title page of a communication addressed to Members of both Houses of Parliament by Edwin Saunders in 1837.

A generation later a more scientific exercise in dental epidemiology with important social implications was conducted by a young dentist, Edwin Saunders. At this time Britain was rapidly becoming industrialized and there was much abuse of child labour in the mines and factories. The great reformers like Sir Robert Peel were striving to have legal restrictions applied to the number of hours per day that young children should be permitted to work, and attempts were made to draw up a scale of permitted working hours according to age. But there was considerable difficulty in ascertaining the true age of children, because the financial interests of parents and employers alike encouraged falsification, and birth registration methods were in their infancy. Measurement of children's height was advised by some, but Saunders strongly condemned such methods and recommended instead an index of maturity, such as would be supplied by the eruption of teeth into the mouth. He carried out what was probably the first systematic dental epidemiology in Britain studying eruption of teeth between the ages of 9 and 13; in 1837 he addressed his findings to Parliament in a report entitled: *The Teeth a Test of Age, considered with reference to the Factory Children* (Saunders, 1837). *Fig.* 3 shows the title page of this report.

A few years later, in 1848, John Tomes, who seemed to excel in every branch of dental science, performed and published a tooth mortality study (Tomes, 1848). He obtained 3000 extracted teeth, classified them by tooth type, and calculated, among other things, the relative frequency of tooth loss and the ages at which the teeth were extracted. The techniques he used in this investigation were similar to those current today.

An interesting early example of clinical data collection is given in the *British Journal of Dental Science* (Atkinson, 1863). The Odontological Society of Great Britain received in this year a request for assistance in scientific dental investigations from the New York Society of Dental Surgeons and the Brooklyn Dental Association. The forms which were sent for distribution to interested dentists include that shown in *Fig.* 4, which is reminiscent of modern data collection methods.

Towards the end of the nineteenth century the public health aspects of dentistry were investigated by William Fisher, a Dundee dentist who qualified in 1877. He was so concerned by the high caries experience and the lack of treatment in the child population that he devoted much time campaigning for compulsory inspection and treatment of children in schools. Following the publication of his paper *Compulsory Attention to the Teeth of School Children* (Fisher, 1885) a Committee was appointed by the British Dental Association to investigate child dental health by epidemiological methods. The studies were carried out between 1890 and 1897, and the subsequent reports were an important step towards the initiation and development of a School Dental Service.

Another historic British study was that conducted by Ainsworth and Young on behalf of the Medical Research Council (1925). This was a nation-wide survey of schoolchildren in which tooth eruption, dental caries prevalence, hypoplasia, gingivitis, and malocclusions were investigated. Apart from being an excellent record of contemporary conditions the report is of particular interest because it indicated the significantly lower caries experience in certain rural schools in East Anglia, a fact not understood at the time but which was to be explained within the next decade.

The story of the association of fluoride in the drinking water first with typical enamel opacities and later with the prevalence of dental caries is an excellent example of epidemiological techniques. The classic procedure of mapping cases, after the example of Snow and others, quickly showed that the enamel condition was associated with water distribution. In Britain Ainsworth's suggestion: 'My own view . . . is that the cause of both mottling and stain will be found in some quality

CASE.					SALIVA IS										TEETH ARE									REMARKS.
									Odour.															
Date.	Age.	Sex.	Nativity.	State of Health.	Abundant.	Deficient.	Aqueous.	Viscid.	Sweet.	Fetid.	Acid.	Alkaline.	Neutral.	Healthy.	Diseased.	Regular.	Irregular.	Normal.	Precocious.	Tardy.	Plus.	Minus.		

Fig. 4. Form for clinical data collection distributed in 1863 by Dr. Atkinson on behalf of the New York Society of Dental Surgeons and the Brooklyn Dental Association.

or impurity of the drinking water not ascertainable by ordinary analytical methods' (Ainsworth, 1928) was strikingly similar to that of McKay in the United States (McKay, 1916). Soon afterwards the trace element responsible for the typical enamel appearance was shown by Churchill (1931) to be fluoride.

The pioneer work in the relationship between caries and fluoride carried out by Dean and his co-workers has been described by Burt in Chapter 3. The effect of all these epidemiological studies was to produce a major public health advance: the control of caries by the artificial adjustment of a fluoride-deficient drinking water to the optimum level. *Fig.* 5 shows some results of Dean's survey (Dean et al., 1942), which demonstrated the relationship between the extent of dental caries in children with the fluoride content of the water they were consuming.

Fluoride was an accidental discovery in the first instance. The difference between dental caries prevalence in certain areas might not have been noticed for many years had not the obvious mottled enamel drawn attention to something worthy of investigation. Current workers in dental epidemiology are not content to wait for the next accidental revelation; they are constantly in the field observing disease and conditions in the population, seeking unexpected differences between groups that may provide another public health advance.

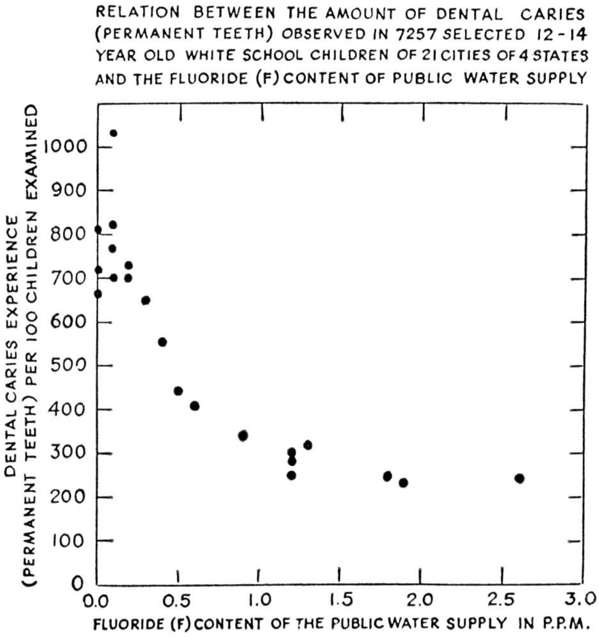

Fig. 5. 'Dean's curve' published in 1942.

SCIENTIFIC METHOD IN DENTAL EPIDEMIOLOGY

An epidemiological investigation should follow a logical scientific pattern, of which the following is an example:

1. Formulation of the hypothesis.
2. Design of the investigation.
3. Selection of the sample.
4. Conduct of the seamination.
5. Analysis of the data.
6. Drawing the conclusions.
7. Publishing the results.

FORMULATION OF THE HYPOTHESIS

The investigator must be absolutely clear about the objects of the investigation before he considers its design as the latter is entirely dependent upon the former. The starting point of a study is frequently the expression of a *null hypothesis*; that is the assumption, for example, that there is no difference in the extent of dental disease between the groups to be investigated; or, in the circumstances of a clinical trial, that one method is no better than another in preventing or treating a disease or condition. The object of the investigation will be to test this hypothesis.

DESIGN OF THE INVESTIGATION

Types of Study There are two main subdivisions of both descriptive and analytical epidemiology. The first is known as the *prevalence study*, also called a point-prevalence or cross-sectional study, where the occurrence of a disease or condition in a population is expressed at a given point in time. This type of study is concerned with the *state* of the population at that time. In a disease such as dental caries, which affects a high proportion of individuals in most communities, it is also necessary to measure the *intensity* or *extent* of individual attack. Prevalence studies are commonly used for making comparisons between two or more populations, or between the same population at different times.

The second type is the *incidence* or longitudinal study, where the amount of new disease in a population is measured over a period of time. This is usually expressed as the proportion of that population which becomes affected per unit time. In contrast to the prevalence study, the incidence study is concerned with *events* which happen during the investigation. In a progressive disease such as dental caries it is necessary to measure the increase by the extent of the new disease, often referred to as the *increment*. This is obtained by observing the same group of individuals on two occasions and subtracting the extent found at the first examination from that observed at the second. This method is usually adopted for conducting clinical trials.

The terms *prevalence* and *incidence* are still used incorrectly at times in the dental literature. The definitions of prevalence, meaning the conditions existing at a particular point in time, and incidence, meaning the change in a condition over a period of time, were accepted by an Expert Committee of the World Health Organization in 1962 (World Health Organization, 1962).

In addition to these two main types of investigation there is, of course, a number of others; correlation studies for example, in which the aim is to investigate the possible relationship between the variables discovered during clinical observation, such as dental cleanliness and gingivitis.

Controls Where an investigation is to be carried out into the possible effects of a factor on the prevalence or incidence of disease in a group of individuals, it is not enough to confine the examinations to the group exposed to the factor under scrutiny. A parallel group *not* exposed must also be studied in the same way; this is called the *control* group and it must be as similar as possible to the test group except in respect of the factor under investigation. This control group is necessary both when the factor under investigation is naturally occurring and when it is under the control of the epidemiologist. Similarly where a group of people known to have a disease is investigated to determine their exposure to factors that may be relevant, the results must be compared with those from a control group in which the individuals do not have the disease in question.

The control group is necessary in order to avoid the fallacious *post hoc* argument, which implies a cause and effect relationship without further substantiation. A reduction in caries following the addition of fluoride to a town's water supply does not prove that the former is the result of the latter; it might be coincidental, due to some other factor. The comparison with a control group which is similar as regards social structure, ethnic background, and geographic position helps to eliminate that possibility.

In the case of a clinical trial, such as the testing of a fluoride dentifrice, the individuals taking part must be assigned to the test or control group at random. In trials of this type it is important to supply the control group with a substance similar in appearance and other properties to that being tested; this is called a *placebo*. In a dentifrice trial the placebo would be a paste having the same colour, texture, and taste as the test paste, but with the test ingredient absent.

In some circumstances it may be possible for the same individual to be both test and control. Where a clinical trial of a measure such as the use of a fissure sealant is to be carried out, one side of the mouth of each subject could be used as the test and the other as the control. However, it is still necessary to assign the test and control sides at random. This method has the additional advantage that paired statistical tests, which are more sensitive, may be used. It must be stressed that this technique is not suitable for all clinical trials. For example, in the testing of a topical fluoride solution it would be impossible to ensure that no fluoride ions crossed the midline in the saliva thus giving the control side the benefit of the test solution.

Blind Studies It is always desirable that the investigator should not know whether a subject is a member of a test or a control group, that is, the study should be 'blind'. If the subject is also in ignorance of whether he is using a test product or a placebo the study is termed *double blind.* This is to avoid unconscious bias in the chain of events or diagnosis.

This condition is sometimes extremely difficult to fulfil, especially in fluoridation studies, where the examiner is almost certain to know where he is and therefore might know the fluoride content of the water. At least one blind fluoridation study has been carried out, however

(Forrest and James, 1965) by taking children from test and control areas to centres where the examination could be conducted without the dentist knowing their place of residence.

Another method of achieving 'blindness' has been used in the Tiel–Culemborg fluoridation study in the Netherlands; here the diagnosis was made from dental radiographs of children from the different areas; the examiner not knowing the place of origin of each set of X-rays. Again, it is possible, after examining subjects in a high fluoride area, to ascertain their individual periods of residence in the district, allocating them to *continuous* and *non-continuous* groups. The caries score can then be expressed for each group separately. This is not the most satisfactory method of obtaining blindness because many of the subjects categorized as 'non-continuous' will have derived benefits from the fluoride proportional to their length of residence, so they do not represent a good control.

Method of Study Some investigations can be carried out as controlled experiments by giving or withholding a specific factor and measuring the effect on the prevention or cure of a disease. For example, a clinical trial may be designed to investigate the efficacy of a fluoride toothpaste. Here a series of prevalence studies may be made at intervals on the *same* group of children to ascertain the incidence of new caries in each child. Comparison with a control group using a placebo dentifrice will enable the effects of the fluoride toothpaste to be assessed.

Other studies necessitate the surveying of groups of individuals without having control of the factors being investigated. These can be regarded as 'nature's experiments' and may be of two types: the case-control study and the cohort study (Armitage, 1971). In the *case-control* study the starting point is a group with the disease under investigation. Assessment is made of the factors which have influenced these subjects in the past and which might be associated with the disease, and the findings are compared with those from a suitable control. The *cohort* study, on the other hand, starts with a population of individuals classified according to the various factors of interest. During a follow-up period assessment is made of the influence that these factors may have on the occurrence of the disease.

Case-control studies are often known as *retrospective* or backward studies, and cohort studies as *prospective* or forward studies. Some workers, however, relate the prospective and retrospective classification to the time of collection of the data, the former being when it is collected by the investigator himself and the latter when he uses previously recorded data. These terms have, therefore, led to some confusion in the past.

In the dental field, the case-control method and the cohort method could both be used for such studies as, for example, the association between the early extraction of first permanent molars and the impaction of the third molars. Unfortunately the study of a disease such as dental caries differs from many other diseases in two important ways.

First, as previously stated, its occurrence is often measured not in terms of the proportion of the population which suffers from it but by the extent to which they are affected. Secondly, each individual provides his own 'retrospective' record of past experience as each affected tooth will either still be carious or have been filled or extracted. Because of these two factors it is impossible to classify the method of study in the same way as for other diseases. It is therefore recommended that studies into the prevalence or extent of dental caries are termed 'retrospective' as they are concerned with past occurrences of the disease, and studies into the incidence or extent of any new caries are called 'prospective' as these relate to its future development.

SELECTION OF THE SAMPLE

When designing a study it is usually impossible to examine every individual in the population or 'universe' under investigation. Resources in terms of time, manpower, and money are not available for the collection and analysis of such vast amounts of data. For this reason a small number of individuals or a *sample* must be chosen from the population.

A *selected sample* is one in which a criterion is set for inclusion in the study and each individual satisfying the criterion forms part of the sample. This type of sample may be self-selected or it may be selected by the research worker. The *self-selected* sample involves volunteers for examination, and they may differ greatly from the rest of the population. In a dental survey subjects might volunteer for an oral examination because they are proud of having a good dentition or, alternatively, because they think that they need treatment and hope that this will be done for them free of charge. The reasons for the self-selection are not known by the investigator but inevitably they lead to bias in one direction or another.

Selection by the epidemiologist may take many forms. It may be haphazard, taking subjects arbitrarily out of a crowd, or it may be systematic, such as by selecting each patient whose registration number ends in 3, whose birthday is on the thirteenth of any month, or whose surname begins with a certain letter. These methods may lead to bias; for example, if the letter M is used for selection by surname the sample may contain a disproportionate number of Scottish people with names starting with Mac or Mc. However, the bias may not always be obvious and care should be taken in using such methods of sampling.

A technique which will provide more valid data is to take a *random sample* from the population. For the sample to be truly random *each individual must have an equal chance of being included in the sample*. One of the easiest ways of doing this is to use random number tables. However, even when using random sampling methods, the sample could be unrepresentative of the population. 'Freak' selections occur occasionally; in card-playing there have been instances where all thirteen cards of one suit have been dealt to one player, and more rarely still, each player being dealt a complete suit. However, the statistical tests used in analysing the data are able to estimate the sampling error.

In some cases it is more convenient for administrative and economic reasons to sample from *clusters* rather than individuals. If a dental officer wishes to examine 10 per cent of the 5-year-old children in his area it may well prove best to sample the schools rather than the individual children. In this case each school forms the appropriate cluster. Using these clusters as sampling units he would make a random selection until the total number of children in the schools selected reaches 10 per cent of the 5-year-old population.

Sometimes a *stratified* random sample is taken. If the condition under investigation is known to be related to various factors such as age, sex, or area of residence the population is first divided into these groups or strata and a random sample taken within each stratum. For example, dental caries is an age-specific disease and so any population in which a survey is to be made into the prevalence or extent of the disease should be stratified by age. The analysis may then be carried out on each stratum separately, or for the population as a whole by weighting the strata to take into account the proportion of each stratum in the population.

Sampling by stages may sometimes be necessary. This technique was used in the Government Social Survey (Gray et al., 1970) in which the aim was: '. . . to provide information about the dental health of the community generally and to establish whether there was any regional variation in dental health'. The inquiry was in two parts, an interview followed at a later date by a dental examination, both conducted in the home.

The population covered was defined as those persons aged 16 and over living in private households. It was found that the Electoral Register provided an adequate *sampling frame* for adults aged 21 or over. A *two-stage sample* design was used. The 547 parliamentary constituencies were first stratified by region and 50 were then selected with a probability proportionate to the electorate on the register. The second stage units were the people over 21 on the register in those selected constituencies. From these was drawn a sample of named people who were selected with a probability inversely proportional to the electorate. In this way the overall probability of selection of each individual over the two stages was equal. The total sample was 3300, that is, 66 subjects per constituency.

The size of the sample is dependent on the statistical characteristics of the data to be collected. Statistical characteristics of sample selection are presented by Osborn in Chapter 10.

CONDUCT OF THE EXAMINATION

For the scientific epidemiological study of dental disease and conditions, three aspects are of great importance: *the examination methods and diagnostic aids*, the *diagnostic criteria*, and the *indices* used for measurement and reporting. These provide between them a very wide area for disagreement and misunderstanding between epidemiological workers and this has made it difficult or impossible to make more than general comparisons between the findings of different research teams in the past. There have been attempts to standardize the various methods at national and international levels but up to the present time international comparisons in particular have been limited and many have been unreliable. The need for standardized procedures was recognized by an Expert Committee of the World Health Organization, which produced the report referred to earlier in this chapter (World Health Organization, 1962). Subsequently, the WHO itself produced a manual entitled *Oral Health Surveys; Basic Methods* (World Health Organization, 1971). It is recommended that this manual should be consulted

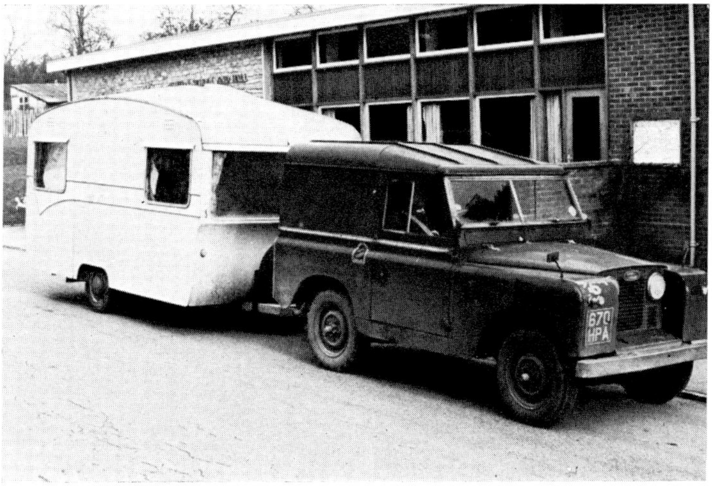

Fig. 6. A typical dental examination unit.

prior to all dental epidemiological studies. It sets out simple procedural and diagnostic systems which, if adopted, would allow comparison of studies all over the world. It is obviously desirable, whatever the purpose of the study, to design it in such a way as to make it contribute to the pool of international information.

Basic requirements for the mouth examination are a chair, preferably with a head rest, on which to seat the subject, a source of illumination, which can either be a separate unit or a light attached to the head of the examiner, and some method of cleaning the teeth to remove loose debris where necessary. There are many refinements designed for the comfort of the subject and convenience of the examiner. Some workers (Slack, 1966) prefer to have the subject in a reclining position on a couch; the dentist can then remain seated at the head and no bending or chair adjustments are required to compensate for the varying size of the subjects. A recorder, live or tape, is necessary for receiving the information called by the examiner; even if a human recorder is available some workers use a tape recorder as well to check possible human errors in the transcription.

It is a great convenience to house the epidemiological team in a mobile unit which is driven or towed to the place of examination. This ensures standardization of the examination environment and also reduces the inconvenience occasioned by the examination at the location visited, an important public relations consideration. *Fig.* 6 shows a typical mobile examination unit and *Fig.* 7 shows an examination in progress.

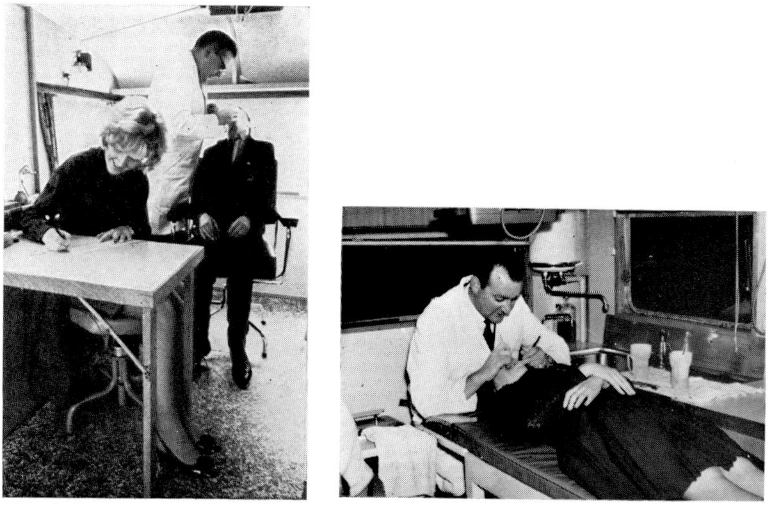

Fig. 7. A dental examination in progress.

The length of time that it takes to examine each subject depends on the extent and detail of the examination and the habits and inclination of the examiner. Times for mouth examination by different workers vary considerably even when exactly the same information is being collected; extremes of two minutes to one and a half hours have been admitted. No rules can be laid down in this matter but two principles should be considered. First, that the examination for epidemiological purposes should be as automatic as possible to obviate excessive intrusion of subjective thought and for this reason it is probably desirable to perform it quickly. Secondly, the object of epidemiological study is to examine subjects in fairly large numbers. Excessive time spent on each individual necessitates a reduction in the number of individuals seen.

The flow of subjects through the examination unit needs careful regulation and should be discussed prior to arrival. When visiting a school it is a daunting experience to find a hundred small children awaiting examination together, and it is not always appreciated that examinations for epidemiological purposes necessarily take longer than a routine school dental inspection, which often merely records whether treatment is required or not. A common practice is obtaining the subjects in groups of about five, and the third member of the group, after examination, is told to ask for another five on his return. In this way a continuous flow can be maintained. Much time is saved if an additional helper is available, apart from the recorder, who can leave the proceedings to investigate and remedy stoppages.

Before any disease or condition can be studied it is necessary to decide on well-defined criteria for its diagnosis and classification. These criteria should be as simple as possible and they should be *standardized and reproducible*; other examiners using the same criteria should diagnose the condition in the same way, and the same examiner should diagnose the condition in the same way on another occasion. A certain degree of diagnostic variation is inevitable and indeed if it does not occur to some extent it probably indicates that the criteria are too crude. Excessive variation indicates that the criteria are ill-defined or too complex. A *reversal* is said to occur when a non-reversible condition is found on one occasion but not on a subsequent one; for example when a tooth has been diagnosed as filled or carious at the first examination and recorded as sound at the second. Further reading Radike (1960).

Examiners should satisfy themselves as to their own ability to reproduce the same diagnosis of the same condition on another occasion. Ideally this should be done both before commencing a study by examining a group of individuals on two occasions separated by a short interval; and during the study by re-examining a sample of the individuals concerned. If more than one examiner is involved in a study they must be carefully standardized in these respects and inter-examiner tests carried out at intervals to ensure that they are diagnosing the same conditions in the same manner (Marken, 1966). As an additional precaution it is advisable, where appropriate, to ensure that all examiners see equal proportions of test and control groups. Standards for diagnosis and indices commonly used for recording dental conditions will be described in the next section for each condition separately.

ANALYSIS OF THE DATA

Data processing and analysis are covered by Osborn in Chapter 10. It is only necessary to stress at this point that the methods of analysis must be considered at the beginning of the investigation, not after it has been completed.

DRAWING THE CONCLUSIONS AND PUBLISHING THE REPORT

These subjects are too large to be dealt with adequately within the framework of this chapter. In general, however, care must be taken that the conclusions are specifically related to the investigation that has been carried out, and that no extrapolation is made to the population as a whole unless the investigation was designed accordingly.

The presentation of the report is, within certain limits, a matter of personal style, but a conventional pattern is summarized as follows:

Introduction Review of the literature. Reasons for conducting the present investigation. Objects of the present investigation, and the hypothesis to be tested.

Material and Methods This deals with the selection and description of the samples and the methods used in diagnosis, together with diagnostic criteria. The whole method and technique of the investigation should be set out clearly.

Results These should be tabulated and illustrated as appropriate, with relevant amplification in the text.

Discussion and Conclusions The investigation, its findings and its conclusions are discussed at the discretion of the author.

METHODS OF EXAMINATION; CRITERIA FOR DIAGNOSIS; INDICES

1. Dental caries.
2. Periodontal disease.
3. Dental cleanliness, stain, calculus.
4. Enamel opacities and fluorosis.
5. Malocclusions and handicapping dentofacial anomalies.

DENTAL CARIES

Examination Numerous methods have been used to examine subjects for dental caries. Some workers use a sharp explorer (Slack et al., 1958), some a blunt explorer (Gray et al., 1970) and some no explorer at all except as a means for cleaning the tooth under observation (Backer Dirks et al., 1961). Some take bite-wing radiographs in a standard manner using a tube-holding device, some take them in a non-standard way, and some omit them altogether. Sometimes the teeth are scaled and polished before examination but usually this is not done, although they are sometimes sprayed and dried. In most cases all the teeth are examined but sometimes half mouth examinations are performed (Marthaler, 1966) and sometimes selected teeth only are examined, representing the various types of sites available for carious attack (Møller, 1966).

It would seem that the type of dental examinations performed depends on many circumstances, not all under the control of the examiner, and that it is difficult to formulate positive rules as to their conduct. In some situations, for example, it is not possible to take bite-wing radiographs, although this method obviously adds to the accuracy of the information. Each study must be considered in view of its objects and the availability of resources on the one hand and the principle of increasing the data pool on the other. With the latter purpose in view it is relevant to quote the WHO report on the subject:

> The appropriate method of examination for public health surveys involves the use of good natural daylight or artificial light, plane mouth mirrors and sharp probes. Radiographs are not recommended for use in this type of examination because of the impracticability of making them a standard requirement. (World Health Organization, 1962).

In practice this means that when reporting the results of a study in which radiographs were taken, the clinical and radiographic data should at some stage be given separately, to allow the clinical results to be compared with those from similar studies elsewhere.

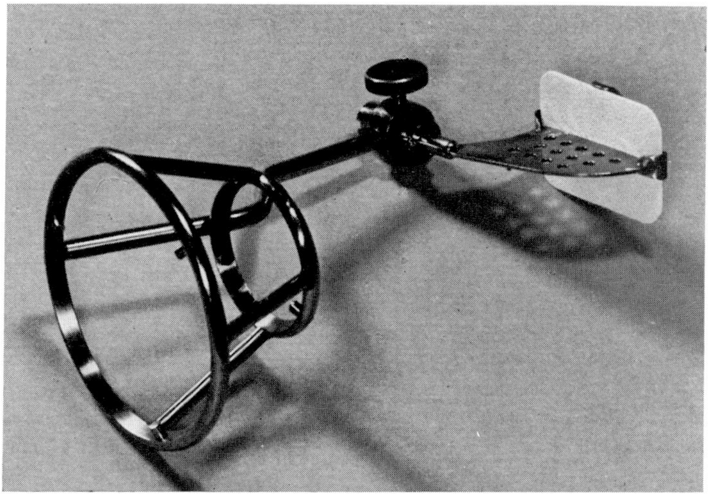

Fig. 8. Film holder and tube positioner used for the standardization of bite-wing radiographs (Backer Dirks et al., 1951).

In certain types of dental caries study radiographs are essential. This is in connexion with the evaluation of the efficacy of caries-preventive measures, such as the use of fluoride-containing dentifrices. Standardization of the technique for taking and processing them is necessary, and the Backer Dirks type of bite-wing holder (*Fig.* 8) ensures that the tube position and distance relative to the tooth and film is the same on each occasion (Backer Dirks et al., 1951).

Because of the different varieties of dental epidemiological studies and the differing circumstances for which they may be designed, a classification of study types has been suggested by the American Dental Association. Dunning (1970) quotes these as follows:

Type 1. This involves a very complete examination, using mouth mirror and explorer, good illumination, full mouth radiographs, and such additional diagnostic methods, where appropriate, as study models, pulp testing, transillumination and laboratory investigations.

Type 2. This is a more limited examination, using mirror and explorer, good illumination, and posterior bite-wing radiographs. Periapical radiographs are included where appropriate.

Type 3. A mirror and explorer examination only, using good illumination.

Type 4. This is a screening procedure only, using a tongue depressor and available illumination.

The commonest type used in Britain for epidemiological surveys is Type 3. Type 2 is used for clinical trials. Type 1 is employed for more intensive clinical studies of special groups, such as the Tristan da Cunha islanders (Holloway et al., 1963). Type 4 is a method employed in some School Dental Service inspections of schoolchildren; its object is to discover quickly the children who require treatment, and to classify the urgency of the treatment necessity.

Classification of study types is a matter of administrative convenience. A similar, though independent, classification to the one just described was made by Chaves (1966).

The question of total or partial recording also depends on the circumstances of the investigation; the World Health Organization (1971) suggests a system of partial examination which can be employed to obtain valid data. The amount of time saved by limitation of a dental examination to part of the mouth depends to a large extent on the total time of each dental examination. Examiners who take only three or four minutes to examine all the teeth in the mouth will save little time while those who take longer will find partial recordings an advantage.

Each tooth or tooth surface should be examined and its status called to the recorder in a descriptive or coded form. Methods of recording are described by Anderson in Chapter 11.

The bulk of British studies, especially those on children, have been carried out using a sharp probe, often with a replaceable point which is changed after every four subjects (Miller and Atkinson, 1951). The experienced examiner, however, finds that he uses the point for 'sticking' into fissures and pits less and less as time goes on, and more in the manner described by Backer Dirks, as a scraper and cleaner of fissures and surfaces and for confirmation or otherwise of a visually suspect area.

Criteria for Diagnosis of Dental Caries Dental caries is already far advanced when the first physical manifestations of it can be seen or felt. Any diagnosis based on visual or tactile methods is therefore recording one of the many gradations in the development of the lesion. In the early stages of development certain diagnosis is difficult to achieve because it may be masked by its position. Early approximal lesions are readily revealed by radiographs but hidden from the explorer. Early occlusal lesions are not readily visible in radiographs and the anatomical nature of the fissure (in which an explorer may stick irrespective of the presence of caries) conceals the earliest manifestations of disease. Therefore at the threshold of positive diagnosis there exists a no-man's-land of uncertainty, and it is in this area that the largest inter-examiner variation occurs and the biggest source of intra-examiner reversals.

For this reason attempts have been made to classify lesions into various categories of certainty or size, so that others who wish to compare their own findings may select the categories most appropriate to their own defined method of diagnosis. White or chalky spots, discoloured or rough areas, and fissures or pits in enamel in which an explorer sticks without further evidence of softening or undermining are included by some as definitive caries. Others, including the Expert Committee of the WHO (1962) and the World Health Organization itself (1971), specifically exclude them in the belief that standardization is more important in public health surveys than absolute accuracy. A third group attempts to achieve safety by including these precavitation lesions but coding them in such a way as to permit their inclusion or exclusion. In general these borderline lesions would then be excluded from public health survey work, recognizing the inevitable understatement, but included in clinical trials. One classification is that given by Slack et al. (1958):

D1 The probe 'catches' in a pit or fissure but does not penetrate to the dentine. (This is a category that, in clinical practice, a dentist might record as suspect but not one that required immediate restorative dentistry.)

D2 There is an obvious carious lesion involving dentine, but cavitation had not proceeded to more than one-quarter of the crown.

D3 Cavitation had proceeded so that more than one-quarter of the crown was involved.

For some research purposes a more detailed examination for caries is required. Such a method is described by Backer Dirks et al. (1961). These authors distinguish four main types of carious lesion occurring respectively in pits and fissures, on approximal surfaces, on free smooth surfaces (buccal and lingual), and at the gingival margin.

Approximal caries is diagnosed entirely by radiographic means, using the standardizing apparatus mentioned previously. Caries 1 indicates a carious lesion in the enamel. Caries 2, 3, and 4 respectively indicate lesions that have penetrated the dentine, which extend into the dentine more than half-way to the pulp, or which have actually involved the pulp.

Pit and fissure caries. The fissures are cleaned with a new sharp explorer, dried with compressed air, and caries is diagnosed visually in four grades. Grade 1 denotes a minute black line at the bottom of the fissure; in Grade 2 there is also a white zone (dark in transmitted light) along the margins of the fissure. Grade 3 indicates the smallest perceptible break in the continuity of the enamel, and Grade 4 is a large cavity more than 3 mm. wide.

Free smooth surfaces. These are initially cleaned and dried. Two stages of caries are recognized; 'caries white' if the surface shows a white chalky opaque lesion and 'carious cavity' if there is a break in the enamel perceptible with an explorer. Gingival margin caries is diagnosed similarly.

It should always be recognized, however, that as criteria become more refined, problems of inconsistency and inter-examiner error will increase. Criteria chosen for any survey will depend to a large degree on survey objective, design of the survey, and uses to which the data will be put.

Indices An index is defined as a numerical value describing the relative status of a population on a graduated scale with definite upper and lower limits designed to permit and facilitate comparison with other populations classified by the same criteria and methods (Young and Striffler, 1969). An index can describe the prevalence of a disease in a population, and also describe the severity, or intensity of the condition.

Prevalence The simplest is 'present' or 'absent'. This is useful mostly when observing and comparing populations with wide differences in caries experience. Modifications of prevalence index include expressing proportions of the population with the minimum of a specified number of affected teeth, often ten.

Intensity The DMF index is the commonest of the current dental caries measurements, first suggested by Klein et al. (1938). Each permanent tooth is considered individually and if it is decayed (D), missing due to caries (M), or filled (F) it scores one. The total of affected teeth is an expression of an individual's dental caries experience, and the average number of DMF teeth for a group is found by dividing the number of individuals in the group into the total number of affected teeth.

The def and *dmf indices* These are indices for the primary dentition. As originally described by Gruebbel (1944) 'd' denoted decayed deciduous teeth indicated for filling; 'e' decayed deciduous teeth indicated for extraction; and 'f' filled deciduous teeth. Teeth missing for any reason were not recorded, and because of this it may be regarded as a measurement of observable dental caries prevalence. Often, however, the index has been used in exactly the same way as the DMF index for the permanent dentition, thus making it a measurement of past and present dental caries experience. When the index is used in this manner the normal exfoliation of primary teeth is a complicating factor: naturally-shed teeth should not, of course, be included. Modifications are sometimes made to allow for this natural loss of teeth; for example it is common practice, after the age of six years, to consider only the primary molars. Even at this age it is difficult, in the course of an epidemiological study, to decide whether a primary tooth has been extracted or shed naturally, and consultation of young children is unreliable. Where the index is used as a measure of past and present caries experience it has been suggested that it should be called dmf to avoid confusion with the original def of Gruebbel, which is still commonly used in some countries.

The World Health Organization (1971) recommendation for primary teeth is to exclude the 'e' component and only express the df score, including under 'd' those teeth regarded as beyond restorative treatment.

Sometimes the caries intensity is expressed, not as an average score per individual, but as the proportion of decayed, missing, or filled teeth per 100 teeth at risk. This is to effect a partial correction of any errors caused by differences in the average eruption dates of teeth between, for example, children of different racial groups. Because all the teeth in any individual are exposed to similar oral environment and caries initiating factors it is important that the unit for calculation of the mean DMF per 100 teeth at risk for a group is the individual and not the tooth. This means that the DMF per 100 teeth for each subject must first be computed:

$$\text{Individual DMF per 100 teeth at risk} = \frac{\text{Individual DMF} \times 100}{\text{Number of teeth at risk in the individual}}$$

The average of these values is then calculated to obtain the group mean. It is not considered correct to calculate this figure by multiplying the total group DMF by 100 and dividing by the total number of teeth at risk in the group.

This index, however, gives no further information than the DMF when comparing groups in which the mean number of teeth at risk are not too different. It is, therefore, only of any value if the groups to be investigated have widely differing numbers of teeth at risk.

DMFS and dmfs indices One of the disadvantages of the DMF method of measurement is that a tooth scores exactly the same under extremes of clinical conditions; a tooth with a small restoration in one pit rates the same as a tooth that has been extracted. A finer measurement than the relatively crude DMF index is sometimes required, especially for public health information and for measurements during clinical trials of caries preventing agents. For these the recommended unit of measurement is not the tooth but the tooth surface. These DMFS and dmfs indices are calculated in the same way as described for the DMF and dmf indices. It has been found (Jackson et al., 1963) that the surface index provides little or no additional information in prevalence studies where the extent of caries is being compared between groups. This index also has the disadvantage of having a wider range of possible values and hence a larger standard deviation and standard error.

Certain difficulties are encountered in the use of surface indices. One is the score to be allocated to extracted teeth, which may have been attacked on one surface only, although its extraction results in the loss of four or five surfaces, according to the tooth. Some workers compromise by scoring an arbitrary three surfaces for an extracted tooth; others prefer to interpret the index literally and score the total four or five. Dunning (1970) states a personal preference for scoring four in every case as he regards this as a realistic average. Another difficulty is the score to be given to two surface fillings in posterior teeth, where the initial attack was probably on one approximal surface and the occlusal surface was involved later, to provide an adequate Class II type of cavity for restoration.

The DMF type indices have other disadvantages, such as the loss of sensitivity in older age-groups due to the saturation of the index, but no better method has yet been reported for public health investigations. The DMF index is the measurement recommended by the World Health Organization (1971).

Treatment Requirements The DMF and dmf indices are useful when broken down into their decayed, missing and filled components in addition to reporting totals. This provides measures such as 'treatment required' (D) and 'treatment carried out' (M and F). Observation of the M and F ratio may suggest the type of dental services and/or attitudes to dental treatment in the group under consideration. The decayed (D) component can also be further broken down and the totals reported as D1, D2, or D3 averages according to the caries classification used. This indicates the urgency of treatment and the type of treatment needs in a group, as well as providing the basis for comparison with other workers as discussed earlier.

Jackson (1961) has described an index for assessing the efficacy of dental treatment in the control of dental caries. He recognizes three grades of treatment: in descending order of success these are a filled tooth (F), a filled tooth that has subsequently become carious (F.C.) and an extracted tooth (M). He weights each of these 3, 2, and 1 respectively according to their estimated 'degree of success' and applies the following formula for expressing a Treatment Index (TI).

$$\text{Treatment Index} = \frac{3(\text{F}/\text{DMF}\%) + 2(\text{F.C.}/\text{DMF}\%) + (\text{M}/\text{DMF}\%)}{3}$$

If all the DMF teeth are filled and otherwise sound the treatment index using this method is 100 per cent, and if all the DMF teeth are extracted the index is 33·3 per cent.

Conversion of survey data into treatment needs is important for adequate public health planning, a problem which is discussed by Sheiham in Chapter 8.

Recording by Particular Sites For research purposes DMF or DMFS indices may not give enough information, and it is often essential to know the type of site attacked by caries as well as the frequency of attack. Information such as the selective nature of protection by fluoride is gained by this method. Caries or fillings are recorded and reported according to their occurrence in pits or fissures, approximal surfaces, or smooth plane surfaces.

PERIODONTAL DISEASE

This important subject has been difficult to study in the past because of the necessity for subjective measurement of the conditions with the resulting wide variations between observers and difficulty in standardizing examination techniques and methods of diagnosis.

Estimations have been made of both gingivitis alone and on the wider range of periodontal conditions.

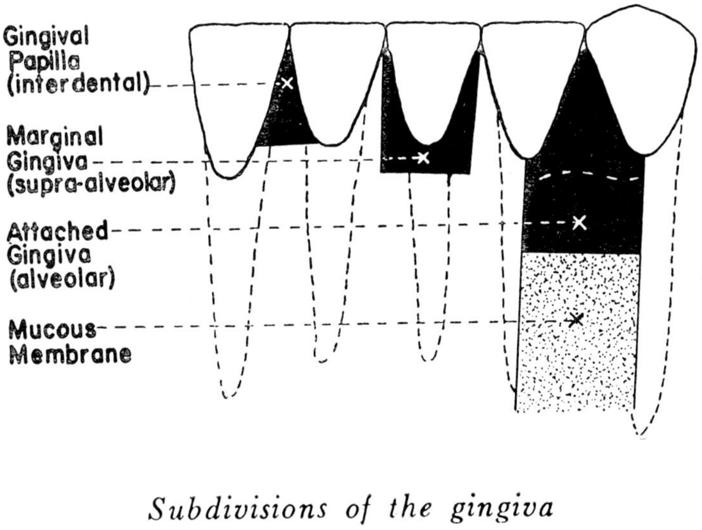

Fig. 9. Areas designated P, M, and A in a gingival assessment (Schour and Massler, 1947).

Gingivitis One of the earliest of the indices for assessing gingivitis is the P-M-A index devised by Schour and Massler (1947). Each tooth has three related gingival areas; the papilla mesial to it (P), the labial or buccal gingival margin (M), and the attached gingivae (A) (*Fig*. 9). The presence or absence of gingival inflammation is recorded in each tooth area and arbitrary ratings of gingivitis prevalence are made for each subject according to the number of areas affected.

A number of workers have modified this index and introduced severity ratings for the degree of gingivitis found in each area, and the areas themselves have been subject to modification. For example, Parfitt et al. (1958) described a method by which a diagnosis was made in each of six areas of the mouth (upper and lower labial, upper and lower, and left and right buccal), taking the worst part of the area as representative of it; and allocating scores for the different degrees of severity. The scores for each area are summed so that totals can be expressed for each individual and averages for the whole group.

A more recent index for gingivitis is the Gingival Index (GI) of Löe and Silness (1963), which has also been used in combination with a Plaque Index and a Retention Index (Löe, 1967). The GI ascribes a score from 0 to 3, depending on severity of the condition, for the gingival tissue in the mesial, distal, buccal, and lingual units. This system is of use in clinical trials, and has demonstrated satisfactory reproducibility.

Some workers have used an arbitrary descriptive classification of gum conditions based on a quick examination and impression of either the whole mouth or part of it, usually the anterior segments. James et al. (1960) defined three standards of gingival health as follows:

Good The gums are healthy. The health line is well marked and stippling is evident. There is no evidence of inflammation.

Poor There is considerable inflammation of the gingival tissues with redness, tendency to bleed on pressure, and engorged dental papillae, and gingival margins.

Fair Any condition that does not fall into either of the other two categories.

The World Health Organization Special Committee (1962) recommended that gingivitis should be diagnosed if there is evidence of any one or more of the following signs around one or more teeth: redness, swelling, ulceration, and bleeding. These criteria have been amplified in the WHO manual (1971), and field experience may demand further investigation.

Periodontal Conditions The examination for gingivitis is visual, but for pocketing some form of measurement is often used. The WHO Committee (1962) advised that pocketing should be determined by exploration with a blunt periodontal probe which has a mark 3 mm. from the tip. Each aspect of each tooth is tested with this probe and in areas where the mark is not visible a pocket is diagnosed as present. Findings can be expressed in two ways: either the simple prevalence report of the proportion of the population with one or more units of gingivitis or periodontal pockets, in which case each examination can be terminated as soon as evidence of gingivitis or one pocket is detected, or by the count of pockets and inflamed gingival units in each individual and an expression of an average number for the group.

Russell's Periodontal Index The best known index for the diagnosis and recording of periodontal disease is that devised by Russell (1956). Gum tissue around each tooth is scored numerically according to its clinical conditions:

Score		
0	*Negative*	There is neither overt inflammation in the investing tissues nor loss of function due to destruction of the supporting tissues.
1	*Mild gingivitis*	There is an overt area of inflammation in the free gingivae, but this area does not encircle the tooth.
2	*Gingivitis*	Inflammation completely circumscribes the tooth but there is no apparent break in the epithelial attachment.
6	*Gingivitis with pocket formation*	The epithelial attachment has been broken and there is a pocket (not merely a deepened gingival crevice due to swelling of the free gingivae). There is no interference with normal masticatory function, the tooth is firm in its socket and has not drifted.
8	*Advanced destruction with loss of masticatory function*	The tooth may be loose; may have drifted; may sound dull on percussion with a metallic instrument; may be depressible in its socket.

The weighting system was designed to place the greater emphasis on advanced disease and to minimize examiner disagreement. The score for an individual subject is the arithmetic average of the scores for the teeth in the mouth, and the population score the average of the individual scores for the subjects examined. Scores may be calculated for populations of particular teeth as well as for subjects. Russell also describes additional X-ray criteria that correspond to the field study categories. He did not use a measuring probe in his diagnosis of periodontal pockets, relying on visual examination supplemented by a straight Jacquette scaler or a chip syringe for demonstrating the lesion. Some workers (Sheiham, 1969) use Russell's method of assessment but have a calibrated periodontal probe (Brinker C.G.B. No. 3) and diagnose the pocket when a 3-mm. depth or more can be demonstrated.

Ramfjord's method This is a system of partial recording based on the findings for six typical teeth; in the upper jaw the right first molar, the left central incisor, and the left first premolar; and in the lower jaw the right first premolar, the right central incisor, and the left first molar.

The clinical examination includes the diagnosis of gingivitis, calculus, pocketing, occlusal and incisal attrition, mobility, lack of contact, and plaque. Classification of gingival findings are as follows:

G0 Absence of inflammation.

G1 Mild to moderate inflammatory gingival changes not extending all around the tooth.

G2 Mild to moderately severe gingivitis extending all around the tooth.

G3 Severe gingivitis characterized by marked redness, tendency to bleed and ulceration.

The measurement of periodontal pocketing was carried out using a special probe ('University of Michigan 0') which is as thin as possible and specially angulated. Ramfjord (1959) states: 'Measuring the depth of the crevice or pocket has limited value unless the measurements are related to fixed landmarks on teeth'. He therefore supplies detailed instructions for measurements in the mouth and the transference of these measurements to schematic teeth on the data collection card. The value of Ramfjord's PDI in making an accurate assessment of treatment needs is discussed by Sheiham in Chapter 8.

Lilienthal et al. (1964) have suggested using Russell's classification of periodontal conditions with a partial recording system; the teeth used by Ramfjord were the ones selected with the difference that second molars replaced the first molars, because of the frequent loss, due to caries, of the latter teeth.

The indices described for gingivitis and periodontal disease are those that have found most frequent use in epidemiological surveys. Numerous others have been described. A description of nearly all indices devised for periodontal conditions is found in part II of the *Journal of Periodontology*, volume 38, Nov.–Dec., 1967.

Care should be exercised in the interpretation of those indices using a numerical score to represent the severity of the condition, especially when these are analysed using statistical tests appropriate to quantitative data. This is because, strictly speaking, a score of 2 should indicate exactly twice the amount of disease as a score of 1, 6 three times the amount of 2, and so on. This is not the case where the numerical score is arbitrary.

DENTAL CLEANLINESS, STAIN, AND CALCULUS

Standards of dental cleanliness are frequently expressed in the routine examination of teeth. The simplest classification is the descriptive one employed by James et al. (1960) and many other workers have used variations on this method (Goose, 1958; Mansbridge, 1960). The teeth are inspected visually, explored with a probe, and the subject's dental cleanliness is arbitrarily classified as good, fair or poor using the following or similar categories:

Good The teeth are clean. There is no sign of food debris or materia alba when examined with an explorer.

Poor The teeth are very dirty. There is considerable food debris of long standing, materia alba, or heavy staining.

Fair This class falls between the two preceding. There is some evidence of debris but not to the degree recognized as poor.

This may be expressed as the impression of the whole dentition, limited to the anterior regions, or used to describe each of the six labial and buccal segments, previously described. As in all such subjective categorizations, standardization and reproducibility are suspect; the examiner tends to be unduly influenced by the first few cases that he examines and to set his standards for that session accordingly.

Stain is not necessarily associated with dental cleanliness. It is possible to have teeth that are extremely clean but with a fine black stain present above the gingival margin. The simplest classification of stain is by 'present' or 'absent' and, if present, according to colour. Calculus may be similarly unrelated to dental cleanliness and may be recorded as 'absent', 'subgingival', or 'supragingival'.

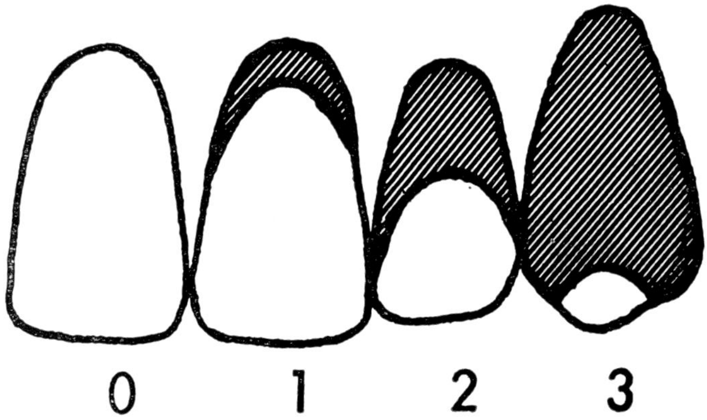

Fig. 10. Diagram showing the varying amounts of oral debris with the appropriate scores (Greene and Vermillion, 1960).

Greene and Vermillion (1960) have described a more definitive method of diagnosing oral debris, stain, and calculus. The upper and lower arches are divided into three segments; anterior and left and right buccal, the latter being defined as the segments distal to the canine teeth. Scores for calculus and debris are recorded buccally and lingually in each segment, giving a total of 12 areas.

Each segment is examined buccally and labially in turn and a score allocated to each, based on the buccal and lingual surface in each area which has the greatest surface area covered by debris. The buccal and lingual scores need not be taken from the same tooth. The surfaces are investigated by running an explorer over them and noting the occlusal or incisal extent of the debris as it is removed from the tooth surface.

The scores allocated for debris are, as shown in *Fig.* 10:

0 No debris or stain present.

1 Soft debris covering not more than one-third of the tooth surface or the presence of extrinsic stains without other debris regardless of surface area covered.

2 Soft debris covering more than one-third but not more than two-thirds of the exposed tooth surface.
3 Soft debris covering more than two-thirds of the exposed tooth surface.

Examination for calculus is carried out in a similar way and the following scoring system is used:

0 No calculus present.
1 Supragingival calculus covering not more than one-third of the exposed tooth surface.
2 Supragingival calculus covering more than one-third but not more than two-thirds of the exposed tooth surface or the presence of individual flecks of subgingival calculus around the cervical portion of the tooth or both.
3 Supragingival calculus covering more than two-thirds of the exposed tooth surface or a continuous heavy band of subgingival calculus around the cervical portion of the tooth or both.

Debris or calculus indices are calculated for each individual by totalling the scores recorded and dividing by the number of segments scored. The two indices are then combined and expressed as an 'oral hygiene index', although the two component parts should also always be given separately as their ratio to the whole is a useful piece of clinical information. Greene and Vermillion (1964) have also described a simplified oral hygiene index halving the number of surfaces examined. Löe (1967) has developed a Plaque Index to match the Gingival Index (GI) previously mentioned. Each of the four gingival areas on teeth are graded from 0–3 according to the thickness of the soft deposit; paying no attention to coronal extension of the plaque.

ENAMEL OPACITIES AND FLUOROSIS

Most fluoridation programmes involve not only the assessment of changes in dental caries experience but also the observation of enamel opacities. Assessment of these causes some difficulty and as observers become more practised at finding and diagnosing minute opacities they naturally tend to find more of them, a fact that sometimes leads to misinterpretation. A complicating factor is that enamel opacities are not all due to fluoride; a high proportion of teeth mineralized in low fluoride areas show opacity levels of greater significance than those found in regions having optimal levels of natural or artificial fluoride in the water.

The classification that is most commonly used for the degree of fluorosis is that of Dean (1942), incorporating a system of scoring for the calculation of an index. A slightly abbreviated form is quoted by Dunning (1970).

Normal enamel	(statistical weight 0·0).
Questionable mottling	Normal translucency of teeth is varied by a few white flecks or white spots (weight 0·5).
Very mild mottling	Small opaque paper-white areas are scattered over the teeth, involving less than 25 per cent of the surface. Summits of cusps of bicuspids and second molars are commonly attacked (weight 1·0).
Mild mottling	The white opaque areas are more extensive but do not involve more than 50 per cent of the surface (weight 2·0).
Moderate mottling	All enamel surfaces are affected and those subject to attrition show marked wear. Brown stain is a frequent disfiguring feature (weight 3·0).
Severe mottling	All enamel surfaces are affected and hypoplasia is so marked that tooth form may be altered. A major diagnostic sign is discrete or confluent pitting. Brown stains are widespread and the teeth often present a corroded appearance (weight 4·0).

Each individual examined is given the appropriate score and the Index of Dental Fluorosis is calculated from the formula:

$$\text{Index} = \frac{\text{Sum of frequency} \times \text{Weight}}{\text{Number examined}}$$

For example if 500 children are examined, and 80 are found to have 'questionable' mottling, 50 'very mild', and 30 'mild' the index is

$$\frac{(80 \times 0{\cdot}5) + (50 \times 1) + (30 \times 2)}{500} \quad \text{which equals} \quad \frac{150}{500} = 0{\cdot}3$$

Zimmerman (1954) has discussed the differences between opacities due to fluoride and those that are not, which he terms 'idiopathic'. He cites three features for differentiation:

Physical appearance of the opacities The idiopathic opacities are usually more oval in shape and more opaque in appearance than questionably fluorosed white spots, whereas the opacities on questionably fluorosed teeth have a tendency to form horizontal striations. On the occlusal surfaces of posterior teeth the non-fluoride lesions involve the cusp tips, similar to snow-capped mountain peaks, while the striae of questionably fluorosed teeth extend down cuspal ridges.

The distribution pattern of the opacities Questionably fluorosed opacities are usually distributed bilaterally in a dentition; idiopathic lesions are not ordinarily found in a definite symmetrical pattern.

The frequency of the opacities per person The questionably fluorosed opacities usually involve several teeth per dentition; idiopathic lesions seldom affect more than one or two teeth.

MALOCCLUSIONS AND HANDICAPPING DENTOFACIAL ANOMALIES

The commonest classification of orthodontic anomalies is that proposed by Angle (1899). There are numerous other methods of recording prevalence and degree of malocclusion, and different skeletal patterns, nearly all of which are more appropriate in clinical orthodontic practice or anthropological research than in the cruder types of public health survey.

The WHO Special Committee (1962) defined a handicapping dentofacial anomaly as one which causes disfigurement or which impedes function, a definition also given in the WHO manual (1971). Since the assessment of such an anomaly depends on the subjective judgement of the examining dentist they recommend that classification of anomalies should be only on the basis of whether or not they require treatment. An anomaly should be regarded as requiring treatment if the disfigurement or functional defect is, or is likely to be, an obstacle to the patient's physical or emotional well-being. The index they recommend is the age-specific percentage of persons who have one or more of the following anomalies requiring treatment: cleft palate, cleft lip, prognathism, retrognathism, deep overbite, open bite, crowding, or spacing.

Prosthetic needs may be recorded for each subject where appropriate. A World Health Organization recommendation is that data pertaining to full dentures should be recorded, for age-groups above 19 years, as follows:

1. No full denture requirement.
2. Requires full denture(s).
3. Has full denture(s).

An assessment that full dentures are required should be made when the patient is edentulous, where all the remaining teeth require extraction, or because the remaining teeth do not provide sufficient function to be of value.

CHOICE OF INDICES

The choice of an index for measuring any condition is dependent upon two main factors. First, the objects of the investigation in which the index is to be used and hence the nature of the information required; and second the ability of the examiner to reproduce consistently the diagnosis on which the index is based. In general the simplest index compatible with the objects of the study should be used, as these are, on the whole, more reproducible, especially where the more subjective judgments are necessary. The desirability of collecting information in a form that can be compared with other workers has already been stressed, and for this reason the indices and criteria recommended by the World Health Organization (1971) should be used whenever possible.

Increasing attention is now being focused on development of indices which can more accurately assess treatment needs. The mere recording of a decayed tooth as 'D' in the DMF index, for example, gives no indication of the treatment time required by the subject. Even more so, an individual who has a mean PI score of 1·8 cannot be assessed at all for treatment needs. This situation arises because the indices were designed to provide a relative comparison of one group with another, and use of any index for a purpose other than the one for which it was designed can be fraught with problems. In programme planning, however, treatment needs require assessment. There is a need, therefore, for development of indices in both of the major oral diseases which provide a more accurate picture of treatment needs. When this development takes place, the dental epidemiologist will have a richer choice of indices to suit his particular objectives.

It is perhaps appropriate to end this chapter with a quotation from W. H. Frost's introduction to *Snow on Cholera* (1965).

> Epidemiology at any given time is something more than the total of established facts. It includes their orderly arrangement into chains of inference which extend more or less beyond the bounds of direct observation. Such of these chains as are well and truly laid guide investigation to facts of the future; those that are ill made fetter progress. But it is not easy when divergent theories are presented, to distinguish immediately between those which are sound and those which are merely plausible. Therefore it is instructive to turn back to arguments which have been tested by the subsequent course of events; to cultivate discrimination by the study of those which the advances of definite knowledge has confirmed.

Acknowledgements We gratefully acknowledge the help given to us by Mr. R. A. Cohen, LDS, FFD, in the section dealing with history. Thanks are also due to Miss J. Davies for preparing the typescript and to the Photographic Department, Birmingham Dental School, for providing the photographs.

REFERENCES

Ainsworth, N. J. (1928), 'Mottled teeth', *R. dent. Hosp. Mag.*, **2,** 2.

Angle, E. H. (1899), 'Classification of malocclusion', *Dent. Cosmos*, **41,** 248.

Armitage, P. (1971), *Statistical Methods in Medical Research*. Oxford and Edinburgh: Blackwell Scientific Publications.

Atkinson, W. H. (1863), Letter, *Br. J. dent. Sci.*, **6,** 554.

Backer Dirks, O., Houwink, B., and Kwant, G. W. (1961), 'The results of artificial fluoridation of drinking water in the Netherlands; the Tiel-Culemborg experiment', *Archs oral Biol.*, **5,** 284.

— — van Amerongen, J., and Winkler, K. C. (1951), 'A reproducible method for caries evaluation', *J. dent. Res.*, **30,** 346.

Chaves, M. M. (1966), 'The W.H.O. approach to dental epidemiology', *Proceedings of a Dental Epidemiology Conference at The London Hospital Medical College Dental School*, November, 1966.

Churchill, H. V. (1931), 'Occurrence of fluorides in some waters of the United States', *Ind. Engng Chem.*, **23,** 996.

Dean, H. T., (1942), 'The investigation of physiological effects by the epidemiological method. Fluorine and dental health', *Am. Ass. Adv. Sci.*, Washington No. 19, 26.

——, ARNOLD, F. A., and ELVOVE, E. (1942), 'Domestic water and dental caries V. Additional studies of the relation of fluoride domestic waters to dental caries experience in 4425 white children aged 12 to 14 years of 13 cities in 4 States', *Publ. Hlth Rep.*, **57,** 1155.

DOLL, R., and HILL, A. B. (1950), 'Smoking and carcinoma of the lung. Preliminary report', *Br. med. J.*, **2,** 739.

— — — — (1964), 'Mortality in relation to lung smoking; ten years' observation of British doctors', *Ibid.*, **1,** 1399 and 1460.

DUNNING, J. M. (1970), *Principles of Dental Public Health.* Cambridge, Mass.: Harvard University Press.

ENGLANDER, H. R. (1962), 'Epidemiology, a fundamental discipline in dental research', *J. Am. dent. Ass.*, **65,** 755.

FISHER, W. (1885), 'Compulsory attention to the teeth of school children', *J. Br. dent. Ass.*, **6,** 585.

FORREST, J. R., and JAMES, P. M. C. (1965), 'A blind study of enamel opacities and dental caries prevalence after eight years of fluoridation of water', in *Advances in Fluorine Research and Dental Caries Prevention* (ed. HARDWICK, J. L., HELD, H. R., and KONIG, K. G.). Oxford: Pergamon.

FROST, W. H. (1965), *Snow on Cholera* (Introduction). New York and London: Hafner.

GOOSE, D. H. (1958), 'The assessment of an oral hygiene campaign', *Publ. Hlth Lond.*, **72,** 20.

GRAY, P. G., TODD, J. C., SLACK, G. L., and BULMAN, J. S. (1970), *Adult Dental Health in England and Wales in 1968.* London: HMSO.

GREENE, J. C., and VERMILLION, J. R. (1960), 'Oral hygiene index, a method for classifying oral hygiene status', *J. Am. dent. Ass.*, **61,** 172.

— — — — (1964), 'The simplified oral hygiene index', *Ibid.*, **68,** 7.

GREGG, N. MCA. (1941), 'Congenital cataract following German measles in mother', *Trans. ophthal. Soc. Aust.*, **3,** 35.

GRUEBBEL, A. O. (1944), 'A measurement of dental caries prevalence and treatment service for deciduous teeth', *J. dent. Res.*, **23,** 163.

GUERINI, V. (1967), *A History of Dentistry.* Amsterdam: Liberac NV.

HOLLOWAY, P. J., JAMES, P. M. C., and SLACK, G. L. (1963), 'Dental disease in Tristan da Cunha', *Br. dent. J.*, **115,** 19.

JACKSON, D. (1961), 'An index for assessing the efficacy of dental treatment in the control of dental caries', *Dent. Practnr dent. Rec.*, **11,** 226.

— — JAMES, P. M. C., and SLACK, G. L. (1963), 'An investigation into the use of indices devised for the clinical measurement of caries degree', *Archs oral Biol.*, **8,** 55.

JAMES, P. M. C., JACKSON, D., SLACK, G. L., and LAWTON, F. E. (1960), 'Gingival health and dental cleanliness in English schoolchildren', *Ibid.*, **3,** 57.

KLEIN, H., PALMER, C. E., and KNUTSON, J. W. (1938), 'Studies on dental caries I. Dental status and dental needs of elementary school children', *Publ. Hlth Rep.*, **53,** 751.

LILIENTHAL, B., AMERENA, V., and GREGORY, G. (1964), 'A comparison of a modified periodontal scoring system with Russell's Periodontal Index', *J. Am. dent. Ass.*, **61,** 172.

LÖE, H. (1967), 'The gingival index, the plaque index, and the retention index systems', *J. Periodont.*, **38,** 610.

— — and SILNESS, J. (1963), 'Periodontal disease in pregnancy I. Prevalence and severity', *Acta odont. scand.*, **21,** 533.

MCKAY, F. S. (1916), 'An investigation of mottled teeth', *Dent. Cosmos*, **58,** 781.

MANSBRIDGE, J. N. (1960), 'The effects of oral hygiene and sweet consumption in the prevalence of dental caries', *Br. dent. J.*, **109,** 343.

MARKEN, K-E. (1966), 'The training of observers', in *Advances in Fluorine Research and Dental Caries Prevention* (ed. JAMES, P. M. C., KONIG, K. G., and HELD, H. R.). Oxford: Pergamon.

MARTHALER, T. M. (1966), 'Partial recording of dental caries in incidence studies', in *Advances in Fluorine Research and Dental Caries Prevention* (ed. JAMES, P. M. C., KONIG, K. G., and HELD, H. R.). Oxford: Pergamon.
MEDICAL RESEARCH COUNCIL (1925), *Reports of the Committee for the Investigation of Dental Disease II. The Incidence of Dental Disease in Children.* London: HMSO.
MILLER, J., and ATKINSON, H. F. (1951), 'A replaceable probe point', *Br. dent. J.*, **90,** 157.
MØLLER, I. J. (1966), 'Clinical criteria for the diagnosis of the incipient caries lesion', in *Advances in Fluorine Research and Dental Caries Prevention* (ed. JAMES, P. M. C., KONIG, K. G., and HELD, H. R.). Oxford: Pergamon.
PARFITT, G. J., JAMES, P. M. C., and DAVIS, H. (1958), 'A controlled study of the effect of dental health education on the gingival structures of schoolchildren', *Br. dent. J.*, **104,** 21.
RAMFJORD, S. P. (1959), 'Indices for prevalence and incidence of periodontal disease', *J. Periodont.*, **30,** 51.
RUSSELL A. L. (1956), 'A system of classification and scoring for prevalence surveys of periodontal disease', *J. dent. Res.*, **35,** 350.
SAUNDERS, E. (1837), *The Teeth of a Test Age.* London: Renshaw. Reprinted in *Am. J. dent. Sci.* (1846–7), **7,** 330.
SCHOUR, I., and MASSLER, M. (1947), 'Gingival disease in post war Italy 1. Prevalence of gingivitis in various age groups', *J. Am. dent. Ass.*, **35,** 475.
SHEIHAM, A. (1969), 'The prevalence and severity of periodontal disease in Surrey schoolchildren', *Dent. Practnr dent. Rec.*, **19,** 232.
SINCLAIR, JOHN (1803), 'An essay on longevity', *Nav. Chron.*, **9,** 388.
SLACK, G. L. (1966), 'The technique of examination in clinical trials', in *Advances in Fluorine Research and Dental Caries Prevention* (ed. JAMES, P. M. C., KONIG, K. G., and HELD, H. R.). Oxford: Pergamon.
—— JACKSON, D., JAMES, P. M. C., and LAWTON, F. E. (1958), 'A clinical investigation into the variability of dental caries diagnosis', *Br. dent. J.*, **104,** 399.
SNOW, J. (1855), *On the Mode of Communication of Cholera.* London: Churchill.
TOMES, J. (1848), *A course of lectures on dental physiology and surgery.* London: Parker.
WORLD HEALTH ORGANIZATION (1962), *Standardization of Reporting of Dental Diseases and Conditions; Report of an Expert Committee on Dental Health.* Geneva: WHO Tech. Rep. Ser. No. 242.
——— (1971), *Oral Health Surveys; Basic Methods.* Geneva: WHO.
YOUNG, W. O., and STRIFFLER, D. F. (1969), *The Dentist, his Practice and his Community*, 2nd. ed. Philadelphia: Saunders.
ZIMMERMAN, E. R. (1954), 'Fluoride and non-fluoride enamel opacities', *Publ. Hlth Rep.*, **69,** 1115.

FURTHER READING

It is impossible, within the limited space of one chapter, to give more than the barest minimum of essential information. Readers may supplement their knowledge of dental epidemiology by studying the relevant section of the following publications:

ADVANCES IN FLUORINE RESEARCH AND DENTAL CARIES PREVENTION (1966), (ed. JAMES, P. M. C., KONIG, K. G., and HELD, H. R.), **4,** 1–92. Oxford; Pergamon.
BACKER DIRKS, O., BAUME, L. J., DAVIES, G. N., and SLACK, G. L. (eds.) (1967), 'Principal requirements for controlled clinical trials; F.D.I. Commission on Classification and Statistics for Oral Conditions', *Int. dent. J.*, **17,** 93.
BAUME, L. J. (ed.) (1962), 'General principles concerning the international standardisation of dental caries statistics; F.D.I. Commission on Oral and Dental Statistics', *Ibid.*, **12,** 65.

CHILTON, N. W. (1967), *Design and Analysis in Dental and Oral Research.* Philadelphia: Lippincott.

DUNNING, J. M. (1970), *Principles of Dental Public Health,* 2nd ed. Cambridge, Mass.: Harvard University Press.

PELTON, W. J., DUNBAR, J. B., MCMILLAN, R. S., MOLLER, P., and WOLFF, A. E. (1969), *The Epidemiology of Oral Health.* Cambridge, Mass.: Harvard University Press; American Public Health Association Vital and Health Statistics Monographs.

RADIKE, A. W. (1960), in *Caries Diagnosis and Experimental Caries Conference* (ed. GREEN, G. E., and WEISENSTEIN, P. R.), p. 201. Ohio: Ohio State University Research Foundation.

Chapter 6

The Administration of Public Dental Treatment Programmes

Brian A. Burt PHD, BDSc, MPH, FRACDS
Lecturer, Community Dentistry Unit, The London Hospital Medical College Dental School

Most public dental programmes concentrate on treating the consequences of disease. While treatment should ideally be offered only as part of an overall programme involving prevention and education, there will be cases where treatment of established dental disease is seen to be the most urgent priority in a community.

Dr. Burt examines the treatment programmes in Norway, New Zealand, and Malaysia, and then describes a planned approach to administering a treatment programme. Where this ideal is not possible, some compromises are suggested. Whatever approach is taken epidemiology remains the key to its successful development.

Dental public health is that branch of dentistry concerned with the dental welfare of the community as a whole, and so includes prevention, education, research, administration, and treatment. The term 'public dental programme' can therefore be used to describe a number of different programmes and without further qualification the term is vague. An Expert Committee of the World Health Organization (WHO) defines public dental health *services* as:

> . . . those dental health services of an educative, preventive, or curative nature, organized by government (central, regional, or local) with its exclusive resources or with participation from other individuals or agencies, or through organized community efforts. (World Health Organization, 1965.)

Traditionally, a public health programme has usually meant a treatment service; meaning repair for the consequences of dental disease.

Despite the growth of programmes in prevention and education, the term 'dental public health programme' probably still most commonly refers to treatment services for specified members of a community. For the sake of clarity, however, a treatment programme should be referred to as such.

The Federation Dentaire Internationale (FDI) has collected information on public dental treatment services from as many as 60 countries in its *Basic Facts Sheets* (1970), and Fisher (1970) states that 39 countries include dental benefits in national programmes of social health insurance. It can thus be seen that public programmes of dental treatment are established in many different parts of the world; ranging in extent from one or two persons conducting a limited service to nationwide programmes involving thousands of dentists and a huge budget. Indeed, the various programmes of public dental treatment show almost as much variety as do the countries themselves.

This chapter aims to examine the scope of a public dental treatment programme by considering in detail some of the public programmes now operating in several different countries. A systematic approach to planning and administration will be presented, and some reasons why few such programmes employ it will be discussed. Some possibilities for modifying this ideal approach in the light of practical limitations will then be suggested.

DEFINITION

A programme of public dental treatment may be defined as one administered at some governmental or community level and supported in whole or in part by public funds, or by funds from organized community groups such as a private company, trade union, or philanthropic foundation. The aim of the programme is to bring recognition and repair of dental and oral disease to a whole community, or to some specified segment of that community.

No attempt is made in this definition to differentiate between local or national administration of the programmes. These terms are found in the dental literature, especially in the USA, and the distinction between them is usually based on the level of programme administration (Easlick, 1963). The increasing role of the federal government in the financing of health services in the USA, however, is tending to blur the distinction between a local and a state or national programme (Cohen, 1967). Probably the last purely local public treatment programmes, in the sense that administration, financing, and community served are all local, are found in philanthropic clinics such as the Mott Foundation Clinic in Flint, Michigan, USA. Even school dental programmes in the USA as described by Dunning (1970), traditionally regarded as local programmes, are being increasingly financed from non-local sources.

In most countries of the world the political tendency appears to be towards increasing central control, a tendency which is developing further in some countries than in others. Even if day-to-day administration of public dental services can remain local, the provision of finance from central sources usually results in ultimate control of the programmes remaining with the central government.

The treatment programmes examined in this chapter are all sponsored by national governments, even though all have aspects of local administration. They are national in the sense that they are planned nationally, have nationally-established priorities, and are financed for the most part from central funds. Their administration is essentially similar in various local districts.

Ideals of programme planning, also to be discussed, are similar whether the programme is for a whole nation or a single school. Most of the discussion in this chapter will be presented with a national governmental programme in mind, but the principles can be applied to a treatment service of any size or content.

GOVERNMENT ROLE IN PUBLIC DENTAL TREATMENT PROGRAMMES

The FDI has stated that government has the responsibility of ensuring that its citizens have the opportunity to achieve an optimal level of dental health, and that the interpretation of this responsibility will vary with the traditions, laws, resources, and social philosophy of the country concerned (Federation Dentaire Internationale, undated). Illustrations of these different interpretations are to be found in the contrasting situations existing in Czechoslovakia and Switzerland. In Czechoslovakia, the state assumes responsibility for the dental health of all its citizens, whereas in Switzerland dental services are hardly a concern of central government at all. In the latter, public dental services are delegated to the cantons, where they play a supplementary role to private practice and are offered only to patients in low-income groups (World Health Organization, 1965). Services in Sweden fall somewhere between these two examples, an extensive public treatment programme which is administered and financed by both central and local government, as well as a large number of private practitioners.

With the growing tendency towards centralization, a large number of countries now accept without question the place of governments in direct or indirect delivery of care. Nations with limited resources for health care provision have little choice but to organize programmes administered by government if any number of their citizens are to receive care, in which case a consideration of alternative systems is irrelevant. By contrast, the debate on systems of health care delivery in the USA, with its wealth of resources, is a lively one indeed. Hillenbrand (1960) stated the traditional view in that country when he placed the responsibility for dental health on '. . . the individual, then the family, the community, the state, and the nation in that order'. American attitudes seem to be changing however in more recent times, as evidenced by the proposals for a form of national health insurance now before Congress.

The increasing role of governments around the world in provision of health care is primarily a reflection of the growth of the philosophy that health care is a fundamental right of all people. Where this philosophy is accepted, the active role of governments in health services is unquestioned. Only the precise nature and extent of this role need to be established.

Dental health services have been grouped into three main categories by an Expert Committee of the World Health Organization (1965) as follows:

Group 1 Dental services provided by the dentists and dental auxiliaries and financed by direct arrangements with the patient or through some form of organization of payment not involving government. In this group would fall prepayment plans, services organized by labour and other consumer groups and by private insurance companies or private philanthropic foundations, and other plans without any governmental participation.

Group 2 Dental services provided by dentists and dental auxiliaries who are partly or entirely remunerated by government, but who are not considered to be government employees.

Group 3 Dental services provided by dentists and dental auxiliaries who are employed by the government.

In many nations, where services are available under all three groups, the dominant group is usually the one which reflects the economic and political organization of the country. For example, Group 1 is dominant in countries where a relatively unrestricted economic system is found, such as the USA and Australia. Countries with an economic system based on free enterprise but where a social philosophy allows a strong governmental responsibility in the provision of health care lean towards the Group 2 type of services. Great Britain is a good example of this type.

Group 3 services predominate in countries with a centrally planned economy where health services are considered a state responsibility, such as the USSR and Hungary.

This system of grouping services is useful to illustrate the point that provision of dental care services cannot be separated from the political system and social philosophy of a country. While some authorities believe that provision of health care, dental treatment programmes included, should not be a subject for the political arena, it is more realistic to accept that, where people demand health care as a right, it has to be a political subject. In addition, the successful administration of public dental treatment programmes must harmonize with a nation's usual administrative methods. A programme which is set up in a manner too far removed from traditional methods of providing care for that country is likely to run into serious difficulties. Of course, nations can change their social philosophy over a period of time, and where this happens so too should the delivery system in dental treatment services change.

TYPES OF PUBLIC DENTAL TREATMENT PROGRAMMES

The public dental treatment programmes in three nations will be considered in some detail as a means of illustrating different approaches to the same problem. The three nations are Norway, New Zealand, and Malaysia. Dental and oral disease is sufficiently widespread in all three to constitute a public health problem. All three nations have some private practice of dentistry, all have treatment services for their armed forces, and all have public treatment programmes of the Group 2 type. Despite these similarities, operation of their public treatment programmes is quite different.

Basic statistical facts for the three nations are given by the Federation Dentaire Internationale in its 1970 edition of *Basic Facts Sheets* (Table 1).

TABLE 1

Manpower resources in Norway, New Zealand and Malaysia (FDI, 1970)

Country	*Population (millions)*	*Qualified dentists*	*Unqualified dentists*	*New Zealand nurses*	*Hygienists*	*Chairside assistants*	*Laboratory technicians*
Norway	3·9	3022	—	—	75	3000	650
New Zealand	2·8	940	—	1330	—	1200	264
Malaysia	9·0	270	566	386	—	296	67

NORWAY

The first public treatment programmes in Norway began in 1910, though private practice was well-established at the time. These programmes were extended into a School Dental Service (SDS) by national legislation in 1917, which set up locally operated programmes of free dental care for schoolchildren aged 7–14. Some localities, where resources were more plentiful, went beyond this basic provision. Oslo, for example, provided care for the pre-school children as well as for the 7–14-year-olds.

By further legislation in 1950, the various school dental programmes then operating were to be expanded and consolidated into a basic uniform system of public dental care, known as the Public Dental Service (PDS). The change from one system to another is developing slowly. The object of the 1950 Act was to absorb the various existing SDS programmes into the uniform programme of the PDS, and it was intended at the time that the change-over would be complete by 1965. More recent estimates, however, put the date for completion at some time after the year 2000. At the present time, 13 out of Norway's 20 local government councils have established a PDS, and one more is about to do so at the time of writing.

Local government units in Norway consist of both county councils and town councils. For the operation of the PDS each county is further divided into separate dental service districts. These districts are defined by the appropriate Ministry of the central government, in consultation with the local councils. Every county must have a PDS established under the 1950 Act, so it is natural to ask why the development of the programme has been slow, and will continue to be slow. The answer appears to be that there is insufficient dental manpower to meet the requirements of the programme and some financial limitations also apply.

Once a county has established a PDS programme, day-to-day administration is undertaken by the county. This administration includes appointing some dentists and the non-professional staff, attending to payment of expenses, and determining programme priorities. Each district has at least one permanent dental clinic, both clinic design and equipment are subject to Ministry approval.

It will be recalled that the Act of 1917 set up the basic provision of free care for schoolchildren aged 7–14 years. It has been estimated that 80 per cent of all schoolchildren aged 7–14 receive all necessary dental treatment under this programme (Federation Dentaire Internationale, 1970). The PDS, established by the 1950 Act, expands this free dental treatment provision to all young people aged 6–17. This priority applies in all dental districts, though, as before, local authorities can grant priority to other groups, such as preschool children, if resources allow. Outside the priority groups, patients pay for treatment in accordance with a scale of fees laid down by the Ministry. Priority groups are entitled to complete and systematic operative and surgical care, prostheses where necessary, and orthodontics where resources allow, all free of charge. Non-priority persons who seek care through the PDS receive it as far as possible after priority groups have been cared for, and as stated, they pay a direct charge for treatment received.

Provision is made in the 1950 Act for each county and town council, except Oslo and Bergen, to have a county dental officer. Oslo and Bergen have a dental officer-in-chief. These dentists have the task of supervising the PDS programmes in the local municipalities. Each district must also have at least one Class A dentist, both the supervising dentists and the Class A dentists are appointed by the Ministry in the central government. Class B and C dentists, as well as ancillaries and non-professional staff, are appointed by the local council. Dentists in the Norwegian PDS are classified as Class A, B, or C, on the basis of hours worked in the service. Class A dentists provide treatment for 1800 hours per year, and class B dentists 1400. Class C dentists are usually local practitioners who treat some 6–17-year-olds in their surgeries and are paid by the government for so doing. There is no PDS career structure for Class C dentists. Salaries for dental staff in the PDS are set by the central government in consultation with the Norwegian Dental Association, these salaries are subject to approval by the Norwegian parliament. Retirement for PDS dentists is at age 65; a pension scheme is in operation. The Ministry appoints a Local Dental Service Committee in each district and sets its duties. Usually they centre around complaints and grievances from both dentist and community. In counties where the SDS has not yet been replaced by the PDS, the municipality makes staff appointments and, in association with other municipalities, negotiates salaries with the Norwegian Dental Association.

County councils receive 60 per cent, and town councils 30 per cent, of the costs of the PDS in a grant from the central government. Each dental district gives the county a token sum of 5 kroner annually for each resident of the district entitled to free care.

Norway has one of the most favourable dentist-to-population ratios in the world, exceeded only by Sweden. From the figures already listed, there is one dentist in Norway for each 1280 persons, and yet this still appears insufficient for the country's needs (Baerum, 1970). Baerum points out that with the excessively high prevalence of dental caries in Norway, it has been estimated that one PDS dentist is required to care for the annual treatment needs of 500 children aged 6–17. The present population in this age-group is 740,000 which theoretically leaves a requirement of 1480 district dental officers to care for them. The 13 countries which have established a PDS have only 417 full-time positions established, and another 250 such positions need to be established in these counties alone to meet estimated treatment needs.

The present rate of expansion of the PDS is about 30 new full-time positions per year. It is estimated that by 1985 the theoretical need for full-time dental officers will have increased from the present 1480 to 1798, but the positions established by then at the current rate will be only 867. Here then is the principal reason for the slow development of the PDS, and why it is stated that the 1950 Act will not be fully implemented until after the year 2000.

Norway presents a fascinating exercise in programme planning. The method chosen to meet all dental needs in the priority age-groups is probably the most expensive one of all, that is the development of a comprehensive dental treatment programme carried out by fully trained dentists. It could be asked that even when the PDS is fully operational, will the nation reach a condition of optimal dental health? Also, will Norway's national resources be unduly strained by the full implementation of this system? There must be the risk that excessive costs will prevent the programme from ever achieving full development.

It has been shown in New Zealand that where treatment needs for caries are reduced by fluoridation, the result is a reduction in manpower requirements in a public treatment programme (Denby and Hollis, 1966). If fluoridation became widespread in Norway, therefore, it could be expected to have a marked impact on the projected manpower requirements. Fluoridation is official policy, but progress to date has been slow.

Another alternative to the development of the estimated dental manpower requirements is the use of operating ancillaries to treat established disease. This approach, however, appears unlikely to be adopted in the near future.

Turning now to another country where prevalence of dental disease is high, one finds a different concept altogether in public dental treatment programmes.

NEW ZEALAND

New Zealand's system of delivery of public dental care has become one of the most widely studied in the world (Gruebbel, 1950; Harris, 1950; UK Mission, 1950; Fulton, 1951; World Health Organization, 1959). The chief reason for this global interest is the utilization of operating ancillaries there, a system which has allowed the term 'New Zealand School Dental Nurse' to find almost universal acceptance in dental terminology. A deeper acceptance of the concept is shown by the increasing number of countries adopting similar or slightly modified schemes (Federation Dentaire Internationale, 1970).

Dental disease emerged as a public health problem in New Zealand during the First World War, when the dental condition of army recruits was found to be appalling. As New Zealand was already moving towards becoming a welfare state, and some precedent had been established with the use of dressers in Great Britain during the First World War (Leff and Leff, 1959), the government's establishment of the scheme to train dental nurses in 1921 was possibly not as revolutionary as it might appear to have been. The government acted with the advice of the New Zealand Dental Association, and the profession generally accepted the scheme, although there was a certain amount of opposition from some members (Editorial, 1921). Perhaps little dental treatment was provided for children by dental practitioners at the time, so the profession at large may not have seen the scheme as any great threat to their livelihood. Most dentists at that time in New Zealand were in private practice, and indeed 85 per cent still are now (Federation Dentaire Internationale, 1970).

There are now three School Dental Nurse training schools in New Zealand, compared with one dental school, and the course of training is two years. The duties of the School Dental Nurse have not altered much down the years. In essence, she may insert fillings in primary and permanent teeth, extract primary teeth, give infiltration anaesthesia, carry out scaling, cleaning and polishing of teeth, apply topical fluorides, and provide dental health education.

Clinics are established in schools, and the nurses, while they remain government employees, are under the jurisdiction of the headmasters in their day-to-day activities. When the scheme began, treatment was offered only to the younger children, but as the system developed more its scope expanded to cover all schoolchildren up to the age of 16. Progress was hampered by the economic depression of the 1930s, and then by the Second World War, but since 1946 the service has continued to show steady growth.

Girls are recruited directly from the sixth form (about 17 years old) for dental nursing. The career is socially acceptable and in recent years there have been around three applicants for each training position available, allowing a high standard of student to be maintained.

Supervision of the School Dental Nurses in their work in school clinics is not close. Each nurse operates under a senior nurse for the district, as well as a district supervisor who is a dentist, in some areas the dentist's visit may be up to two months apart. In theory at least he is always available for advice and assistance when required. A nurse is trained to refer to a dentist anything she sees that is outside her legally defined range of treatment.

New Zealand is divided into 13 dental districts, each district has a Principal Dental Officer. This dentist's responsibility is the administration of the National Dental Service, as the public treatment programme is known, in his area. The National Dental Service is organized in three sections:

The School Dental Service, staffed by the School Dental Nurses, who treat primary schoolchildren and preschool children between the ages of $2\frac{1}{2}$ and 13. This upper limit is approximate because the eligibility ends at the finish of primary school. There are about 600,000 children in these categories.

The Adolescent Dental Service, established in 1946. Schoolchildren who leave the highest class treated by the School Dental Service may enrol with a private practitioner of their choice, and are entitled to treatment free of charge up to the age of 16. The dentist is paid for his care by the government. Younger children who are seen by the School Dental Nurse, and who require treatment which is beyond her training to provide, are also usually treated under this system. The Adolescent Dental Service provides care for about 150,000 children. It was originally intended to man this service with salaried staff, but this development was halted in favour of using private practitioners in the scheme.

The Hospital Service is a dental service for patients in hospital attached to the Division of Mental Health, staffed by dentists.

Adults receive care only through private practice, where the patients bear the complete charge. Supplementary benefits are available to a patient in a case of proven need.

The New Zealand system of public dental treatment has been widely studied, there is no need to reiterate the findings of the study groups here. It is enough to say that the principle of utilizing operating ancillaries has been shown in New Zealand to be a workable, safe, and reasonably economic method of bringing dental care to priority groups within the population. It does not appear to have affected the growth of the dental profession, nor has it been shown to have an adverse effect on the income of practitioners. It is now estimated that some 93 per cent of primary schoolchildren are being treated in the School Dental Service, and many of the remaining 7 per cent are treated by private practitioners at the parents' expense. Quality of care, in so far as it can be judged at all, has generally been regarded as excellent by the study groups, the most notable exception being Gruebbel's report in 1950.

The School Dental Nurse scheme was never intended to be just a treatment service and nothing else. Dental health education has always been part of the nurses' duties, though it was until recent years a fairly nominal duty. In recent years topical fluorides have been regularly applied in non-fluoridated areas.

Prevalence of dental caries appears to be as high in New Zealand as it is in Norway, though direct comparisons are difficult because of the absence of comparable data. In New Zealand, unlike Norway, fluoridation is progressing steadily despite the usual opposition. Public water supplies reach 71 per cent of the population and two-thirds of these supplies are now fluoridated (Walsh, 1970). Following some torrid legal battles, local authorities now have the power to fluoridate water supplies. There is an economic problem, however, in that many public water supplies serve only small communities and without financial aid from central sources fluoridation can be relatively expensive in these circumstances.

Although fluoridation by itself will never be the complete answer to the high prevalence of dental caries in New Zealand, its impact is being seen there as elsewhere. One measurable effect has been seen in the School Dental Service already and is described by Denby and Hollis (1966). Their study found that a dental nurse, who was usually able to treat about 450 children per year, was able to care for 690 per year after ten years of fluoridation. Walsh (1970) put the number of schoolchildren a dental nurse could treat as 'somewhere in the order of 800' after fluoridation. It is obvious that manpower requirements, and hence costs, of the School Dental Service in New Zealand are likely to be further reduced in the future.

Administrators of the School Dental Service consider that only in the last ten years has the service truly been offering full and necessary care to every child in the target group. Despite the comprehensiveness of the service and the experience gained in nearly 50 years of development it became evident that a treatment service alone was not going to allow complete control of dental caries in New Zealand. With fluoridation now reducing the treatment needs for caries, however, a goal which appeared utopian may now be seen as rather more realistic. Authorities in New Zealand may soon have to decide whether to scale down the School Dental Nurse scheme as fewer nurses become required to care for the child population, or whether to turn the nurses' activities towards other areas of dental needs, in particular towards periodontal disease.

The New Zealand system is now being seen in a number of countries, one of which is Malaysia, a nation where the practice of dentistry is at a completely different stage of development.

MALAYSIA

Malaysia provides an example of a developing country making a planned deployment of its limited resources to achieve maximum effect. The nation is a confederation of the 11 states of West Malaysia (formerly known as Malaya) together with Sarawak and Sabah in the northern part of the island of Borneo. The population is a little over 9 million. Most of the population and administrative expertise is in West Malaysia; both Sarawak and Sabah lagging behind in general development.

Malaysia's first dental school is still not complete, and unqualified dentists have traditionally carried out most treatment. However, the dental register was closed to these unqualified practitioners in 1952, and now one-third of the 836 registered dentists are qualified graduates of dental schools. Unqualified dentists are in private practice only, they may not be employed in the public dental service at all. About half of the qualified dentists are employed by the government in the public dental treatment service.

In addition to these two types of dentists, there are 386 New Zealand-type dental nurses on the register, plus about 300 government-trained chairside assistants and 67 government-trained technicians. The majority of all types of dental personnel are in West Malaysia (Federation Dentaire Internationale, 1970).

The dental nurses are trained at one school in Penang, which was established in 1949. The training is for two years and each nurse undergoes a 16-month period of field probation after graduation. Her duties are very similar to those of the New Zealand nurses, but Malaysian nurses are subject to closer field supervision by dentists than are their New Zealand counterparts. This supervision is especially close in the probationary period, less so afterwards. Each Malaysian nurse maintains the dental health of 550–650 children, aiming for a monthly output of 15 new patient completions, 50 recall completions, and 200 fillings (Abdul Karim, 1965).

Each of the 11 states of West Malaysia has a Principal Dental Officer or an Acting-Principal Dental Officer, who supervises the activities of his dental officers operating in the various types of clinical facility. These facilities consist of main health clinics, subsidiary health centres, school clinics, and hospital clinics. There are a number of specialist dental officers (oral surgeons and orthodontists) who operate in these facilities, these specialists are also under the general supervision of the Principal Dental Officer.

Malaysia has formidable problems of transport and communication in many areas, but the dental service is planned at a local level so that even the most remote area receives at least a part-time service. This is mainly being organized by the development of rural health centres, designed to meet the needs of rural populations of 50,000. These centres consist of one main centre and four sub-centres, each to serve 10,000 people, and each with provision for a comprehensive range of health services. The main centres, and some sub-centres, also contain living accommodation for the staff.

For health care administration, each of West Malaysia's 11 states is further divided into districts, the number of districts per state varies from 3 to 12. For the delivery of dental care, the dental team is regarded as a basic unit, there is at least one dental team in each health district. The dental team consists, at a minimum, of one qualified dentist, one dental nurse, one assistant, one technician, and one attendant. Many teams have more members, such as two or three nurses and up to four assistants. The main health centres have a full-time dental staff providing care. Sub-centres are usually manned full-time only by general nursing staff, sometimes by dental nurses as well if resources permit. The sub-centres are visited regularly by the dental teams and by the other health care teams.

The dental treatment services in all clinical facilities operate to a system of priorities. First priority is given to schoolchildren aged 6–17, who are entitled to routine care without charge. A recall system operates for this age-group, and the only direct patient charges made are nominal ones for dentures and orthodontic treatment. In this age-group, the dental nurses may treat children aged 6–12. The next priority is for preschool children, who are treated by both nurses and dentists. These groups are followed by expectant mothers and hospital patients. The very poor may receive emergency care, for which they pay a nominal sum. All others outside the priority groups must receive their care through private practice. A government dental officer is considered to spend about 70 per cent of his time treating schoolchildren.

It has been estimated that the public treatment services cover 10 per cent of the population, and 30 per cent of the school-going population (Federation Dentaire Internationale, 1970). Fluoridation has been instituted in some communities and there are plans for further fluoridation projects. There is some application of topical fluoride by the dental nurses (Federation Dentaire Internationale, 1970).

A developing country like Malaysia must have a severe manpower shortage for some time yet and it will be a long time before it can hope to approach a goal of universal dental care. The shortage of dentists has led to the adoption of operating ancillaries as a means of providing dental care, and with the closing of the register to unqualified dentists and the establishment of a dental school, the dental profession and a corps of ancillaries are being developed simultaneously. Development of dental teams, planned dispersal of health centres in rural areas, and training of senior dental administrators in postgraduate dental public health courses are further areas of health service administration which other countries could well emulate.

Disquiet has been expressed in some quarters about the development of operating ancillaries before the dental profession has established itself as a body of some strength. The fear is that emphasis on the use of these ancillaries may appear more politically attractive than strengthening the dental profession and that consequently the profession may suffer in the future. With the obvious political desire to develop the dental service as quickly as possible, the results of Malaysia's policy will be watched with interest.

A SYSTEMATIC APPROACH TO PROGRAMME PLANNING AND ADMINISTRATION

The ideal systematic method of operating a public dental programme has been described in a number of different ways, essentially it consists of six steps, which are:

1. Assessment of dental treatment needs.
2. Assessment of available resources.
3. Determination of priorities in the programme.
4. Establishment of objectives.
5. Operation of the programme.
6. Evaluation of the programme.

A similar approach to the practice of dental public health has been described in Young and Striffler (1969).

In an ideal situation, a public dental treatment programme would never be proposed without supporting programmes of prevention and education, for as Davies (1965) has said: '. . . the long-term aims of a public dental health programme will not be fulfilled by treatment alone'. But, as stated earlier, public dental health programmes have traditionally meant treatment services, and certainly the three programmes discussed all began as treatment services with little genuine support for education and prevention. The same comment could be made about the European dental programmes described by Kostlan in Chapter 4, and to the British National Health Service described by Renson in Chapter 7.

It is now necessary to examine some of these steps towards planning and administration in more detail.

ASSESSMENT OF DENTAL TREATMENT NEEDS

A dental administrator should first of all know his community as well as he can, whether it is a small district or a whole nation. The distribution of population, its age structure, rate of growth, regional variations, its culture, diet and nutritional levels, standard of living, development of public services and utilities, and patterns of general health are all basic knowledge.

The extent of dental disease is most accurately obtained by epidemiological survey techniques. The most common dental and oral diseases are caries and periodontal disease, others which occur to a varying extent in most societies are malocclusions, oral cancer, and cleft lip and palate. Prevalence of these diseases needs to be assessed against some of the demographic factors just listed. The patterns of treatment already being received can also be disclosed, these can vary among age-groups, socio-economic groups, or localities. Even though a dental administrator feels that he knows the dental disease patterns in his community from personal experience, surveys can often disclose conditions that have not been previously thought to exist, such as severe caries in a particular racial group or lack of treatment facilities in a certain area.

It must not be forgotten that as population grows so do the total dental needs. In addition, the prevalence of caries in many nations appears to be increasing, a situation especially likely in the so-called 'developing' nations, where rapid social and cultural change often includes the adoption of dietary habits which can promote caries (World Health Organization, 1971b). Where rapid population growth coincides with an undesirable change in dietary habits, a sharp increase in dental treatment needs can be expected over a relatively short period of time.

Figures related to the extent of dental disease may require translation into figures for treatment needs, for the two are not necessarily the same. Some ways of translating disease figures to treatment needs are given by Sheiham in Chapter 8.

ASSESSMENT OF AVAILABLE RESOURCES

Once the dental administrator has secured a knowledge of the dental needs of his community, he is in a position to assess the manpower, surgery facilities, equipment, and finance required to meet those needs.

These resource requirements can also be projected into the future. The term 'resources' includes dentists, auxiliaries, ancillaries, administrative personnel, surgery and clinic facilities, equipment and supplies, and finance for programme operations. Projecting likely requirements for the future would include assessing the estimated production of personnel from dental and auxiliary training schools, and assessing the likely level of expenditure for personnel and facilities. Future needs in manpower and facilities must always be assessed against population growth, change in population age-structure and estimated increases or decreases in prevalence of caries.

Where an assessment of resources is being carried out, it must be remembered that a programme usually requires a long time to reach its full potential. New Zealand's School Dental Nurse scheme is now 50 years old, and only recently has it been reaching almost all schoolchildren in the target group. Manpower limitations have forced a slowing-down in Norway's Public Dental Service programme and Malaysia cannot hope to approach its projected manpower requirements for many years. In New Zealand an end to continuous growth of the programme can be seen, especially with advances in fluoridation. In Norway, the end of programme expansion is less clear unless fluoridation becomes established.

DETERMINATION OF PRIORITIES IN THE PROGRAMME

There are very few examples of a public treatment programme being able to reach all cases of dental need in a large population. Practically every assessment of needs, and resources available to meet those needs, shows that resources are insufficient. It then becomes necessary to establish priorities in the programme so as to allow the most efficient deployment of the available resources. The rationale for using a priority approach is that it is better to give one or more sections of a population an efficient service rather than to spread resources too thinly over a whole population. Also, lack of a priority system may result in dental treatment not being adequately provided to those persons or groups who need it most.

Children are most frequently the main priority group. Norway, New Zealand, and Malaysia all have their public dental treatment services aimed at children in the first instance, so do a number of other countries. Expectant and nursing mothers and preschool children are other groups given priority in many programmes. Again, survey techniques are the best method of identification of community groups most in need of treatment services. Careful surveying can disclose unmet needs in groups that are frequently neglected, such as the chronically ill and the mentally and physically handicapped.

One method of delivering priority dental care to a group of schoolchildren is the incremental care scheme. This system is not new, for Davis (1969) records that it was proposed by George Cunningham in

England in 1907. Basically, it consists of providing necessary dental care for the lowest age-group in the priority scale in one year, then adding a new age-group to the group receiving care each year. As an illustration, suppose that a programme with limited resources is proposing to provide dental care to the 6–12-year-old age-group. The first year would see complete care for the 6-year-olds. The following year this group, now aged 7, would receive necessary dental maintenance and the new group of 6-year-olds would receive complete care. The third year would see maintenance care for the first two groups, now 7- and 8-year-olds, plus complete care for the new 6-year-olds. By this system, all ages in the priority group would be reached within seven years, and probably more efficiently than by haphazard treatment of the whole 6–12-year-old group initially. This system has been used in some school dental treatment programmes (Dunning, 1970), and has been proposed in others (McKendrick, 1970).

When needs, resources, and priorities have been determined, objectives can be established for short-term or long-term achievement. Objectives provide 'markers' against which effectiveness of the programme can be evaluated.

EVALUATION

Evaluation of a programme should be considered at the planning stage. When an objective is set, so should a method of determining whether the objective has been reached. In a public dental treatment programme, epidemiological surveys are the fundamental form of evaluation.

Evaluation, or analysis, is one of the basic applications of epidemiology that Dunning (1970) has described, and as he also points out, it is one of the most neglected applications of the science. Data obtained in evaluation surveys can be assessed against the original data collected for the assessment of needs, assuming that it is collected in as similar a way as possible to that employed in the original survey. A regular system of evaluation surveys can indicate:

1. Whether prevalence of a disease condition is changing.
2. Whether existing disease is being treated at a greater or lesser rate than new disease is commencing, or whether the two factors are balancing each other.
3. If any sub-group within the priority section, such as an age-group or persons living in a particular area, is not receiving the service it should be.
4. Whether re-assessment of objectives and priorities is indicated.
5. If any dental operators are inefficient, or not concentrating their efforts towards the right groups.
6. Whether any preventive or educative measures being operated are proving effective in reducing needs or promoting demands for treatment.

Many treatment programmes confine their evaluation to an assessment of dental treatment statistics. Evaluation of this nature is of dubious value, as it would only evaluate the efforts of the treatment operators, as in point (5) above, and possibly whether demands for care are increasing. Treatment statistics give no real information on the other points listed. Other programmes go a little further and conduct surveys among those in the priority groups who present for treatment. This procedure may provide more useful data, but as it would apply only to those who present for treatment the data could not be applied to the community at large. The only true evaluation is a system of surveying the community, or at least the whole of the priority groups, on a standardized basis at fairly regular intervals. The survey conducted in New Zealand by Beck (1968) is an example of an evaluatory survey of a high order.

Evaluation of public dental treatment programmes has been a neglected aspect of programme operation in the past, it seems that only in recent years has the value of treatment services been seriously examined. Careful evaluation must allow improvement in programme efficiency, as well as indicating methods of controlling the costs of programme administration.

WHY IS THIS MODEL APPROACH NOT USED MORE OFTEN?

The assessment–planning–evaluation approach to a public dental treatment programme is simple enough in concept, so it is logical to ask why it has not been used more often. There seem to be a number of reasons, probably the major ones are political pressures and the fact that no one thought of applying the concepts to a treatment programme.

It must be accepted that public dental treatment programmes are inherently political in nature. They are initiated by politicians at some level, presumably because a demand for them is seen to exist. The politicians also allocate finances for them, and set the programmes at an order of importance in relation to other socially-oriented programmes. This will mean that time and resources, especially finances, awarded to the programme will have some ceiling set by the politicians concerned. The dental administrator and the politician therefore may well look at the programme from totally different points of view, and each can have a set of goals which they see the programme achieving. Occasionally these goals may coincide, but frequently they do not.

Traditional methods of providing care are often hard to change, especially when the programme is operated by a well-entrenched bureaucracy. A more scientific approach to administration may be difficult to initiate in these circumstances. New Zealand, however, provides a good example of a long-established treatment programme which is in the process of evaluating itself. Political response in that country appears favourable because the evaluation may be leading to ways of reducing the costs of the service.

Where programmes are administered by laymen, or even by dentists who have no special qualifications or experience in public health, it cannot be expected that a model approach will be adopted, simply because these persons may not grasp its significance. Even if they do, they may not feel qualified to follow it through. Leaders of public dental treatment programmes should receive postgraduate training in dental public health wherever possible (World Health Organization, 1965); deputies and potential leaders would also benefit. Trained personnel should be able to collect the most reliable data in the assessment of needs and evaluation sections of the programme, and should also be capable of reaching the most logical conclusions from their data.

In situations where there is a complete lack of resources, where the few available dentists and auxiliaries are literally swamped by overwhelming demands, then little more than an emergency service can be operated. There is no question of an ideal approach here.

It is likely that most programmes do not use the systematic method for some combination of these reasons discussed, and because the practical limitations involved never make it feasible to do so. The final part of this chapter examines some possible ways of operating an efficient programme under less than ideal circumstances.

MODIFICATION OF THE IDEAL APPROACH WHERE PRACTICAL LIMITATIONS DICTATE

Political pressures of all kinds on a public dental treatment programme are unlikely ever to go away, so the dental administrator has to learn to live with them. Reliable data, especially on costs, may be one hedge against undesirable political action, such as a reduction in the scope of a programme which is developing well. Data to assess dental needs and for evaluation may be of more use to the administrator than simply to help him operate an efficient programme, they can also be invaluable in making a case to politicians.

But what if the administrator cannot obtain reliable data on the prevalence of dental disease? He may have insufficient staff, feel inadequately trained, or find that the treatment time lost by surveying may bring him into disfavour. Until the situation can be rectified, he will have to use whatever data he can. He probably has a reasonable idea of the worst dental disease problems in his community, and rapid screening campaigns of convenient population groups such as schoolchildren, armed forces, or factory personnel may give him further information. Data from surveys of this kind must be recognized as inadequate, but they can serve to promote a programme until better data can be obtained. Barmes (1968) has outlined how a country's dental manpower planning may be advanced in the absence of reliable epidemiological data.

Priorities will have to be set on some arbitrary basis. Children are traditionally the first priority, though it could be argued that there is little point in providing a children's service if reasonable follow-up facilities are not available. Some communities again have priorities set by political decisions, groups such as armed forces, factory workers, or police receiving high priority. Where social conditions dictate, the programme may be directed only at lower-income groups in the community, a tradition still seen in the public treatment programmes in the USA (Hollinshead, 1961; Young and Striffler, 1969).

Evaluation is especially challenging in conditions of limited resources, and in these circumstances the desire to ignore it altogether can be strong. The programme administrator should at least be able to assess what proportion of this target group is being reached by the programme, and how many of those reached are receiving complete treatment. Treatment needs of patients presenting for the first time may give some idea of disease prevalence and extent of previous treatment in the community, although it must be remembered that those who present for treatment may show different patterns from those who do not. A shrewd administrator may be able to use his absence of reliable data as a lever to obtain an increased allocation of resources to his programme. But again, evaluation of this limited variety must always be seen only as a temporary measure. Surveying the community, or at least its priority groups, is the only genuine and thorough way to obtain reliable data with which to evaluate a programme.

Even with limited resources, there is much in the way of surveying that can be done. A major barrier to surveying in the past has been the inability of administrators to develop a suitable record form and to process the data obtained. Now, however, the Dental Health Unit of the World Health Organization in Geneva has developed a simple system of recording and processing dental survey data. This system is described in the publication *Oral Health Surveys; Basic Methods* (World Health Organization, 1971a), which is obtainable from the Dental Health Unit, World Health Organization, Geneva. So long as the record form is marked correctly, all processing of the data is carried out in Geneva, and the administrator receives back the information he needs. The development of this system has greatly simplified surveying in areas where resources are limited, and has brought the possibility of obtaining dental survey data within the reach of most administrators.

SUMMARY

Public dental treatment services are but one aspect of a total dental public health programme, and should be allied to programmes of prevention and education as far as possible. For reasons usually associated with politics and tradition, however, dental treatment programmes may be initiated in isolation. Most of these programmes are administered by government at some level, and in all of them governments have the duty to ensure that all citizens have access to dental care as far as possible. The way in which this duty may be interpreted will vary, for any programme to be successful must conform to the social, cultural, and political traditions of the country concerned. The concept of health care as a fundamental human right has promoted the growth of public dental treatment programmes.

Dental public treatment programmes in Norway, New Zealand, and Malaysia provide examples of various approaches to the same problem. There is a systematic method of planning and administering such a programme, it involves an assessment of dental needs and available resources, setting priorities and objectives, and evaluating the operation of the programme. None of the programmes discussed conformed completely to this ideal because political needs, lack of finance and absence of trained personnel have acted as barriers.

Even when resources are lacking, there are some modifications to this systematic approach which will assist in establishing an efficient programme. Surveying has been made simpler and more feasible through the efforts of the World Health Organization in providing facilities for recording and processing data. Even if with this assistance reliable epidemiological data cannot be obtained, that in itself should not prevent satisfactory planning and operation of the programme.

Planning and administration of a public dental treatment programme, to be efficient, requires careful and rational thought. It is an advantage if programme administrators can receive postgraduate training in dental public health. In the planning and operating process, reliable data is the most valuable aid available to an administrator. These data should cover dental needs, operating costs, and allow an evaluation of the programme to be made. Careful application of these data, both before and during a programme, will help ensure the most efficient use of the resources available to bring maximum benefit to the community.

REFERENCES

Abdul Karim, B. N. D. (1965), 'Public dental health services in Malaya', *J. dent. Aux.*, **3,** 4.

Baerum, P. (1970), 'Folketannrøkta-20ar', *Norske Tandlægeforen, Ibid.*, **80,** 755.

Barmes, D. E. (1968), *Manpower Planning with and without Epidemiology; Flexible Definition of Categories of Dental Personnel. Inter-Regional Seminar on Training and Utilization of Dental Personnel in Developing Countries at New Delhi, Dec. 1967.* Geneva: WHO. Mimeograph.

Beck, D. J. (1968), *Dental Health Status of the New Zealand Population in Late Adolescence and Young Adulthood.* Wellington, NZ: National Health Statistics Centre, Department of Health, Special Report Series No. 29.

COHEN, W. J. (1967), 'Challenge and opportunity: Meeting the health needs of the American people', in *Sesquicentennial Symposiums*. Ann Arbor: University of Michigan School of Dentistry.

DAVIES, G. N. (1965), 'Planning a public health programme', The Annie Praed Oration, typescript.

DAVIS, H. C. (1969), 'George Cunningham: The man and his message', *Br. dent. J.*, **127,** 527.

DENBY, G. C., and HOLLIS, M. J. (1966), 'The effect of fluoridation on a dental public health programme', *N.Z. dent. J.*, **62,** 32.

DUNNING, J. M. (1970), *Principles of Dental Public Health*, 2nd ed. Cambridge, Mass.: Harvard University Press.

EASLICK, K. A. (ed.) (1963), *The Administration of Local Dental Programs*. Ann Arbor: University of Michigan School of Public Health.

EDITORIAL (1921), 'The State Dental Scheme and the New Zealand Dental Association', *N.Z. dent. J.*, **16,** 145.

FEDERATION DENTAIRE INTERNATIONALE (1970), *Basic Facts Sheets*.

———*Commission on Public Dental Health Services. Programme for Public Dental Health Services*. Undated, mimeograph.

FISHER, M. A. (1970), 'The costs of delivering dental services', *J. Publ. Hlth Dent.*, **30,** 76.

FULTON, J. T. (1951), *Experiment in Dental Care*. Geneva: World Health Organization Monograph Series, No. 4.

GRUEBBEL, A. O. (1950), 'Report on the study of dental public health services in New Zealand', *J. Am. dent. Ass.*, **41,** 275.

HARRIS, R. (1950), 'The New Zealand experiment in dental services', *Dent. J. Aust.*, **22,** 437.

HILLENBRAND, H. (1960), 'The 1960 workshop of prepaid dental care; part II', *J. Mich. St. dent. Ass.*, **42,** 366.

HOLLINSHEAD, B. S. (ed.) (1961), *Survey of Dentistry*. Washington DC: American Council on Education.

LEFF, S., and LEFF, V. (1959), *The School Health Service*. London: Lewis.

MCKENDRICK, A. J. W. (1970), 'Control of dental caries by the school dental service', *Br. dent. J.*, **128,** 185.

UNITED KINGDOM MISSION (1950), *Report on the New Zealand School Dental Nurse*. London: HMSO.

WALSH, JOHN (1970), 'The changing face of dentistry in New Zealand', *N.Z. dent. J.*, **66,** 214.

WORLD HEALTH ORGANIZATION (1959), *Expert Committee on Auxiliary Dental Personnel*. Geneva: WHO. Tech. Rep. Ser. No. 163.

——— (1965), *Organization of Dental Public Health Services*. Geneva: WHO Tech. Rep. Ser. No. 298.

——— (1971a), *Oral Health Surveys; Basic Methods*. Geneva: WHO.

——— (1971b), personal communication.

YOUNG, W. O., and STRIFFLER, D. F. (1969), *The Dentist, his Practice and his Community*, 2nd ed. Philadelphia: Saunders.

Chapter 7

The Administration of Dental Services: The Example of Great Britain

C. Edward Renson PHD, DDPH, BDS, LDSRCS
Senior Lecturer in Conservative Dentistry, The London Hospital Medical College Dental School, Honorary Consultant Dental Surgeon, The London Hospital

Following the description of public treatment programmes, the system of dental care services in Great Britain is described in detail. Here is a delivery system which has evolved over many years, which attempts to bring dental care within the reach of all citizens, and which is still evolving. How well has it succeeded in reaching its goals?

Dr. Renson describes the tripartite system of the National Health Service, and examines the administration of the dental services. He looks at the obligations of both dentist and patient under the Service, and considers the economics of the Service, dentists' remuneration, patient grievances and reviews the role of the British Dental Association in the administration of the dental services. He concludes by examining the need and demand for dental care and some possible future developments.

The National Insurance Bill is the most decisive step yet taken upon the path of social organization. . . . The force of science is brought to the defence of health. The force of numbers is enlisted in aid of the individual. When *all* stand together, how much better it will be for each!' (Briggs, 1965). Thus, wrote the young Winston Spencer Churchill of the Bill which became law in mid-December, 1911. Even a Churchill, however, could not have foreseen that it was to be thirty-seven years later, with two World Wars intervening, before his words could be accepted as a reference to a real situation.

Though a great advance, Lloyd George's National Health Insurance Act of 1911 was deficient in two main ways. Because there was an income limit and dependents of insured persons were excluded from benefit, only about one-third of the population was covered and it was therefore far from national; in addition, because hospital and specialist treatment including dental treatment until 1922 were also excluded, it was far from being a complete health service even for those it did cover. Nevertheless, the passing of the National Health Insurance Act in 1911, together with certain events which had taken place four years earlier, may be regarded as important milestones in the evolution of the tripartite structure of the dental services as they exist today in Great Britain.

THE EVOLUTION OF THE TRIPARTITE STRUCTURE OF THE DENTAL SERVICES IN GREAT BRITAIN

Dental care under the National Health Service in Britain is provided in three ways. The main one is the General Dental Services, in which nearly 11,000 dentists operate as independent practitioners working under contract to statutory bodies, the National Health Service Executive Councils. This work-force constitutes nearly 80 per cent of Britain's total dental manpower.

Secondly, the Hospital Dental Service provides specialist advice and treatment for cases of special difficulty, referred by dental and medical practitioners, or for patients admitted for emergency or accident treatment. It also provides dental care for long-stay hospital in-patients, emergency care for short-stay in-patients and out-patient dental care, in

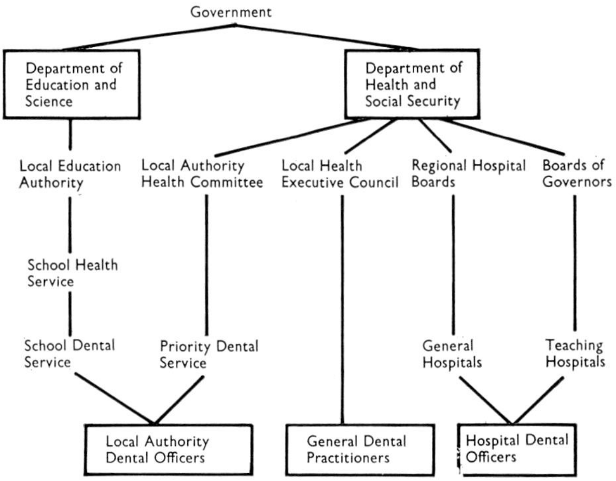

Fig. 1. Administration of the Dental Service in the National Health Service, 1971 (Department of Health and Social Security, 1971).

K

the case of teaching hospitals, to the extent required for student instruction.

The third way is through the Local Authorities: the county councils, and county borough councils. These bodies run salaried dental services and provide care in their clinics for expectant and nursing mothers and preschool children. The same salaried dental officers also man the School Dental Service, which aims to examine all schoolchildren at least once a year, and to offer treatment to those schoolchildren who require it and who are not receiving care elsewhere.

The basic administration of the dental services of the National Health Service, and the chain of administrative responsibility is shown in *Fig.* 1. It should be noted that the Ministry of Health, set up in 1919, was absorbed into the Department of Health and Social Security in 1969. Hence the duties of the Minister of Health passed to the Secretary of State for Social Services in 1969.

THE LOCAL AUTHORITY SERVICE

This service was originally designed as a service for schoolchildren only. The first treatment centre was established in the university city of Cambridge in 1907, and was a gift from a grateful patient (Davis, 1969). The 1907 report of the Board of Education, the central educational authority at the time, stated that in that year examinations by school medical officers (without the use of dental mirrors or probes) had revealed that 20–40 per cent of all schoolchildren examined had four or more carious teeth, it was also noted that the degree of carious destruction increased with age. Following these findings the Board of Education was persuaded to sanction an arrangement permitting local government spending on the dental treatment of schoolchildren for a limited period. The civic authority of Cambridge assumed responsibility in 1909 for the clinic, which had opened two years earlier. For the first time local government was concerned with dental health and dental treatment.

By July 1912 twenty-nine authorities had received sanction for their arrangements but only six employed a full-time dentist. Expansion after this was rapid and by the beginning of the First World War dental treatment had been sanctioned in 130 areas which were staffed by 250 dental surgeons of whom 52 were full-time officers.

In 1918 the Education Act made it a duty rather than, as hitherto, a permissible arrangement, of local education authorities to provide treatment in public elementary schools, and authorities were empowered to provide treatment facilities in other schools. The period between the wars saw some expansion in the number of dentists employed by local authorities and the number of treatment centres. The type of service offered was governed by the prevailing standards and attitudes. Conservation was the exception rather than the rule, and large numbers of extractions were carried out.

In 1919, Mr. (later Sir) Norman Bennett, Chairman of the Representative Board of the British Dental Association, inspected a number of school clinics at the invitation of the Board of Education. His later report dealt with regular school inspections and treatment programmes.

A detailed study of ten local authority dental services was carried out by A. T. Pitts, a well-known children's dentist, in 1929 at the invitation of the Board of Education. Many of Pitt's recommendations with regard to working conditions, the need for adequate numbers of dental surgery assistants and the appointment of senior dental officers within the service were accepted and supported by the Board of Education. Sir George Newman, Chief Medical Officer at the Board stated in his report of that year: 'of all the routine activities of the School Medical Service, the Dental Service having regard to its importance is the least fully developed'. He suggested the employment of more than 2100 whole-time dentists, an increase over the existing numbers of 1600. However, at the time that the suggestion was made the financial climate was not right for the additional expenditure which would have been involved. The depression years of the 1930s put paid to many social welfare schemes and this was but one of them. Then came the Second World War and shortly after the war ended came the National Health Act (1946), which had the effect of diverting dentists from the school dental service into the better-paid area of general practice.

The local authority service of today has a whole-time equivalent of about 1400 dental officers, about 9 per cent of all professionally employed dentists in the UK, and over 200 dental auxiliaries, who were first introduced to the UK in 1960. The training and utilization of these auxiliaries, known as New Cross auxiliaries from the location of their training school in South London, is discussed at length by Elderton in Chapter 9. There are over 1900 dentists altogether in the local authority service, many of them part-time. They operate in over 2000 dental surgeries in fixed clinics and in more than 200 mobile clinics.

The School Dental Service The Education Act (1944) states that local education authorities have a duty to provide for the dental inspection of pupils attending maintained schools or county colleges. The Education (Miscellaneous Provisions) Act, 1953, requires the local education authority to make available for such pupils comprehensive facilities for free dental treatment. The 1944 Act states that the aim of the School Dental Service is to 'inspect every child annually, offer care to those who need it and to provide care for all who accept this offer'. The service does not seem to be achieving this aim, largely because it is chronically undermanned (Burt, 1971).

No one local body is responsible for administrative arrangements in all places. These arrangements can be looked after by the Education Committee, Health and Welfare Committee, or split between various committees which are part of the local government organization.

Each local education authority is responsible for appointing a Principal School Dental Officer; almost invariably the local health authority's Chief Dental Officer is appointed to this post. The Principal School Dental Officer is subordinate to the Principal School Medical Officer and this vestigial reminder of medicine's former dominance over dentistry in the UK still rankles in some situations.

Full-time or part-time dental officers work under the Principal School Dental Officer. Many children inspected under the auspices of the School Service receive treatment from general practitioners in the General Dental Service, but no statistics exist on this aspect of treatment.

Maternity and Child Welfare Dental Services Local authorities, in this context county councils or county boroughs, also have the duty, under the National Health Service Act (1946), of making arrangements for the free dental care of expectant and nursing mothers and children of pre-school age. This area of the service usually makes use of the School Dental Service facilities and the same salaried officers treat these priority classes.

Health Centres A small, but increasing, number of health centres, provided by local health authorities under the provisions of the NHS Act, provide dental services. Dentists employed in Health Centres are paid by NHS Executive Councils. These dentists do not deal directly with the Dental Estimates Board (*vide infra*), but the approval of a Regional Dental Officer is required before certain 'prior approval' items of treatment are commenced. Schoolchildren, nursing, and expectant mothers are treated at Health Centres without charge.

THE HOSPITAL DENTAL SERVICE

When the National Health Service began on the appointed day, 5 July 1948, the existing property, premises and equipment of all voluntary and public hospitals were transferred to Government ownership. Although the Minister of Health (as he then was) has a general duty under the terms of the Act to provide hospital and specialist-care services of all kinds, organized on a national scale, the actual administration of the services is delegated to Regional Hospital Boards, Hospital Management Committees, and Boards of Governors. At the time that the NHS Act was passed England and Wales were divided into fourteen regions, each based upon a university medical school whose influence it was anticipated would do much to promote higher standards of professional work throughout the region. The hospital boards were appointed by the Minister of Health after consultations with the universities, the medical and dental profession, the local health authorities, and the (at that time) voluntary hospitals. These boards, as agents of the Minister and in collaboration with the teaching hospitals, carried out the planned co-ordination of hospital and specialist services for their regions. The day-to-day management of hospitals or a related group of hospitals is carried out by Hospital Management Committees working under the control of Regional Hospital Boards. In its task of appointing the members of these committees, the Regional Hospital Board must consult with organizations representative of general medical and dental practitioners, with the senior medical and dental staff of the hospitals concerned, and with those local government bodies which have been given powers as local health authorities (*vide supra*).

Hospitals or groups of hospitals that are designated as teaching hospitals are not under the control of the regional boards or local management committees. For each such hospital or group a Board of Governors is constituted which includes members nominated by the university, the regional board, and the senior staff of the hospital or hospitals concerned.

The endowment funds of the teaching hospitals passed to the new boards of governors; the endowments of other voluntary hospitals were placed in a central Hospital Endowment Fund and then were re-apportioned.

Hospital Staff Medical and dental specialists in consultant appointments in the hospital service may give either full- or part-time service and private practice is therefore still open to them. Although they are attached to the staff of particular hospitals they receive their appointments from, and are the employees of, the regional hospital boards or the boards of governors in the case of teaching hospitals. The appointments are made on the advice of expert professional advisory committees and only after public advertisement of the vacancy in the manner customary for such posts in Britain.

Private accommodation for patients who wish to pay the whole cost of their treatment continues to be provided, subject to the over-riding right of other patients to be admitted to such accommodation if clinical consideration urgently requires it. This arrangement has given rise to complaints of 'queue-jumping' from time to time, that is, the ability to pay has enabled certain patients to obtain treatment quickly. These complaints have been surprisingly few over the years. The existence of provident and private patient schemes allow many people to receive private health care treatment and the number appears to be increasing.

The functions of the Hospital Dental Service have been referred to earlier in this chapter. In 1963 the Standing Dental Advisory Committee, a group of prominent dentists whose function is to advise the Minister of Health, issued a report on the development of the Hospital Dental Service. The slow development of the service was emphasized and its expansion was recommended. The committee concluded that one dental consultant (consultant in this context means a specialist) should be appointed within the Hospital Service for every 250,000 of the population. At the time of the report it was shown that the teaching hospitals were providing about half this desired ratio.

Each consultant dental surgeon should be supported by appropriate staff and should have all the requisite ancillary staff and services. Even today in many regions these desiderata do not prevail.

The Orthodontic Services were also considered and the recommended ratio was one consultant orthodontist to every 500,000 population with similar conditions as apply to specialists in general dentistry. It is worth noting here that to date only two types of specialist appointments within dentistry are recognized by the NHS authorities, these are specialist in (a) dental surgery and in (b) orthodontics. In the former case, until very recently, only dental surgeons recognized as primarily trained in oral surgery have been appointed. This situation is now slowly changing and specialists in restorative dentistry (operative/prosthetic/periodontology) are beginning to receive recognition and appointments. Honorary consultant appointments have been conferred upon senior University teachers in all the dental disciplines for many years, but the appointments are always technically in dental surgery or in orthodontics.

In 1970, there were 249 full-time equivalent consultant dental surgeons in the Hospital Dental Service (Department of Health and Social Security, 1971a). Dentistry in hospital is regarded as a speciality of medicine and the staffing structure and conditions are similar to both. The grades of appointment include House Officer and Senior House Officer, Registrar and Senior Registrar, Assistant Dental Surgeon, and Consultant. House officer and registrar are regarded as training grades prior to higher qualifications, a senior registrar is normally recruited from the registrar grade and will usually have a higher qualification. The senior registrar is a full-time training post intended to lead to consultant grade and normally tenure is limited to a maximum of four years. Appropriately, more senior registrars exist than there are consultant posts for them to fill and the post of Assistant Dental Surgeon may be used as a device for keeping a senior registrar ‘marking time’. The Assistant Dental Surgeon (ADS) may also be recruited from the ranks of experienced general practitioners. The post is of unlimited tenure and is below that of the grade of consultant under whom the ADS nominally works, providing treatment not considered to be of consultant level, such as routine dental treatment of long-stay hospital patients.

The consultant dental surgeon (or consultant orthodontist) is normally recruited from the senior registrar/assistant dental surgeon grades at around age 32, after a minimum of eight years’ full-time training following graduation. Consultants may be honorary or paid in the dental teaching hospitals. Honorary appointments are usually held by university staff who are paid by the university.

In 1970, the full-time equivalent of 714 dentists including consultants were employed in the hospital dental service (Department of Health and Social Security, 1971a) and an estimated £1 million was spent on the service in 1966 (Office of Health Economics, 1969). This figure, however, does not include expenditure on dental services, including training, in dental teaching hospitals. It has been estimated that this would have involved an additional £3 million (Allred, 1969). These figures must be contrasted with the £9 million spent by local health and local education authorities in the same year and the total expenditure of an estimated £89 million on the dental services in the United Kingdom in 1966 to obtain comparative estimates of the quantities of services involved. Quantification in this way may be considered unreasonable, but it is difficult to offer any other useful comparative figures.

THE GENERAL DENTAL SERVICE

The shortcomings with regard to dental benefits under the National Health Insurance Act of 1911 have already been noted. An oblique reference was made to these shortcomings by Sir William Beveridge in his Report of 1942. He stated:

> There is a general demand that dental services should become statutory benefits available to all under health insurance. There appear to be grounds for regarding a development of preservative dental treatment as a measure of major importance for improving the health of the nation. This measure involves, first, a change of popular habit from aversion to visiting the dentist till pain compels into a readiness to visit and be inspected periodically. It involves, simultaneously, with creation by these means of a demand for a larger supply of the service. That the insurance title to free dental service should become as universal as that to free medical service is not open to serious doubt. The only substantial distinction which it seems right to make is in the supply of appliances. To ensure careful use, it is reasonable that part of the cost of renewals of dentures should be borne by the person using them. This might possibly be extended to the original supply. (Beveridge, 1942.)

Two years after the Beveridge Report the Government published a White Paper, which is a statement of intended legislation published to allow discussion prior to the legislation being brought before Parliament. It outlined proposals for a National Health Service. There was to be no compulsion to join the Service for either patient or practitioner, but it was to be available to all. Taking up the Beveridge theme the White Paper stated:

> A full dental service for the whole population, including regular conservative treatment, is unquestionably a proper aim in every health service and must be so regarded. But there are not at present and will not be for many years enough dentists in the country to provide it. Until the supply can be increased, attention will have to be concentrated on priority needs. These must include the needs of children and young people and of expectant and nursing mothers. The whole dental problem is a peculiarly difficult one, and a committee under the chairmanship of Lord Teviot has been set up to consider and report on it. (Ministry of Health, 1944a.)

In a review of the then existing arrangements, the White Paper stated that 30 per cent of the 21 million then insured persons were eligible for dental benefit, and yet in any one year only 6–7 per cent claimed it. The

Teviot Committee published two reports, the first in 1944 recommended, among other things, that:

1. A comprehensive dental service should be instituted as an integral part of the National Health Service at its inception.

2. The General Dental Service should be broadly analagous to the General Medical Service.

3. Dental health centres should be developed in conjunction with general health centres.

4. There should be freedom for dentists and patients at their own wish, to participate in the dental services (Ministry of Health, 1944b).

In the final Teviot Report in 1946, manpower problems were investigated and it was recommended that:

1. The intake of dental students should be stepped up to 900 a year (a number not achieved at time of writing).

2. Dental curricula should be as short as possible compatible with a satisfactory standard of training.

3. Dental schools should be an integral part of a university.

4. A close relationship with a medical school would benefit both medical and dental students (Ministry of Health, 1946).

The National Health Service Act, 1946, placed on the Minister of Health the duty of promoting for the people of England and Wales (Scotland and Northern Ireland have similar but separate legislative instruments) the establishment of a comprehensive health service. The service was to include general practitioner services provided by medical and dental practitioners, pharmaceutical services and an ophthalmic service. The service was also to include local health services, hospital and specialist services to which reference has already been made.

The Administration of the General Dental Service The inter-relationship of bodies with administrative responsibility in the operations of the General Dental Service is shown on *Fig.* 2. This diagram does not include the various advisory bodies.

Department of Health and Social Security It has been mentioned previously that the Ministry of Health was absorbed into the Department of Health and Social Security in 1969. The habit of years still sometimes causes the Secretary of State for Social Services to be referred to as 'the Minister' but this title is no longer strictly correct.

The Chief Medical Officer has an overall responsibility for the coordination of all the activities of the staff who are members of the health professions in the Department, and conjointly in the Department of Education and Science. However, the Chief Dental Officer is wholly responsible for clinical and other professional advice to the respective Secretaries of State on the dental aspects of national and local authorities health services and for advising other Crown Departments on dental matters. The Secretary of State for Social Services may also seek the advice of the Central Health Services Council, with three dental members, or the Standing Dental Advisory Committee, which has a predominantly dental membership. The Dental Staff of the Department of Health consists of a Deputy Chief Dental Officer, eight Senior Dental Officers, and thirty-two Dental Officers. In addition, there are three Dental Officers at the Department of Education and Science, all of whom are under the direct control of the Chief Dental Officer.

Executive Councils The National Health Service Act provided that Executive Councils should be set up for the area of each local authority, but in the interest of efficiency the Secretary of State has the power to set up single Executive Councils for the area of two or more health authorities. Such a council is known as a 'combined' council. There are 163 Executive Councils in England and Wales and Scotland. Only 8 in

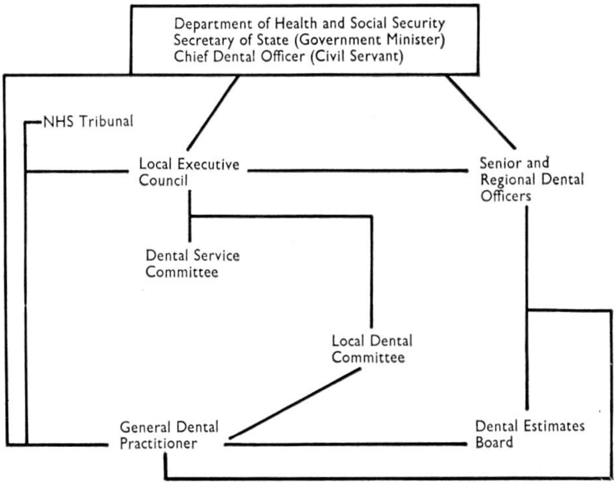

Fig. 2. The inter-relationship of official bodies with administrative responsibility in the General Dental Service, 1971. Advisory bodies are not included (Department of Health and Social Security, 1971).

England and Wales are combined councils, whereas in Scotland 16 out of 25 are combined councils.

An Executive Council consists of 25 members. There are three dental members, who are elected by the Local Dental Committee for the area. The Executive Council also is responsible for local arrangements for medical, pharmaceutical, and ophthalmic services. The main duty of the Executive Councils, as far as the General Dental Services are concerned, is to ensure that local arrangements are adequate to meet the needs of the public. In areas short of dentists, the local Executive Council can make arrangements to provide housing at economic rates to dentists.

When a dentist wishes to practice in the Health Service in a certain area he applies to the appropriate Executive Council asking to be included on its list of practitioners. If he wishes to practice in different areas covered by more than one council he must apply separately to each one concerned. When a dentist wishes to withdraw from a Council's list he must give three months' notice in writing, although on occasions the Council may agree to a shorter period.

Much of the work of Executive Councils is done by small committees, but all decisions must be ratified by the full Council. These full Council meetings are open to the Press.

Dental Service Committees These committees consist of a lay Chairman and six members. Three of these members are appointed from the lay members of the Executive Council and three by the Local Dental Committee.

It is the duty of the Service Committee to investigate cases in which a dentist is alleged to be in breach of his terms of service. Proceedings commence on a complaint from a patient or on the initiative of the Executive Council or Dental Estimates Board. The majority of cases begin with the Dental Estimates Board, but Executive Councils settle many of these disputes without recourse to Service Committee proceedings.

When a Service Committee has investigated a case, it comes to a decision and recommends appropriate action to the Executive Council. The actions the Executive Council can take against a dentist include: (1) recovering from the practitioner and repayment to the patient, of expenses reasonably incurred by the patient owing to the practitioner's failure to observe his terms of service; (2) recommendation to the Secretary of State that a given amount of remuneration should be withheld; (3) to require that all estimates, other than those for emergency treatment or examination, be submitted to the Dental Estimates Board for prior approval; (4) refer the case to the National Health Service Tribunal; or (5) the dentist may be simply warned by the Executive Council. The dentist may appeal to the Secretary of State if he feels unjustly treated.

Local Dental Committees These are committees of, and elected by, local dental practitioners. They nominate three members of the Executive Council, but are basically the expression of local professional opinion. They play a part in maintaining the standards of professional practice. Local Dental Committees are elected by practitioners in every Executive Council area; they are recognized by the Secretary of State and Executive Councils are required to consult them on matters connected with the administration of the General Dental Services.

Regional Dental Officers England and Wales are divided into 15 regions (coincident with Regional Hospital Board areas). These regions are in two divisions, each division under a Senior Dental Officer. There are 32 Regional Dental Officers in England and Wales; Scotland has one Chief Dental Officer and four Regional Dental Officers. Regional Dental Officers (RDOs) are recruited from among practitioners of at least 10 years' experience. Their duties consist almost entirely of clinical examinations of patients and the giving of advice as a result of those examinations. It is a General Dental Services condition that a patient must submit for such an examination if required. RDOs may also, at the request of the Executive Council, inspect accommodation provided by dentists if there is reason to suspect that it is unsatisfactory, or visit a dentist suspected of keeping inadequate records. Ninety per cent of referrals to the RDO come from the Dental Estimates Board, comprising 'estimates' references where the Board wants a second opinion prior to approving a course of treatment (there were 6655 such cases in 1970) and treatment references which arise from the Board's work in investigating practices. 'Treatment' references are the most frequent. In 1970, there were 19,531 treatment references from 18,539,423 completed courses of treatment in England and Wales; that is, slightly more than 0·001 per cent of the total. In only 0·2 per cent of these, that is in 31 cases, did the Dental Officer express complete dissatisfaction with the treatment given. Sixty per cent were entirely satisfactory, and some minor degree of dissatisfaction was found in 39·8 per cent (Department of Health and Social Security, 1971b).

Referrals to the RDO by the Executive Council usually follow patients' complaints. The Executive Council can, if the RDO so advises, institute Service Committee proceedings, in which case the RDO would be an important witness. Referrals from practitioners are usually requests for a second opinion. In 1970, the total of cases referred by Executive Councils to practitioners was only 1201 in England and Wales (Department of Health and Social Security, 1971a).

Dental Estimates Board There is one Dental Estimates Board (DEB) for England and Wales situated at Eastbourne, and one for Scotland at Edinburgh. The DEB is responsible for the professional and financial scrutiny of the claims for payment of fees submitted by dental practitioners and for the approval of treatment, and supplies the Executive Council with the necessary authority for payment. For both Boards, the Chairman and Vice-Chairman are both dental practitioners, and five of the remaining seven members must also be dental practitioners. In England and Wales the Board has four full-time members including the Chairman. The Board employs 28 other dental advisors who are also dental practitioners, and 1100 other non-dental staff. Scotland has the Chairman only as a full-time member, it employs three dental advisors and 170 other staff. The work of the DEB may be divided into two categories:

1. Routine work of sanctioning estimates and authorizing payment of fees.
2. Compiling statistics and detection of possible frauds and malpractice.

About 3·8 per cent of the estimates submitted are of 'prior approval' type (Department of Health and Social Security, 1971c). Approval from the DEB prior to commencement of treatment is required for more complex and expensive treatment such as gold inlays, crowns, bridges, metal dentures. The prior approval list is revised from time to time.

Orthodontic treatment must have prior approval, and pre- and post-treatment models are required by the DEB. Orthodontic cases are considered by a special committee which includes two orthodontic consultants.

Dentists or patients may appeal against decisions of the DEB. Appeals are heard by independent dentists appointed by the Secretary of State.

The Secretary of State is supplied with a list of dentists, by the Local Dental Committees and the British Dental Association, who are willing to act as referees. Usually the two selected are from another area and are not immediate neighbours of the dentist concerned. Appeals are usually heard in the evenings and all interested parties are asked to attend. If the Board has acted on the advice of the RDO he will attend to support his own case, but for decisions made by the Board it may send its own representative. The decision of the referees is final and there is no 'higher court', but a dentist cannot be compelled to carry out treatment with which he does not agree. In such circumstances the Executive Council would usually allow him to withdraw from the case. Appeals can only be made against decisions of the Board where it has discretion in a clinical or financial matter, appeals cannot be made against the regulations under which the service works.

Excessive Dental Treatment Where there is a *prima facie* case for considering that a practitioner has regularly carried out excessive dental treatment the case can be referred by the Secretary of State to the Local Dental Committee for consideration. Such a reference is made, when after investigation of estimate forms submitted by the practitioner to the DEB the Secretary of State is of the opinion that the character and volume of treatment gives reason to consider that the practitioner may have regularly provided treatment in excess of what was reasonably necessary to secure the dental fitness of his patients or that the cost incurred by the Executive Council may have been in excess of what was reasonably necessary to secure proper treatment.

The practitioner is sent a statement of the matters on which an explanation is required and he has the right to attend a hearing before the Committee. If the Committee decide there has regularly been excessive treatment or cost they must tell the Council, the practitioner, and the Secretary of State.

The practitioner can appeal against the Committee's decision within one month of its receipt. The appeal is then heard and determined by referees appointed by the Secretary of State, normally three in number, of whom at least one must be a dental practitioner. Similarly, if the Secretary of State is dissatisfied with the Committee's decision he may arrange for referees to hear and determine the matter in the same manner. If the decision of the Committee, or of referees on appeal, is that there has been excessive treatment or cost, the Secretary of State must require the practitioner to submit all his estimates or estimates of a particular type to the DEB for prior approval for a period of 12 months After six months the practitioner may apply for the period to be reduced.

The Dental Practitioner A dentist who elects to practice under the General Dental Services enters a contractual agreement with the local Executive Council. He may then practice in his own surgery and he agrees to abide by the specified terms of service. His name will then appear on the list of the local Executive Council.

It should be made clear that practitioners are not 'employees' of Executive Councils; they manage their own practices and meet their own expenses. They are paid, in respect of items of treatment, fees which are designed to cover both expenses and their remuneration.

The dentist submits his claim for payment, and treatment plans for prior approval when necessary, to the DEB under a number allocated by the Executive Council. The DEB process these claims and inform the Executive Council of the amount which the dentist should be paid each month. The DEB can ask the RDO for a second opinion if it so wishes, prior to approving any particular plan of treatment.

If a patient wishes to complain about a dentist, he approaches the Executive Council. The Executive Council often settle such disputes directly with the dentist, but they can institute Service Committee proceedings if this is deemed advisable. The Service Committee in turn recommends a course of action to the Executive Council. The dentist may appeal, past the Executive Council to the Secretary of State if he wishes.

The Patient Anyone may apply for dental treatment to any dentist whose name is on a dental list maintained by local Executive Councils and available at Executive Council Offices, post offices, or public libraries. The dentist has the right to accept or reject the patient for treatment under the service.

A course of treatment is normally completed when the practitioner has carried out all the treatment necessary for dental fitness that the patient is willing to receive. When further treatment becomes necessary it is open to the patient to apply for treatment to his previous practitioner, who may refuse if he wishes, or to any other practitioner. A patient does not register with a dental practitioner as he does with a medical practitioner under the terms of the General Medical Service.

The term 'dental fitness' is defined in the regulations as 'Such a reasonable standard of dental efficiency and oral health as is necessary to safeguard general health.' All treatment must be completed with reasonable expedition but in any case within 6 months for those treatments not requiring prior approval. In the case of extractions followed by dentures the time is extended to 12 months and in the case of orthodontic treatment the DEB has discretion as to the length of time of treatment. To obtain extensions on these time limits the practitioner has to resubmit a form with an explanation.

The National Health Service Tribunals There are two National Health Service Tribunals for dental matters, one for England and Wales and one for Scotland. These Tribunals are responsible for deciding whether or not a dentist should be permitted to remain on the Executive Council list.

Both Tribunals are independent bodies, consisting of a legally qualified chairman, a lay member of the Executive Council, and a dental practitioner. The Tribunal considers representations that a dentist is not fit to continue to practice in the General Dental Services. Such representations usually come from the Executive Councils following Service Committee proceedings, but they may follow prosecution of a dentist in the courts. Legal representation is allowed at Tribunals and witnesses may be subpoenaed. The Tribunal decides whether to direct that the practitioner's name should be removed from the dental list and debarred from inclusion in the list of other Executive Councils. If the decision goes against the practitioner he may appeal to the Secretary of State within 14 days. If this appeal fails he may appeal to the High Court.

Remuneration of Dentists in the General Dental Service In determining dentists' remuneration two standing bodies, the Review Body and the Dental Rates Study Group each play a part. Both were set up in accordance with recommendations made in the 1960 Report of the Royal Commission on Doctor's and Dentist's Remuneration (Royal Commission, 1960), known as the Pilkington Report.

Remuneration in the Health Service has always been a vexed question. In 1948, the chronic backlog of treatment required produced an acute demand on an understaffed profession, resulting in a rapid increase in the quantity of dental treatment carried out. The much wider availability of a dental service combined with the contact with dentistry experienced by many thousands of young adults during the World War led to a greatly enlarged demand for treatment. Dentists worked long and hard to satisfy this demand and in consequence their incomes were on average much higher than had been anticipated. A Report of an Interdepartmental Committee on the Remuneration of General Dental Practitioners, the Spens Report, published in 1948, recommended specific levels of remuneration in relation to a 33-hour working week (Ministry of Health, 1948). However, in the following year a Working Party studied the chairside times taken in carrying out treatment in the General Dental Services, and published its findings as the Penman Report (1949). The report stated that a very large proportion of the profession were working 25 per cent longer than the 33 hours weekly envisaged by Spens and that this was the reason for the relatively large incomes, in excess of the Spens' proposals, which were being currently earned by dentists. Nevertheless, in February 1949, a 'ceiling' on incomes for dentists in the GDS was imposed so that when a dentist's gross monthly earnings exceeded £400 the government retained 50 per cent of the figure above £400. In June 1949, this 'ceiling' was ended but a new scale of fees, which represented a 17 per cent reduction compared to the former scale, was introduced. In May 1950, the fees were again cut by an additional 10 per cent. Exactly a year later in an effort to further reduce dental costs the government imposed a patient's contribution for the supply of dentures, approximating to 50 per cent of the scale fee. Thus ended the concept of a 'free' service. Just over a year later, in June 1952, a maximum patient contribution of £1 was introduced for a course of dental treatment not involving dentures. This charge remained unaffected for sixteen years when, in 1968, it was increased to £1·50. The 'priority classes', that is expectant and nursing mothers, preschool children, and schoolchildren were exempted from these charges and continued to receive free treatment.

In 1956, a Report by a Committee of Enquiry into the cost of the National Health Service, the Guillebaud Report, advocated the retention of charges for dentures because it was felt that its removal might lead to an increase in the amount of denture work at the expense of conservative work (Ministry of Health, 1956a). However, the Report's recommendations had been largely overtaken by events before they saw the light of day. From the early 1950s partly as a result of the measures described above and also because of the exhaustion of the reservoir of unsatisfied demand for dentures, the cost of the GDS started to decline. It fell dramatically up to 1953, reaching a figure of £30 million (Office of Health Economics, 1969) but since then has risen steadily to some £90 million by 1970 (Department of Health and Social Security, 1971b). In 1949 constant price terms this last figure is slightly lower than the cost of the service in 1949.

An examination of the Ministry of Health Annual Reports for the years 1949–66 reveals that the fall in expenditure on the General Dental Services is emphasized when the expenditure is measured as a proportion of the total NHS expenditure. In 1949, the General Dental Service expenditure accounted for 10 per cent of the gross NHS figure, but by 1953 it accounted for only 5·5 per cent. No other branch of the health service has seen such a large proportionate change. Since 1953, the proportion has remained steady at around the 5 per cent level dropping to 4·6 per cent in 1970. The UK now spends about 5·25 per cent of its National Income on health services, and dentistry accounts for 0·25 per cent of National Income (Office of Health Economics, 1969).

Mounting anxiety on both the part of the doctors and dentists that their incomes were at the mercy of 'the whim of the Minister of Health' was somewhat allayed following the publication of the Pilkington Report in 1960. Both professions and the government accepted its findings, and it is on these that methods of remuneration for the General

Dental Service and the Hospital Service are presently based. In reference to the General Dental Service the Report states that:

> In the absence of any effective machinery to see that general dental surgeons earned what had been intended, they have consistently earned more. There have never yet been enough dentists to ensure prompt treatment within the National Health Service of all patients on the basis of a free or very heavily subsidized service. For this reason general dental practitioners have worked longer hours than were envisaged by the Spens Committee, and have not only earned more than was intended, but have earned more than general medical practitioners—in a sharp contrast to the position in all other countries of which we have knowledge. (Royal Commission, 1960.)

The Commission recommended the setting up of a Review Body, 'to watch the levels and spread of medical and dental remuneration and to make recommendations to the Prime Minister'. This last phrase was considered to be of much significance since it interposed the Prime Minister between the Minister of Health and practitioners working within the NHS. The main task of the Review Body:

> Will be the exercise of the faculty of good judgement, and it must be composed of individuals whose standing and reputation will command the confidence of the profession, the Government and the public.
>
> It must be regarded as a better judge than either the Government or the representatives of the profession as to what level and spread of medical and dental remuneration should be. (Royal Commission, 1960.)

Special importance was attached by the Commission to prompt action by the government in dealing with any recommendations made by the Review Body, which was composed of seven eminent individuals representative of various sections of public life—such as the professions, banking, and universities, headed by Lord Kindersley, and for 10 years reasonably prompt action was in fact forthcoming.

The Pilkington Report also states:

> Now that the vast majority of their earnings come from the State, a monopoly employer for practical purposes, doctors and dentists should have their remuneration settled by external comparison, principally, though not necessarily exclusively, with professional men and others with a university background in other walks of life in Great Britain. Earnings ought not to be determined by short-term supply and demand. The level of demand is artificial and is easily increased or reduced by Government action, whereas the supply of skilled people cannot be quickly adjusted.
>
> Dentists have earned more than had been expected. They were able to work more chairside hours than had been assumed by the Spens' Committee, and during such hours to get through more work than had been indicated by the Penman Committee's statistics. We view with disfavour the failure of the profession and the Government to establish a method that would ensure that dental earnings match intentions. (Royal Commission, 1960.)

In this somewhat condemnatory reference to the profession the Pilkington Report adopts a different stance to that of a report published some four years earlier. In 1956, a committee under the chairmanship of Lord McNair was set up to ascertain the reason for the lack of candidates of suitable calibre for training as dentists and to indicate possible solutions (Ministry of Health, 1956b). This committee agreed with the Penman Committee that the profession appeared to have been harshly treated by the Press, and they could not help feeling that had the true facts been more readily available to the public in proper form and at the right time, much of the adverse criticism might have been avoided.

The 1960 Pilkington Report went on to recommend that a permanent study group should assess and keep under review rates for items of service, based on proved performance of dentists. This recommendation stated:

> It will be for the Review Body to say what dentists in the future ought to earn. It will be for the study group to arrange that this is what they do earn. Doctors and Dentists in public service should not be used as a regulator for the national economy. Their earnings should not be prevented from rising because of the fears that others might follow. This does not mean that we consider that either doctors or dentists should ever have a fixed place in a changing world. Over the years in this country and in others the financial position held by doctors or dentists may rise in relation to some fall in relation to others, and in relation to each other, for various reasons including the maintenance of a proper balance of recruitment between these and other professions. (Royal Commission, 1960.)

The Review Body and the Dental Rates Study Group were set up in 1961, and the machinery for determining dentists' and doctors' pay envisaged by the Royal Commission came into being. In the period 1961–70 the Review Body issued twelve reports. The recommendations of the report issued in 1970 (Review Body, 1970) were not accepted by the Government of the day and this led to the resignation of the chairman, Lord Kindersley, and the entire membership of the Body. Following the 1970 General Election the new administration implemented, in part, the recommendations of the last Review Body report and in addition appointed a new Review Body, which published its first report in 1971.

THE ROLE OF THE BRITISH DENTAL ASSOCIATION IN THE ADMINISTRATION OF DENTAL SERVICES

Throughout the 25 years which have elapsed since the commencement of the National Health Service the British Dental Association has consistently represented the interests of the dentists working in the Service. Before the Service began the BDA concept of a national dental health service was that it should begin with a comprehensive service to all children and be extended to older age-groups as that became practical. This concept was not acceptable to the government which insisted on making the dental service available immediately to all. The BDA advised its members, before the Health Service came into being, not to enter the Service. The membership, in large measure, rejected this advice. However, the BDA has continued to serve the profession in an endeavour to obtain maximum benefit both for dentists and their patients.

The tripartite structure of the public dental services is reflected by the structure of the BDA's political committees, i.e., the Public Dental Officers' Group Committee (which represents the interests of dentists employed by local authorities), Central Committee for Hospital Dental Services, University Dental Teachers' Group Committee, and the General Dental Services Committee.

Members of these committees are elected by democratic process. They function in numerous ways but can chiefly be said to exercise powers of persuasion, advice, and negotiation. Persuasory powers are used in connexion with formal and informal contacts with Members of Parliament, deputations to Government Departments, public relations activities and the like.

Advisory powers are used via formal resolutions, policy documents and memoranda, representation on official advisory committees (e.g. Central Health Services Council, Standing Dental Advisory Committee, Dental Rates Study Group), evidence to Royal Commissions and Interdepartmental Committees, deputations to the Secretary of State, and by continual, person-to-person exchanges with senior civil servants of the appropriate Government Departments.

Negotiation in connexion with remuneration is carried out via the largely formalized machinery of the Review Body and the Dental Rates Study Group for general and hospital practitioners and a body called the Whitley Council for local authority employed dentists.

Negotiation on such matters as the interpretation of Health Service regulations is a continuous process largely carried on with the Department of Health and the Dental Estimates Board. These negotiations are conducted through joint working parties, deputations, and day-to-day correspondence.

Many dentists have felt that the BDA has been insufficiently pressing in its negotiations. The passage of time has made it clear, however, that a threat of withdrawal of services, which could only be made if there was evidence of a unity of purpose, is never likely to be made. Persuasion as to the justice of claims made on behalf of the profession is regarded as a much more realistic approach.

SUPPLY AND DEMAND IN RELATION TO DENTAL CARE

The demand for treatment has continued to increase since the inception of the health service. In 1949, less than seven million courses of treatment were supplied under the General Dental Services, in 1970 the figure was approximately 21 million for England and Wales (Department of Health and Social Security, 1971b). However, even this figure indicates that only about one-quarter to one-third of the total population is likely to be receiving regular dental treatment. Annual reports from the Ministry of Health and the Department of Health and Social Security indicate that this large increase in courses of treatment from 1949 to 1970 has been achieved by little more than the original number of practitioners (approximately 9400 in 1949 and 10,800 in 1970).

Dentists are paid on an 'item of service' basis, that is, the dentist is paid a fixed fee for each operation he performs. The Dental Rates Study Group from time to time reviews the fees in the light of prevailing practice expenses. The Review Body sets a target average net income for a dentist working a specified number of hours and the scale of fees drawn up by the Study Group is governed by this target figure.

This method of remuneration has been derisively termed the 'treadmill' and the output of the individual dentist has increased markedly with the passage of the years because of improvements in technology, equipment, and practice organization, but his return has not increased to the extent that would be expected in other fields of endeavour when improved productivity is achieved.

Curiously, an attempt to offer the practitioner an alternative pay structure in 1964 failed because it was rejected by practitioners. This was the British Dental Association's Tattersall Report (British Dental Association, 1964), which suggested a capitation fee, plus fees by scale for certain items, following the achievement of dental fitness. In 1965 a survey carried out by the British Dental Association indicated that 73 per cent of practitioners favoured remuneration by scale of fees.

Until 1968, no attempt had been made to assess the demand and need for dental care on a national basis. There had been what in effect was a pilot study of the dental health and attitudes towards dentistry of two different communities in Salisbury and Darlington (Bulman et al., 1968), however, the authors of that paper were naturally reluctant to draw national conclusions on this basis. As a consequence, in 1968 a national survey of adult dental health in England and Wales was carried out for the Department of Health and Social Security by the Government Social Survey and The London Hospital Medical College Dental School (Gray et al., 1970).

A random sample of some 3000 adults over the age of 16 were interviewed and dentally examined. The authors of the resulting publication point out that dental treatment patterns affect the state of dental health for very long periods. Although the survey was carried out twenty years after the beginning of the NHS, 45 per cent of all the people who were found to be edentulous had lost their teeth before 1948 and had therefore no opportunity of restorative dentistry in the NHS.

A definite regional variation in dental health was revealed by the survey. In England and Wales as a whole the proportion of adults aged 16 or more who had no natural teeth was 36·8 per cent. In London and the South East, however, the proportion was 28·4 per cent, while in the North the proportion was 45·5 per cent. No explanation was put forward for this particular difference, but evidently it is possible that regional differences in attitudes and behaviour can affect dental health.

Although some people obtained conservative dental treatment prior to the NHS, many people did not, and the resultant attitudes and behaviour towards dental treatment are not likely to change in a relatively small number of years. Among the younger group (16–34 years) who had had virtually free treatment available to them for all or almost all their lives nearly half (45 per cent) claimed to be regular dental attenders, but an almost equal number (41 per cent) said that they attended a dentist only when in dental trouble.

A factor which would obviously influence attendance is accessibility to dental care. The survey showed that whereas the population per dentist in the London and South East region was about 3290, in the North it was 5750. It is obviously difficult to separate the supply of dentists, the prevalence of disease, and the attitudes to dentistry as causal factors in the maldistribution of manpower.

A clear association between social class structure of the population in an area and the ratio of dentists to population in that area has been shown by Cook and Walker (1967). The higher the proportion of persons in higher social classes in an area, the higher the proportion of dentists. The distribution of dental manpower could be improved by government intervention but this would entail a drastic alteration to the present arrangements, which make no provision for the direction of dental manpower but which do make provision for the direction of medical manpower.

The authors of the survey referred to above (Gray et al., 1970) point out that there are circumstances in the general dental services which tend to perpetuate the differences between regular dental attenders and irregular attenders. Foremost are the provisions in the regulations for 'emergency treatment of casual patients'. These regulations state that practitioners may accept casual patients for specified items of treatment only, without incurring the obligation to carry out all necessary treatment. These items are: (1) Denture repairs; (2) the following items of emergency treatment: (a) not more than two extractions, (b) anaesthetic, (c) dressing teeth, (d) arrest of haemorrhage, (e) radiological examination, and (f) domiciliary visits (Gray et al., 1970). In the financial year 1969–70, of the £84 million spent on the GDS in England and Wales, emergency treatment accounted for £1·4 million (Department of Health and Social Security, 1971a).

Dental health education is not an item for payment under the General Dental Service, hence dentists face a financial disincentive when they consider spending time in trying to persuade people to change their dental attitudes. It could obviously take a very long time to persuade someone who had never had a filling to have one. Such dentist–patient problems must be particularly acute in parts of the country where the population per dentist rate is nearly twice as high as in other areas.

A complementary survey of the dental health of schoolchildren aged 5–16 is now progressing. These surveys should be regarded as base-lines for future studies to gauge the response to dental treatment over a period of time.

Recent and forecast government changes are bound to lead to changes in attitudes, behaviour, and dental treatment patterns. During the Labour administration of 1964–70, two Green Papers were published (Ministry of Health, 1968; Department of Health and Social Security, 1970) in which fundamental changes to the existing National Health Service, including changes in the tripartite structure of the dental services, were recommended. These changes were not effected in that government's term of office. In May 1971 the Secretary of State for Social Services, Sir Keith Joseph, published a Consultative Document on *National Health Service Reorganization* which again attacked the present tripartite structure as being outmoded and called for integration of the health services (Department of Health and Social Security, 1971a). Green Papers and Consultative Documents are statements of proposed future legislation, introduced to allow public feeling on a particular subject to be expressed. They are both less firm statements of intent than are White Papers. The Green Paper of 1968 was actually withdrawn when public reaction to the proposals it suggested was unfavourable, the 1970 Green Paper contained some fresh proposals.

In April 1971, the government introduced a new system of increased contributions from patients. In place of the maximum £1·50 towards the cost of a course of treatment which did not include dentures, patients must now pay *half the cost* of a course of treatment, up to a limit of £10. The priority classes and old age pensioners still remain exempt from charges.

In many ways this is reminiscent of the arrangements for dental benefits under the National Health Insurance scheme which existed prior to 1948, persons entitled to dental benefit then had to pay about half the cost of treatment. It is to be hoped that in the 25 years during which the General Dental Services have been available, sufficient impact has been made so that there will not be a return to the attitudes and treatment patterns which existed then.

The wheel has turned full cycle from the days in 1942 when Sir William Beveridge wrote: 'That the insurance title to free dental service should become as universal as that to free medical service is not open to serious doubt'. The dental care services now face problems in the supply of dental manpower, economic pressures and forthcoming changes in the structure of local government and the National Health Service. These factors lead many to regard the future of the General Dental Service—as an integral part of the National Health Service—with uncertainty and foreboding.

CHRONOLOGY OF MAJOR EVENTS IN THE EVOLUTION OF THE DENTAL SERVICES IN GREAT BRITAIN 1907–1973

1907 Dental school inspections carried out for the first time under the provisions of the Education (Administrative Provisions) Act. Medical officer inspections (without mirror and probe) revealed that 20–40 per cent of the children examined had 4 or more carious teeth. Dental treatment centre established in Cambridge, as an act of philanthropy, and taken over in 1909 by the Cambridge Corporation.

1911 NHI Act. Financial assistance, for medical care for lower paid workers, from Friendly Societies.

1912 Board of Education 'Recommendations for the Basis of a Satisfactory School Dental Scheme'.

1918 Education Act made it a duty (instead of a power as previously) of local education authorities to provide treatment.

1918 Maternity and Child Welfare Act established 'priority classes' for dental treatment.

1919 Report of Mr. (later Sir) Norman Bennett, Chairman of the Representative Board of the British Dental Association on the state of a number of school clinics.
Creation of a Ministry of Health.

1921 Dentists Act. Over 7000 previously unregistered dentists admitted to Register.

1922 Financial assistance for dental care, for lower paid workers, through Friendly Societies under the NHI Act.

1927 Appointment of Regional Dental Officers to advise Dental Benefit Joint Council.

1929 Report of Mr. A. T. Pitts on ten local authority dental services.

1942 Beveridge Report (Social Insurance and Allied Services Command 6404, 1942).

1944 White paper on *A National Health Service* (Command 6502, 1944).

1944 Education Act (Section 48 (1)) provides a legal basis for local authority dental service for pupils of maintained schools and county colleges.

1944 Interim Report of the Interdepartmental Committee on Dentistry (Teviot Committee) Command 6565, 1944.

1946 Final Report of the Interdepartmental Committee on Dentistry, Command 6727, 1946.

1946 National Health Service Act (with amendments in 1949, 1951, 1952, 1957, 1961, 1965, 1966).

1948 Report of the Interdepartmental Committee on the Remuneration of General Dental Practitioners (Spens Report), Command 7402, 1948.

1948 The National Health Service comes into being, including General Dental Services.

1949 Report of the Working Party on the chairside times taken in carrying out treatment in the General Dental Services (Penman Report).

1949 February. Ceiling on income for general dental practitioners.

1949 June. Ceiling ended but new scales of fees represented a 17 per cent reduction.

1950 May. Scale of fees reduced by a further 10 per cent.

1950 Report of UK Dental Mission on New Zealand School for Dental Nurses.

1951 May. The 'free' service ended with the imposition of a fee for dentures.

1952 June. Maximum patient charge of £1 instituted (for patients not exempted) for treatment which did not include dentures.

1953 Education (Miscellaneous Provisions) Act provides that local education authorities shall make available to its pupils comprehensive facilities for free dental treatment which may be given by dentists employed by the authorities or by the Regional Hospital Board.

1956 Report of the Committee of Enquiry into the cost of the National Health Service (Guillebaud Report) Command 9663, 1956.

1956 Report of the Committee on Recruitment to the Dental Profession (McNair Report) Command 9861, 1956.

1957 Dentists Act (replacing Dentists Act of 1878, 1921, 1923, and 1956).

1960 Report of the Royal Commission on Doctor's and Dentist's Remuneration (Pilkington Report) Command 939, 1960.
Review Body.
Dental Rates Study Group.

1961 Platt Report on Medical Staffing Structure in the Hospital Service.

1962 Dental Rates Study Group first report.

1963 Standing Dental Advisory Committee Report on the Hospital Dental Service.

1963 Review Body, First Report on Doctor's and Dentist's Remuneration (with eleven subsequent reports up to 1970).

1964 Report of the BDA Ad Hoc Sub-Committee on Methods of Remuneration (Tattersall Report).

1968 Patient charges up from £1 to £1·50.

1968 First Green Paper (*The Future Structure of the Health Service*).

1970 Adult Dental Health Survey in England and Wales 1968 published.

1970 Review Body (12th Report) recommendations not implemented by the Wilson administration. Review Body resigns.

1970 Second Green Paper.

1970 Review Body (12th Report) recommendations partially implemented by Heath administration. New Review Body set up.
1970 Patient charges up to 50 per cent of cost.
1971 National Health Service Re-organization Consultative Document.
1971 First report of new Review Body.
1972 National Health Service Reorganization White Paper.
1973 NHS Reorganization Bill proceeding through Parliament.
1974 NHS Reorganization effective from 1 April (see Appendix II).

REFERENCES

ALLRED, H. (1969), 'Appendix 3: Material resources', in *The London Hospital Medical College: The future of Dental Education. Proposals for Planned Change in Dental Education.* London: mimeograph.

BEVERIDGE, W. (1942), *Social Insurance and Allied Services.* Command 6404. London: HMSO.

BRIGGS, A. (1965), 'Public health: the health of the nation', in *The Origins of the Social Services.* London: New Society.

BRITISH DENTAL ASSOCIATION, 'General Dental Services Committee (1964). Report of the Ad Hoc Sub-Committee on methods of remuneration (Tattersall Report)', *Br. dent. J.*, **117**, 331.

BULMAN, J. S., RICHARDS, N. D., SLACK, G. L., and WILLCOCKS, A. J. (1968), *Demand and Need for Dental Care.* London: Oxford University Press.

BURT, B. A. (1971), 'Present and future needs in the Local Authority Dental Service', *Br. dent. J.*, **131**, 492.

COOK, P. J., and WALKER, R. O. (1967), 'The geographical distribution of dental care in the United Kingdom', *Ibid.*, **122**, 494.

DAVIS, H. C. (1969), 'George Cunningham: the man and his message', *Ibid.*, **127**, 527.

DEPARTMENT OF HEALTH AND SOCIAL SECURITY (1970), *The Future Structure of the National Health Service* (Green Paper). London: HMSO.

———— (1971a), *Digest of Health Statistics 1970.* London: HMSO.

———— (1971b), *Annual Report 1970.* London: HMSO.

———— (1971c), *Annual Report of the Dental Estimates Board, 1970.* Mimeograph.

GRAY, P. G. et al. (1970), *Adult Dental Health in England and Wales, 1968.* London: HMSO.

MINISTRY OF HEALTH (1944a), *A National Health Service* (White Paper). Command 6502. London: HMSO.

—— (1944b), *Interim Report of the Interdepartmental Committee on Dentistry* (*Teviot Report*). Command 6565. London: HMSO.

—— (1946), *Final Report of the Interdepartmental Committee on Dentistry* (*Teviot Report*). Command 6727. London: HMSO.

—— (1948), *Report of the Interdepartmental Committee on the Remuneration of General Dental Practitioners* (*Spens Report*). Command 7402. London: HMSO.

—— (1956a), *Report of the Committee of Enquiry into the National Health Service* (*Guillebaud Report*). Command 9663. London: HMSO.

—— (1956b), *Report of the Committee on Recruitment to the Dental Profession* (*McNair Report*). Command 9861. London: HMSO.

—— (1968), *The Administrative Structure of the Medical and Related Services in England and Wales* (*Green Paper*). London: HMSO.

NATIONAL HEALTH SERVICE ACTS of 1946, 1949, 1951, 1952, 1957, 1961, 1965, and 1966. London: HMSO.

OFFICE OF HEALTH ECONOMICS (1969), *The Dental Service.* London: HMSO.

PENMAN REPORT (1949), *Report of the Working Party on the Chairside Times Taken in Carrying Out Treatment in the General Dental Services*, pp. 32–393. London: HMSO.
REVIEW BODY (1970), *Review Body on Doctors' and Dentists' Remuneration: Twelfth Report*. Command 4352. London: HMSO.
ROYAL COMMISSION (1960), *Report of the Royal Commission on Doctors' and Dentists' Remuneration (Pilkington Report)*. Command 939. London: HMSO.

Chapter 8

Planning for Manpower Requirements in Dental Public Health

Aubrey Sheiham BDS, PHD
Senior Lecturer in Periodontology, Department of Oral Medicine, The London Hospital Medical College Dental School

The heart of a dental public health programme is the manpower required to carry it out. There are many factors involved in assessing manpower needs, and a number of them can inter-relate to produce complex situations. As the expenditure of money and effort in developing a programme is often heavy, these factors must be carefully considered.

This thought-provoking chapter, with an introduction to different kinds of delivery systems, then goes on to consider needs and demands, the translation of epidemiological data to treatment needs, the role of ancillaries, motivational forces, policy formulation, manpower planning, and evaluation.

The objective of the dental profession should be the attainment by all peoples of the highest level of dental health. For such an objective to be approached requires thorough planning on a nationwide basis and the rational and efficient utilization of resources. Considering that both the major dental diseases, periodontal disease and dental caries, are preventable, dental services should be developed primarily on the basis of the preventive approach both for the community and the individual. From a survey of the literature on dental services, however, it is apparent that the vast majority of services are concerned with the curative and reparative aspects of dental disease rather than prevention, a theme which was developed by Burt in Chapter 6. In addition, the individual has been the main focus of attention whereas the community needs have been sadly neglected. For a better understanding of the reasons why dental services have developed in this way we must consider the factors acting upon the community and the dental profession.

POLITICAL, SOCIAL, AND ECONOMIC FACTORS IN THE DEVELOPMENT OF HEALTH SERVICES

The control of general and dental health services never takes place in a vacuum but in a given political, social, and economic setting; the way in which a given country serves its people in the field of health can only be understood in the light of those factors. Because countries differ widely in their political policies, economic standing, and social structure, no two countries have an identical organization of health services. However, there are three broad socio-political categories of health services.

THE WESTERN EUROPEAN TYPE

This type developed in its original form in central, continental Europe but gradually involved the Nordic countries and Great Britain. The economic system is based upon free enterprise but the social and political philosophy encourages increasing governmental responsibility in the provision of health services. An example of this is seen in the welfare state idea which exists in Great Britain, a system of health care which was discussed fully by Renson in Chapter 7. There the National Health Service Act, 1946, established three main objectives:

1. To ensure that everybody in the country irrespective of means, age, sex, or occupation should have equal opportunity to benefit from the best and most up-to-date medical and allied services available.
2. To provide for all who want it, a comprehensive service covering every branch of medical and allied activity, from care of minor ailments to major medicine and surgery, which would include the care of mental as well as physical health, all specialist services, all general services and necessary drugs, medicines, and a wide range of appliances.
3. To divorce the care of health from questions of personal means or other factors relevant to it and thus encourage the obtaining of early advice and the promotion of good health rather than only the treatment of ill health.

This system embodies many of the basic principles for the development of national health services resolved by the Twenty-third World Health Assembly in 1970 (World Health Organization, 1970) and is founded on the principle that good health is a social concern. As early as 1932, Sir Arthur Newsholme summed up this principle as follows:

> In the first place, the health of every individual is a social concern and responsibility and secondly, as following from this, medical care in its widest sense for every individual is an essential condition of maximum efficiency and happiness in a civilised community. (Newsholme, 1932.)

In the Western European Type countries dental health services are offered to the population under different types of health insurance, financed to a greater or lesser extent from government funds. These systems have been described by Kostlan in Chapter 4.

THE AMERICAN TYPE

This is found in its characteristic form in the United States of America and partly in countries ideologically close to the United States. The health services are guided by the idea of free enterprise and free competition and citizens are encouraged to use their own initiative in obtaining and financing their health care.

Recently, following the marked rise in medical and dental care costs combined with some shift in traditional social attitudes, the Federal Government has begun to finance health care for specific groups of poor and aged Americans. The current feeling among health planners in the United States is that there is a state of 'crisis and despair' at this stage in the development of the health system. It is felt by many that unless the prevailing delivery method is fundamentally overhauled, health services will be priced out of the market (National Advisory Commission on Health Manpower, 1967).

There are specific problems in the delivery of dental services to the whole community under this system. One problem is that typically private practitioners define as patients those who seek their services; they do not encourage people to come for services nor do they feel responsible for the assessment of the needs of the whole population. Services tend to be fragmented and unevenly distributed, and many services are not available to large sections of the population. Another shortcoming is the financial barrier created by the high cost of dental services when provided through the individual private practitioner, for although 64·3 per cent of persons enjoying family income of \$10,000 or more visited a dentist in 1963–4, where family income was below \$2000 only 22·7 per cent made a dental visit in the same year (Chulis, 1966).

Alternative systems of financing dental care have begun to develop in the USA in recent years, however, mostly they involve dental services for defined groups in attempts to spread the burden of the costs of care at the time of need. These schemes are developed by trade unions, by insurance companies, and by the dental profession. The current increase of dental prepayment schemes in the USA is of interest because the evolution of the dental service there is similar to what occurred in Europe seventy years ago. Briefly, what happened in Austria and Germany and much later in the United Kingdom was the development of numerous fragmented insurance schemes each offering limited benefits. These were later amalgamated and rationalized; in the case of the United Kingdom there was over 20,000 approved societies before 1948, financed by the central government (Honigsbaum, 1970). National health insurance had been introduced in Germany in 1883 by Bismarck.

In the United States this pattern is being repeated to such an extent that in 1971 there were at least three Bills before Congress outlining some form of national health insurance.

THE SOVIET UNION TYPE

This was introduced through the Russian Revolution in 1917 and spread from the USSR to the Eastern European countries and later to China and certain countries in Asia and Africa. The dominating health philosophy under this system is that health and disease cannot be regarded as private affairs, and that society must take full responsibility for organizing health services from planning and co-ordination to execution.

ATTITUDES OF THE HEALTH PROFESSIONS

It is apparent that the question of what type of health service, how much to spend for which health services, and for whom, remains a political question for the society concerned. This problem is further complicated by the politics of the health professions themselves. For example, the vested economic interests of the dental profession could hinder progress by not allowing paradental personnel to carry out simple dental procedures. There are many examples of opposition by dentists to the introduction of dental hygienists and dental auxiliaries. This attitude tends to increase the cost and reduce the availability of dental care. Secondly, the profession shows little interest in the administrative aspects of dental health services thereby abdicating the planning role to non-dental administrators who are more concerned with efficiency than efficacy. Thirdly, the profession has shown little interest in the prevention of dental disease. One has only to look at the apathy and in some cases antagonism of the profession towards the subject of water fluoridation for evidence to support this statement.

PATTERNS OF ORGANIZATION OF DENTAL HEALTH SERVICES

Within these three broad groups of health services there are various combinations of types of dental health services. The World Health Organization (1965) has categorized dental health services as follows:

Group 1 Dental services are provided by dentists and dental auxiliaries and financed directly by the consumer or through a non-government organization. Prepayment plans, insurance plans, and other philanthropic foundations are the main examples of non-government organizations involved in financing the services.

Group 2 Dental services provided by dentists and dental auxiliaries who are partly or entirely remunerated by government but who are not considered to be government employees.

Group 3 Dental services provided by dentists and dental auxiliaries who are employed by the government.

These groupings are mainly based on the method of payment of the provider of dental services and the grouping is important because it may affect the types of services provided. However, the financial arrangements are not necessarily the most important factor affecting the services; the provider–consumer relationship is also an important factor. In order that the provider–consumer relationship is considered in addition to the method of financing, Rudko (1970) has suggested the following classification of dental systems:

	Provider		*Consumer*
1.	Individual	to	Individual
2.	Individual	to	Group
3.	Individual	to	Society
4.	Group	to	Group
5.	Public Service	to	Group
6.	Public Service	to	Society

This wider classification can be used to characterize dental services more adequately.

It is not surprising that the types of services which are more concerned with the group or society as a whole, as consumer of dental services are found more frequently in countries with the welfare state or communist political philosophies. In the USSR and China, for example, the public services provide dental services for the whole society (Rudko's point 6) while in the United Kingdom the whole society is provided for by individuals (Rudko's point 3). In the USA however, the individual has to make his own arrangements for health care and the predominant type of dental service is individual to individual (Rudko's point 1).

THE CONCEPT OF PRIORITIES

Because the financial barriers to receiving dental care have deterred patients from using the dental services, attempts have been made firstly by government to provide dental services for particular groups of the population. The most common group which is singled out for this type of care is schoolchildren. However poorly developed the dental services in a country may be, an attempt is frequently made to get dental care to schoolchildren because of the belief that (1) the community has a social responsibility for its children; (2) if the children can be maintained in a state of good dental health it will be relatively easy to maintain their dental health in adult life; (3) a regular dental attendance pattern in early life will be continued after school age. This concept of dental care for priority groups has been discussed more fully by Burt in Chapter 6.

A critical analysis of the development of dental services will show that dental services for children have not come about by efforts of the body of the profession. On the contrary, children have been neglected by the profession to such an extent that either philanthropic groups or government have been forced to accept the responsibility for the dental care of children and to allow governments to introduce paradental workers to treat them. The long-established New Zealand dental service for children was introduced despite some opposition from sections of the dental profession, and the profession there still wishes to restrict the dental nurse to operating in schools only. If dentists really believed in the maintenance of teeth for life, efforts should be diverted from the large number of adults with advanced dental disease and concentrated on long-term prevention of dental disease in the young.

THE DEVELOPMENT OF DENTAL MANPOWER

It has already been said that the form of the health services of a nation is determined by its prevailing social values, historical precedents, and its educational and fiscal resources. Whilst differences do exist between nations several features are common to health service systems; it is important to have a detailed knowledge of these features before embarking upon dental health manpower proposals. These include the relative priority given to good health, and dental health in particular, the amount and source of financial support for health services, and the amount and type of legislative power exercised by politicians.

Against this background the more detailed aspects of planning may proceed. The World Health Organization (1969) has suggested that the following framework be considered important in formulating plans:

1. Analysis of the existing situation
   a. dental health needs and demands for services
   b. dental health manpower supply
   c. utilization of dental health manpower
2. Policy formulation
   a. dental health manpower planning
   b. incentives and controls
   c. levels of decision making

This framework involves an assessment of the existing situation which includes the social, cultural, and political environment and the identification of factors which may positively or adversely influence the planning process. Information on levels of dental health, the effectiveness and efficiency of dental health services and the views of the consumers must be obtained. Subsequently an estimate of the dental needs of the population must be assessed and costed. Furthermore, attempts must be made to do a census of all dental health workers, taking into account the type of work they do and the growth and organization of the profession.

The utilization of dental health services by the public will vary according to the availability, accessibility, and acceptability of the services. In addition, attributes of the population such as its educational system and economic status will affect utilization.

If the above-mentioned information is available and estimates of future manpower requirements have been established and some form of action is contemplated then an overall plan must be outlined. Dental manpower planning must be based upon rational foundations and there must be a commitment to make necessary changes in policy, even if the proposed changes meet opposition among sections of the profession.

The over-riding principle governing manpower development is that the service has a commitment to improve the dental well-being of the population it is serving. If the services are not achieving that objective alternative solutions should be considered, but the planner should avoid the common failing of viewing the alternative method only in terms of other ways of increasing the supply of a given type of dental health worker. Instead he should, for example, consider relating the services to dental health control; to increasing efficiency and productivity of dental health workers or to changing the dental health manpower profile by changing the proportions of different grades of worker.

The dental health planner must also consider incentives and controls to achieve the specified objectives of his programme. The types of incentives and controls will vary according to the local or national circumstances. Incentives may be based upon promotion, monetary bonuses, and other fringe benefits. Controls may be imposed by national, professional, or consumer groups. The effects of various forms of administering the controls should be closely scrutinized. Controls are more likely to be accepted by dental health workers if they have been closely involved in each stage of the decision-making process of the dental health plan. Ideally the public, professional associations, dental public health workers, civil servants, and senior politicians should be involved in making decisions.

The framework suggested by World Health Organization in 1969 for formulating manpower plans will now be considered in more detail.

ANALYSIS OF THE EXISTING SITUATION

DEFINITIONS

The need for dental care must be distinguished from the demand for care and from the use of services or utilization. A need for dental care exists when an individual has dental disease or disability for which there is an effective and acceptable treatment. It can be defined either in terms of the type of dental disease causing the need or of the treatment or facilities for treatment required to meet it.

A demand for care exists when an individual considers that he has a need and wishes to receive care. Utilization occurs when an individual actually receives care. Need is not necessarily expressed as demand and demand is not necessarily followed by utilization.

DENTAL HEALTH NEEDS AND DEMANDS FOR SERVICES

The dental health survey is an essential means of establishing the incidence and prevalence of dental diseases in a population, of gauging patterns of utilization of dental health services, and of serving as a basis of determining priorities for dental health.

In several countries large scale dental health surveys have been conducted but most of them suffer from a lack of information on some aspects of dental disease, and few actually report the dental health status of individuals in terms which can readily be converted into overall dental treatment needs. For example, a person with a Periodontal Index (Russell, 1956) of 1·5 may have a simple gingivitis or periodontitis; each of these conditions may require different forms of treatment. Similarly a decayed tooth may indicate the need for a restoration or an extraction, depending on the extent of the destruction. To make matters even more complicated there is the problem of assessing dental needs not only on an individual tooth basis, but also on a group of teeth, each of which can be sound, decayed, restored, periodontally involved, non-vital, malposed, or missing. Therefore, converting findings into needs must take into account not only the condition of the individual tooth but also the number and condition of all the teeth in one mouth, their relationship to each other in each arch, and the relationship of the teeth in the upper and lower arch to each other.

Another difficulty in converting dental findings into needs is the wide variations in the methods and types of treatment for a given dental condition. For example, a person with three missing posterior teeth may be considered not to be in need of dental treatment, or to require an acrylic denture, a chrome/cobalt denture, or a fixed bridge depending on the clinical judgement of the examiner. Another example of this problem is found in assessing the need for orthodontic treatment (Brown, 1967; Summers, 1971). Here the decision whether there is a need for treatment is made even more difficult because psychological, social, and cultural considerations are very important factors in determining what type of occlusion is considered 'normal' for that family, town, or country (Moyers, 1956; Ballard and Wayman, 1964).

One further important reason why it is difficult to assess the true dental needs is that the strong traditional emphasis on dental caries leads many dental examiners to pay insufficient attention to other oral and dental conditions in the mouth, particularly periodontal disease. This failure to diagnose obvious dental disease leads to gross errors in the assessment of need.

With due regard for the shortcomings of the findings, some idea of the extent of the dental health problem can be assessed from various survey findings. The two most prevalent dental diseases are dental caries and periodontal disease. Malocclusion, handicapping dentofacial anomalies, and oral cancer are other important oral and dental diseases.

Some methods by which epidemiological survey data on these conditions can be converted to manpower requirements will now be considered.

Dental Caries

Dental caries poses an immense dental health problem in most developed countries. Caries is prevalent in young children, and the extent of the disease increases steadily with age in children of western countries. Beck (1968) has reported that 15-year-old New Zealanders had an average of 17·27 decayed, missing, or filled teeth (DMFT) each; at that age 99·3 per cent of children showed evidence of dental decay at some time in their lives. At 21 years-of-age the average DMFT was 20·39. Reports from the United States (Johnson et al., 1965) and Great Britain (Sheiham and Hobdell, 1969) indicate a lower caries prevalence than in the New Zealanders, but it still is sufficiently high to create a public health problem.

The extent of the problem in western countries may be assessed from two nationwide surveys. The first showed that the 111 million adults in the United States had 2¼ billion decayed, missing, or filled teeth. Of the average 20·4 DMF teeth per person: 13·5 were missing, 5·7 filled, and 1·2 decayed (Baird and Kelly, 1970). In England and Wales the DMFT was 19·2: 2·2 decayed, 10·1 missing, and 6·9 filled (Gray et al., 1970). In contrast to this high dental caries rate, the prevalence of caries in parts of Africa and Asia is often remarkably low. Sheiham (1967) reported that 98·5 per cent of Nigerians of all ages showed no signs of having had dental caries; the average DMF at ages 20 to 24 years was 0·10. Similar findings have been recorded in Thailand (Leatherwood et al., 1965), Ghana (Houpt, et al., 1967), and South Vietnam (Russell et al., 1965), whilst East African countries have a slightly higher caries prevalence (Akpabio, 1966).

Two methods of conversion of dental caries prevalence and severity findings into treatment needs have been commonly used. The first is based upon the assumption that carious teeth should be filled, whilst the second and more elaborate method involves conversion of findings into either time taken to carry out the procedure or into units based upon fees for different treatment items; the fees in turn are usually related to timing of procedures. The longitudinal study of Fanning et al. (1969) of the treatment requirements of South Australian schoolchildren illustrates the first method. There a count was made of the numbers of decayed, filled, extracted because of decay, extracted because of crowding, and unerupted teeth. Findings are recorded as numbers of decayed and unfilled teeth, and percentages of children requiring fillings. By re-examining the children every year Fanning was able to estimate the average number of new carious teeth per year. She found that between the ages of 14·5 and 15·5 years the mean number of decayed teeth increased by 1·83 in boys and by 1·72 in girls. These annual caries increments can be used to estimate projected needs.

The second method uses timings of either total patient care or individual procedures in treatment for caries. Two illustrations of this method will be discussed, one described by Ast and the other by Beck in his Dental Services Index.

In the study conducted by Ast et al. (1965; 1970) in fluoridated and non-fluoridated areas of New York State the amount of treatment required was assessed by survey (Table 1).

TABLE 1

Dental caries experience of initial care groups by age, Newburgh and Kingston, NY, 1962 (Ast et al., 1965)

Age	*Per cent caries free*	*DMFT per child*	*Per cent DMFT requiring treatment*	*df teeth per child*	*Per cent df teeth requiring treatment*
Newburgh					
5	47·9	0·03	100·0	2·5	89·0
6	33·9	0·09	87·5	2·8	94·7
Kingston					
5	14·2	0·12	66·7	5·7	94·0
6	16·4	0·65	100·0	5·6	89·4

Thereafter the treatment was carried out by the study team under standardized conditions thus converting the findings for disease into actual treatment (Table 2).

TABLE 2

Total services and mean number of services per child (Ast et al., 1965)

	Newburgh		*Kingston*	
	No.	*Percentage*	*No.*	*Percentage*
Number of children	182	—	141	—
Total services*	425	100·0	757	100·0
Restorations	379	89·2	603	79·7
One surface fillings	171	40·2	160	21·1
Two surface fillings	184	43·3	340	44·9
Three or more surface fillings	24	5·6	103	13·6
Pulpotomy or pulpectomy	—	—	3	0·4
Extractions	46	10·8	86	11·4
Miscellaneous treatments†	—	—	65	8·6
Mean number of services per child	2·3	—	5·4	—

* Excluding clinical examinations, X-rays and prophylaxis

† Cement bases, sedative fillings, and postoperative care

The actual amount of chair time for each child was also recorded (Table 3). This included nonoperating time which was mainly taken up

TABLE 3

Mean chair time (minutes) per child by race, Newburgh and Kingston, NY (Ast et al., 1965)

Race	*Newburgh*	*Kingston*
White	86·6	118·4
Non-white	65·6	114·7
Total	76·9	117·3

by child management and the individual services were priced according to the New York State Department of Health scale of fees prevailing at the time. This allowed the conversion of treatment needs into dollar costs (Table 4). The monetary values of course change rapidly, but different countries or communities can make their own conversions.

TABLE 4

Mean cost (dollars) according to prevailing fees at the time, per child by race, Newburgh and Kingston, NY (Ast et al., 1965)

Race	*Newburgh*	*Kingston*
White	14·48	32·79
Non-white	11·37	28·85
Total	14·16	32·38

The Dental Services Index devised by Beck (1968) is an attempt to overcome the shortcomings of dental surveys which only record dental disease findings. It provides an indication of the amount of dental treatment required in a given individual or population. The magnitude of the index is directly proportional to the amount of dental treatment required to make the individual or population dentally fit. On the individual basis, it is directly related to the cost of dental services required and assumes a standardized or agreed scale of fees. On a population basis, the index is directly related to dental manpower and facilities necessary to make the population dentally fit.

The Dental Services Index (DSI) will be affected by both the annual caries increment of age-specific populations, and the amount of dental treatment received before the examination. If any two of the three factors, the DSI, caries increment, or dental treatment received is known the third can be estimated.

The DSI has been related to the scale of fees because the relative size of the fee is usually directly related to the time, effort, skill, and materials required to carry out a procedure. The basic aim was not to relate the index to the actual cost but to produce an arbitrary scale which will allow comparisons to be made between individuals or groups.

Before using this method of assessing requirements the following information must be compiled:

1. A coding system composed of three symbols: a major symbol, a minor symbol and a qualifying symbol. These are defined below:

Major Symbol (Treatment Required)	
None	0
Class I	1
MO	2
DO	3
MOD	4
Class III	5
Class IV	6
Class V	7
Crown	8
Bridge	9
Extraction	10
Minor Symbol	
Buccal or lingual extension to Class I or II	—A
Cusp restoration	—B
Endodontia	—C
Qualifying Symbol	
New filling (or crown or bridge)	—X
Replacement filling (or crown or bridge)	—Y
Extension of existing filling	—Z

2. A conversion table based upon a fee scale and giving relative values to each of the codes mentioned above remembering that the values will differ according to the tooth type and the type of material used. For example, in the study conducted by Beck treatment code 1X (Class I restoration on a previously unfilled occlusal surface) the value for a premolar is 100 and for a molar is 125. Table 5 illustrates some of the values given to Beck's DSI as he applied it in New Zealand.

3. A dental examination using well-defined criteria for each of the codes.

Periodontal Diseases

Unlike dental caries, which is a major dental health problem in developed countries, periodontal diseases are a universal problem and tend to be more severe in the poorer developing countries where they constitute the major dental health problem (Ramfjord et al., 1968; Pelton et al., 1969).

When discussing the needs for periodontal treatment consideration is often only given to chronic periodontal disease. However, acute ulcerative gingivitis (AUG), a condition prevalent in young children in Nigeria (Sheiham, 1966), India (Pindborg et al., 1966), Gambia (Malberger, 1967), and China (Fu-Tang Chu and Chuan Fam, 1963), and some South American countries, is often a more seriously felt need by the population. This is mainly because cancrum oris is often associated with the severe forms of AUG (Emslie, 1963; Sheiham, 1966; Malberger, 1967). Surveys in Nigeria have shown that 11·5 per cent of children aged 2–6 years had AUG and 0·74 per cent had cancrum oris (Sheiham, 1966).

TABLE 5

Conversion table, dental services index: the value of the dental services index for different treatment needs as recorded by treatment codes (Beck, 1968)

Treatment code	*Dental services index*		
	Premolar		*Molar*
1X	100		125
1AX	100		125
2X	150		190
2Z	100		125
3X	150		190
4X	230		290
4CY	635		695
		Anterior teeth	
5X		175	
5CY		630	
6CX		1035	
9CX		1605	
10	150		175
Examination, prophylaxis and X-rays		210	

Chronic periodontal disease commences as gingivitis and progresses to periodontitis and ultimately leads to the loosening and loss of teeth. The condition is prevalent in young children; over 95 per cent are affected (Jamison, 1963; Sheiham, 1967). Indeed Jamison's study showed that destructive periodontal disease with alveolar bone loss occurs around deciduous teeth. The prevalence remains over 95 per cent for children of all ages, and increasing age the severity also increases in a linear fashion. Pocketing around the permanent teeth is found in 11-year-old English (Sheiham, 1969) and African children (Sheiham, 1968; Skougaard et al., 1969), and by the ages 20–29 years over 70 per cent of these persons have one or more teeth with pockets (Sheiham, 1968).

The conversion of periodontal findings into treatment needs poses an even greater problem than the similar conversion of dental caries. The problem was recognized by Russell (1956) when he developed the Periodontal Index. He carried out a full clinical and radiographic analysis of a group of persons and then tabulated them according to the stage of periodontal disease; the ranges of Periodontal Index scores within each clinical group was then estimated.

Persons with a clinical diagnosis of gingivitis and requiring no more than a single prophylaxis scored in the PI range of 0·1 to 1·0; those for whom minimal periodontal treatment was necessary to treat severe gingivitis and incipient destructive periodontal disease, from 0·5 to 1·9; persons with scores in the range 1·5 to 5·0 had frankly established destructive periodontal disease requiring elaborate and perhaps protracted periodontal treatment, whereas for those with the terminal of periodontal disease (scores 4·0 to 8·0), full mouth extraction was the most rational treatment.

On the basis of these findings Russell (1967) has estimated that about 5 million of the 90 million United States adults who have natural teeth had periodontal disease so advanced that extractions were indicated; a further 30 million required highly skilled and elaborate treatment; 25 million required a simple prophylaxis. Using the same method of assessment Sheiham (1968) estimated that the periodontal treatment needs of British populations were greater than were those in the United States. Firstly the mean Periodontal Index was much higher, and secondly the percentages in each of the periodontal disease categories were higher in the British population. Sheiham (1971) estimated that 42 per cent of British adults aged 16–65 years required extractions for the treatment of their advanced periodontal condition 44 per cent needed highly skilled and elaborate periodontal treatment and the remaining 14 per cent a simple prophylaxis.

Going by these estimates from highly industrialized countries with better dentist : population ratios than the majority of developing countries, and knowing that the severity of periodontal disease is less in the United States than in the majority of developing countries (Pelton et al., 1969), the estimates of needs for periodontal treatment are even higher in India, Africa, Asia, and South America than those reported here. In the case of Nigeria (Sheiham, 1968), 11·5 per cent of 3842 persons aged 6 months to 84 years were in the terminal stages of periodontal disease, 69 per cent had destructive periodontal disease, and 19 per cent had gingivitis only.

In Nigerian males aged 20 to 24 years, 18 per cent were in the terminal stages of disease and 45·5 per cent of 40–44-year-old males were similarly affected (Table 6).

These estimates of periodontal diseases are underestimates of the true need because the examination for the PI is a quick scanning rather than a detailed clinical diagnosis. If more detailed diagnosis is required then the Periodontal Disease Index (PDI) (Ramfjord, 1959) should be used. This method measures (1) plaque, subgingival and supragingival calculus, teeth present, and gingivitis; (2) depth of periodontal pockets; (3) alveolar bone height, and (4) mobility. All these are essential factors in making a more accurate estimate of treatment needs.

Although this scoring method, and a recent modification of it developed by O'Leary (1967), has been used for over 10 years, no large-scale study has been carried out to assess periodontal needs, and the time and personnel necessary to treat those needs. This neglect may be largely attributed to the preoccupation of public health dentists with the treatment of dental caries.

TABLE 6

Periodontal treatment needs in Nigerians by age and sex (Sheiham, 1968)

Age in years	*Simple prophylaxis (percentage)*		*Skilled and elaborate treatment (percentage)*		*Extractions (percentage)*	
	Male	*Female*	*Male*	*Female*	*Male*	*Female*
10–14	12·5	31·3	86·1	67·1	1·1	0·7
20–24	13·3	18·3	80·1	63·5	6·6	18·2
30–34	4·2	7·1	49·0	62·5	46·8	29·4
40–44	1·4	9·1	43·5	45·4	55·1	45·5
50+	1·2	5·1	36·7	42·3	62·1	52·6

Malocclusion

The estimates of needs for orthodontic treatment vary considerably because of a lack of uniformity in diagnosis. Estimates of the prevalence of malocclusion vary from 0·6 in New Zealand (Beck, 1968) to 82·5 per cent in the United States (Mills, 1966). Ballard and Wayman (1964), in a detailed study of army apprentices aged 15½–16 years, estimated that 25 per cent of the British population might require orthodontic treatment, and that if the treatment were supervised by an orthodontic specialist then much of it could be carried out by general dental practitioners. Based upon these findings they estimate that if there were 700,000 British schoolchildren in each age year then the maximum number who could possibly require orthodontic treatment in any one year would be 22·2 per cent (155,400) and of this group a percentage will be satisfied with their appearance and not request treatment.

Methods of Assessing Orthodontic Needs

Angle's classification is the best known classification of malocclusion and is still widely used, although not in its original form. Later, Moore (1948) developed a classification of malocclusion for survey purposes based on orthodontic needs and the time required for correction of the abnormality. The classification was divided into three parts: a statement of functional status; a list of oral habits, and a classification for cases, graded according to diagnostic, clinical, and laboratory time required for treatment. Van Kirk and Pennell (1959) brought out the Malalignment Index which is based on the deviation of individual teeth from the normal arch alignment. Another useful index of need was developed by Draker (1960). This index known as the Handicapping Labio-lingual Deviations Index (HLD) provides a score denoting priority for treatment and permits the selection of a cut-off point for treatment dictated by the treatment resources available in the community. Seven conditions are noted and by weighting each condition an index of severity is obtained. Cleft palate and severe traumatic deviations are given the highest scores characteristics such as overbite, overjet, and mandibular protrusion are noted.

The method of assessment of need for orthodontic treatment used by Ballard and Wayman (1964) is a modification of Angle's classification using criteria which they attribute to Backlund. In addition there is a questionnaire asking about the subject's own assessment of his appearance.

In an attempt to develop an assessment procedure which would objectively express the severity of malocclusion in clinical terms and which could be used to assess the severity of the common forms of malocclusion, Grainger (1967) proposed the Orthodontic Treatment Priority Index. This method, and its modification by Summers (1971), is applicable to surveys of assessments of needs. The methods suggested by World Health Organization (1971), Salzmann (1968), and Björk et al. (1964) are also useful methods which require further testing.

Dental Prosthetic Needs

The failure to prevent and control dental caries and periodontal disease ultimately leads to tooth loss. The unenviable record of toothlessness in developed countries such as Great Britain, United States, and Denmark reflects the failure of the dental profession to respond to the dental needs of the population. This failure in turn creates a need for dentures especially among the middle-aged and older members of the community. In England and Wales where almost 4 out of every 10 adults aged 16 years and over had no natural teeth (Gray et al., 1970), the need for new or replacement full dentures is considerable. Add to that the need for partial dentures and one finds that almost 70 per cent of the adult population had some form of dental prosthetic need.

Estimates of need for dentures are difficult to make unless one makes the unrealistic assumption that every missing tooth must be replaced. However, some idea of the need can be assessed by assuming that anterior teeth and gaps of three or more adjacent teeth should be replaced. Using these criteria Gray et al. (1970) calculated that almost

20 per cent of the adult England and Wales population required some form of partial prosthesis.

Congenital Malformation and Neoplasms

In addition to the massive needs already described, one in a thousand live births (Greene, 1963; Carter, 1967) have congenital clefts of the lip or palate which require treatment. Greene (1963) has estimated that 6000 new cases of lip and palatal clefts occur each year in the United States of America.

There is also the need for early detection and treatment of oral neoplasms, the most serious oral condition in terms of mortality risk. Oral cancers have a relatively high prevalence in some countries (Anderson, 1968; Mehta et al., 1969; Tan, 1969; Binnie et al., 1972) and specific types of cancer, such as Burkitt's lymphoma, are problems in others (Burkitt, 1964).

In summary, it can be said that dental caries and periodontal disease present the major dental treatment needs in populations. The need for orthodontic care remains difficult to define, prosthetic needs are frequently high, while cancers and congenital malformations require special consideration.

THE DEMANDS FOR DENTAL SERVICES

Dental care programmes have little chance of success, regardless of how effective the treatment is, if individuals do not recognize their own dental needs and translate them into a demand for service. Unfortunately, whilst effective methods of prevention and treatment of dental diseases exist, public acceptance of these treatments is often poor and there is a wide disparity between the need for dental care and the amount of care actually sought and received.

As the leaders of the dental profession are concerned about promoting regular dental attendance, it is important to know the characteristics of those people who do attend, the reasons why most people do not attend, and barriers to utilization of dental health services. This information is essential for the planning of dental services.

Characteristics of Persons Attending for Dental Care

Age and Sex The extent of dental visits varies with age and sex. Very young children and old persons in the under-5 years and the over-64-year-olds had the lowest annual rates of dental visits in the United States. In 1963–4, persons under 5-years-old visited their dentist 0·3 times and persons aged 65 years and older 0·8 times per year, whilst 15–24-year-olds went on average 2·0 times per year (Alderman, 1965) (Table 7). Only 11·1 per cent of under-5-year-olds attended in the last year before the survey whereas 55·2 per cent of 15–25-year-olds and 20·8 per cent of 65 years and older attended (Chulis, 1966). Tables 7 and 8 illustrate these patterns.

The dental attendance patterns may be a reflection of the system of dental care in the country rather than inherent differences in demand for dental care related to age. If a system of annual school dental inspections, similar to that in New Zealand, existed in the United States then an entirely different pattern of demand amongst young children could

TABLE 7

Number of dental visits per person per year by age and sex: United States, July 1963–June 1964 and in 1969 (Alderman, 1965; Blanken, 1971)

Age and sex	*No. visits per person per year*	
	July 1963–June 1964	*1969*
All ages, both sexes	1·6	1·5
Under 5 years	0·3	—
5–14 years	1·9	—
15–24 years	2·0	—
25–44 years	1·9	1·6
45–64 years	1·7	1·6
65+ years	0·8	1·0
Male	1·4	1·4
Female	1·7	1·6

TABLE 8

Percentage distribution of persons by time interval since last dental visit according to age: United States, July 1963–June 1964 (Chulis, 1966)

Age	*Time interval since last dental visit*						
	Under 6 months	*6–11 months*	*1 year*	*2–4 years*	*4 years and over*	*Never*	*Un-known*
All ages	28·7	13·3	12·6	13·3	14·0	16·6	1·4
Under 5 years	8·1	3·0	1·5	0·3	—	86·9	—
5–14 years	38·0	16·9	12·1	7·0	1·1	24·5	0·4
15–24 years	36·5	18·7	17·1	14·4	4·5	7·1	1·8
25–44 years	32·6	15·9	16·9	18·8	12·2	2·0	1·6
45–64 years	26·9	11·5	13·1	18·5	26·9	1·3	1·8
65+ years	14·4	6·4	7·7	15·2	51·7	1·5	3·1

exist there. In New Zealand (Beck, 1968) 94 per cent of 15-year-olds attend for regular dental treatment, a figure far in excess of the United States attendance for that age.

In most countries females attend the dentist more frequently and regularly than males (McFarlane, 1965; Chulis, 1966; Beck, 1968).

Family Income Dental treatment is the most sensitive of all the available health services to variations in the family income of North Americans (Anderson, 1957; Anderson and Anderson, 1967). One-fifth of Americans from families with an income of less than $2000 had never visited a dentist whilst 7 per cent of individuals from families earning $10,000 or more had never had dental treatment (Chulis, 1966). In Canada, four times as many children under 15 years in the upper income group as in the low income group received dental care (McFarlane, 1965). Family income remains an important factor in determining whether individuals attend for dental care even when the financial barrier to receiving care is removed. This indicates that socially defined patterns of behaviour associated with high income are often related to high-status occupation and good educational background, because these three factors are often positively associated with each other.

Occupation and Education American figures show that there is a direct relationship between occupational status and frequency of dental visits (Koos, 1954; Kegeles, 1961). Persons in professional occupations visit their dentists more frequently than semi- or non-skilled manual workers (Nikias, 1968). Members of professional families are more likely than manual workers to go for preventive visits. Differences in pattern of dental attendance and reasons for attendance are found when individuals are classified according to the educational attainment. In the United States, in families in which the head of the family had completed one year or more at college, approximately three out of every five persons had seen a dentist within the past 12 months. By comparison, only one out of every five persons from families where the head of the family had less than five years of education had visited a dentist during that period (Chulis, 1966).

Race Differences exist between the non-white and white families in the United States with respect to the regularity of attending for dental care and the type of treatment received. A larger percentage of white than non-white persons visit their dentist each year. The average number of visits per year was 1·7 for whites and 0·9 for non-whites, while 33 per cent of non-whites and 14 per cent of whites had never visited a dentist (Chulis, 1966). Non-whites tended to have an equal number of tooth extractions and filling visits whilst whites had three times as many fillings than extraction visits.

Residence Proportionally more persons in urban than in rural areas visit the dentist, and the urbanites visit the dentist more regularly. In Canada, the utilization of dental services varied with the size of the community; the larger the community the greater was the utilization and the smaller the size of the community the less likely the treatment was to be fillings (McFarlane, 1965). This difference in utilization is mainly due to the difficulty of getting to the dental services and introduces barriers related to transportation. One illustration of this problem comes from Uganda where the number of visits to a hospital were shown to vary according to the distance of the patient's home from the hospital. Thus persons living within two miles made five visits, those living four miles away 1·3 visits and those living 12 miles away only 0·1 visits annually (Jolly and King, 1970).

The number of dental visits made per year can differ from one geographical area to another within the same country. In the north-east United States the average number of dental visits per year was 2·1, compared with 1·1 in the south, and 12·8 per cent of persons in the north-east compared to 22·6 per cent in the South had never visited a dentist (Alderman, 1965). Dental attendance patterns also vary by region in England and Wales where Gray et al. (1970) reported that 51 per cent of persons in London and the South East attended the dentist regularly compared to 38 per cent in the North.

Comments on Methodology in Studies on Dental Demands

The majority of the studies referred to here relied upon the individual's assessment of when he last went for dental treatment and what treatment was carried out. The accuracy of their statements were not verified by checking their actual dental records. Two studies in which statements were verified indicate that wide discrepancies can exist between what was reported and what happened. Draker et al. (1965) found that respondents tended to overestimate the lapse of time since receiving dental care. Only 26 per cent were accurate in recalling the correct year of their dental care (Table 9) and the respondent's attitude towards

TABLE 9

Verification of treatment data: dentist's record versus patient's statement (Draker et al., 1965)

Recollection	*Percentage of total group*
Date recalled within 1 year	25·7
Date recalled within 3 years	59·6
Date recalled within 5 years	74·4

dental service was considered to have a bearing on his ability to recall accurately.

There was also poor agreement between reported dental treatment and the dental treatment actually carried out. Extractions were recalled correctly in only 44 per cent of cases and fillings, which were performed more frequently, were only recalled by 66 per cent of respondents (Table 10).

Chatwin et al. (1968) also found considerable errors in reporting simple dental information about services received by servicemen during the previous year. They found that whereas the dentists' records indicated an annual average of 1·52 visits, the servicemen questioned in the survey recalled on average 1·69 or 11 per cent in excess of actual visits. The majority (55·2 per cent) did not remember the correct number of visits made in the previous year and of these 60·7 per cent overestimated the number of visits made.

TABLE 10

Agreement between types of services (patients' recall versus dentists' records) (Draker et al., 1965)

	Fillings	*Extractions*	*Dentures*	*Cleaning*
Percentage of dentists' records agreeing with patients' statements	66·4	44·2	39·5	50·5

These errors in reporting dental attendance may jeopardize the validity of dental information especially since the attitude of the respondents towards dental care is considered to affect their ability to recall accurately.

Barriers to the Utilization of Dental Services

From the foregoing discussion it is apparent that some individuals find that there are barriers to attendance for dental care. The importance of the barriers varies according to the social system of the country. The barriers can be categorized as psychological, educational, social, economic, and geographic.

The first three categories are closely interrelated. Thus the decision to seek dental care is affected by the socially defined view of what is appropriate behaviour, and the knowledge about the disease and its treatment. Whether the individual finally presents for treatment will depend on anxiety, fear of the dentist, and other psychological factors. Suchman (1965) maintains that the sequence of decision making points in the illness behaviour spectrum are: the decision that something is wrong (symptom experience); the decision that one is sick and needs professional care (assumption of sick role); decision to seek medical or dental care (medical/dental care contact); decision to transfer control to the physician (dependent patient role); decision to relinquish the patient role (recovery and rehabilitation).

This theory of illness behaviour is one of a large number of theories which have been postulated to explain why individuals seek medical or dental care. These theories have been reviewed by Rosenstock et al. (1960), and by Young (1967). Rosenstock, Hochbaum, and Kegeles warn the dentist against interpreting the public's behaviour in terms of his own frame of reference. They state:

> We usually describe a person's behaviour as 'apathetic' if he is doing something other than what we wish him to do. Yet, this apparent apathy towards what *we* want him to do may simply reflect the fact that he is trying urgently and actively to obtain *what he* wants. We must keep constantly in mind that the individual's behaviour is determined by *his* motives and by *his* beliefs regardless of whether the motives and beliefs correspond to our notion of reality or our notion of what is good for him.

It is important, therefore, to distinguish between objective health needs and subjective health needs. Objective health needs correspond to the professional judgement of a person's state of health, whilst a subjective need exists as a function of the beliefs of each individual. For example, if a group of individuals have periodontal disease some will be aware of it and may do something about it; these persons have a subjective dental health need. Others may be aware of the disease but not troubled by it, either because they believe periodontal disease is inevitable and incurable or because they have little discomfort. Such people do not experience a subjective need. Other people will not believe that there is periodontal disease in their mouths because they have no pain, and so they too have no subjective need. Another group may be concerned that their healthy gums may become diseased and take preventive action; although there may not be an objective basis for their concern there exists a subjective need.

Before taking action the individual must consider that health is important to him, that he is susceptible to the disease, and that the disease is serious. The degree of seriousness of the threat will often affect the health related action that is taken. Then the action taken will depend upon the beliefs about the effectiveness of various actions. At this stage the barriers to utilizing the health services become important, for if he considers the treatment too expensive, too far away, or otherwise inconvenient to get to no action may be taken. If all the conditions favouring health action, namely the presence of a threat which is moderately intense and highly important, the belief that there is a relevant means of reducing the threat then a 'cue' is often necessary which triggers off action. This cue may be internal in the form of a symptom or it may be external like a poster or social pressures.

THE SUPPLY OF DENTAL HEALTH MANPOWER

Few countries in the world, if any, have currently sufficient qualified dental manpower to satisfy their own demand for dental health services. In many countries a high proportion of dental care is carried out by non-qualified persons (Fendall, 1968).

The measurement of dental manpower supply involves a number of variables that determine the validity of the measurement. Among these variables, the most important is the personnel who are included and the functions that they perform, because in different countries, different job titles are attached to personnel carrying out similar functions. For example, in Papua, New Guinea, dental technicians and orderlies are

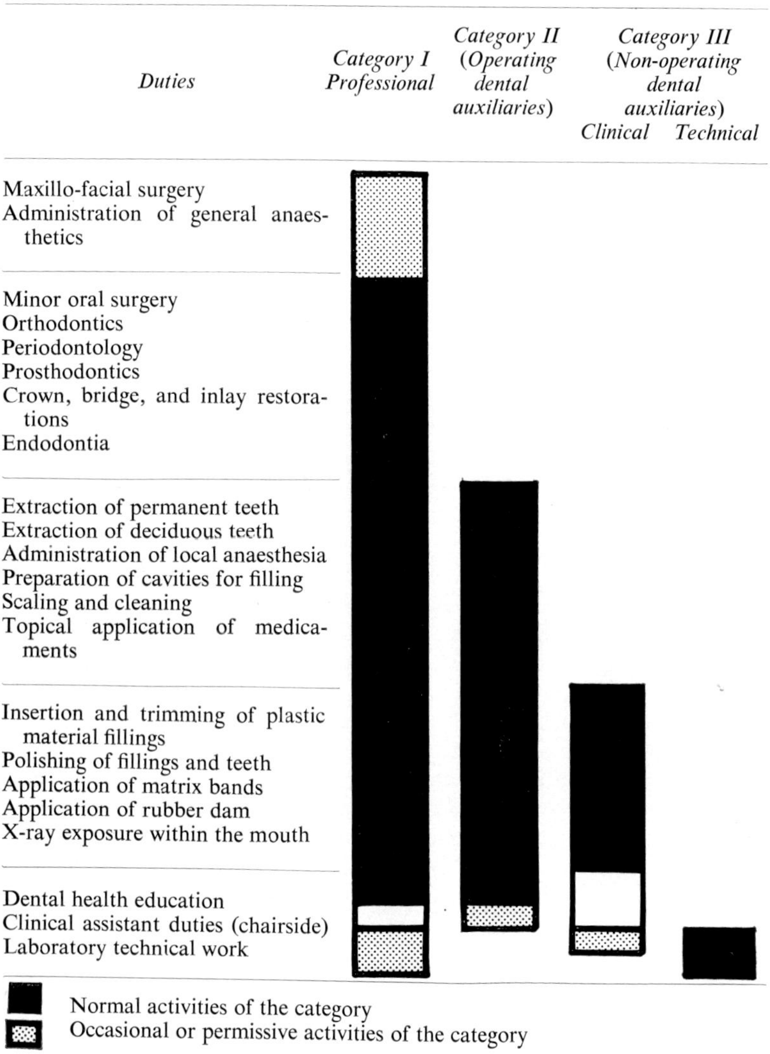

Duties
Category I Professional
Category II (Operating dental auxiliaries)
Category III (Non-operating dental auxiliaries)
Clinical
Technical
Maxillo-facial surgery
Administration of general anaesthetics
Minor oral surgery
Orthodontics
Periodontology
Prosthodontics
Crown, bridge, and inlay restorations
Endodontia
Extraction of permanent teeth
Extraction of deciduous teeth
Administration of local anaesthesia
Preparation of cavities for filling
Scaling and cleaning
Topical application of medicaments
Insertion and trimming of plastic material fillings
Polishing of fillings and teeth
Application of matrix bands
Application of rubber dam
X-ray exposure within the mouth
Dental health education
Clinical assistant duties (chairside)
Laboratory technical work
Normal activities of the category
Occasional or permissive activities of the category

Fig. 1. Delineation of recommended scope of clinical and laboratory of various categories of dental personnel.

trained to carry out dental hygienist functions (Schamschula and Barmes, 1966). The nomenclature and function of the various types of dental ancillary is discussed by Elderton in Chapter 9.

Therefore, unless standard definitions are provided of what constitutes a dentist, a dental auxiliary, or any other dental health worker, national and international statistics cannot be meaningful and comparable. Standardization of definitions of health workers has been initiated by the International Labour Organization (International Labour Office, 1969), and by the World Health Organization (1968). Classifications of dental health workers were suggested at the World Health Organization conference in New Delhi in 1967, these will be described by Elderton in Chapter 9. *Fig.* 1 presents an illustration of these duties. It should be realized that these categories are by no means mutually exclusive and a certain amount of overlap does exist (Barmes, 1969).

The measurement and analysis of present dental health manpower supply provide a profile of the amount and type of skills available for dental health work at a given time and demographic information such as age and sex distribution, deployment, retention rates and speciality growth. Such knowledge is essential for the projection of requirements and for outlining future policy: it also provides information for recruits to the dental health field about opportunities open to them and the working conditions and prospects that exist.

The primary source of information on dental manpower varies according to country. The most frequent sources are professional registers, licensing institutions, dental societies, and census data.

INTERNATIONAL MANPOWER VARIATIONS

The most commonly used approach to gauging dental manpower supply is the dentist:population ratios. However, this ratio often conceals more than it reveals. There is little doubt that the better the ratio the more likelihood there is that the demand for dental care can be met. In addition, the comparison of ratios between countries with similar social structure at the same stage of economic development can give some indication of the relative position of individual countries with respect to adequacy of supply. On the other hand the ratio does not indicate the volume, nature, and quality of dental care provided. Nor does it allow for social, economic, and political characteristics; patterns of dental disease; paradental personnel, and regional variations in manpower distribution within a country. Therefore, the ratio should be used with caution and as a very rough guide to the supply of dental manpower.

The dentist to population ratio varies from 1:1126 in Sweden to 1:1,100,000 in Nigeria (Federation Dentaire Internationale, 1970). Other dentist:population ratios are provided by the USA (1:2043), USSR (1:3200), South America (1:3200), Europe (1:3600), Asia (1:8700) and lastly Africa (over 1:100,000). Within each of these areas the ratio varies. For example in South America, Brazil and Chile have ratios of about 1:2400 whereas Paraguay's ratio is 1:48,562.

These widely varying ratios *may* be a reflection of the need and demand for dental care in each country, and its economic status. The former explanation is true for the Scandinavian countries compared to African countries. Caries is widespread in the former and relatively uncommon in Africa (Akpabio, 1966; Sheiham, 1967). It is also true that the poorer and less developed countries have poorer manpower ratios. Table 11 illustrates this fact by correlating health manpower availability with national income.

TABLE 11

Health manpower and economics (Kaprio, 1967)

Country	*Gross national product per head (US dollars)*	*Level of human resource development*	*Physicians and dentists per 10,000 population*
Nigeria	78	Underdeveloped	0·2
Colombia	263	Partially developed	5·0
Turkey	220	Partially developed	3·5
Chile	379	Semi-advanced	7·5
USA	2577	Advanced	18·0

GEOGRAPHICAL DISTRIBUTION OF DENTAL MANPOWER WITHIN COUNTRIES

The availability of dental services within a country varies considerably. Table 12 shows that in Guatemala, for example, 81 per cent of the dentists practise in the capital city which contains 15 per cent of the population. Variations in availability are almost universal (McFarlane, 1965; Cook and Walker, 1967). In England and Wales, the range is from one to just under six dentists to every 10,000 persons. Areas like Chester (5·93), Bournemouth (5·54), and London (4·18) have relatively good

TABLE 12

Number of dentists in country and per cent practising in capital (Fendall, 1968)

Country	*No. of dentists*	*Per cent of dentists in capital*	*Per cent of population in capital*
Jamaica	117	63	25
Guatemala	176	81	15
Senegal	19	79	12
Kenya	35	52	4
Thailand	378	79	8

ratios whereas Norfolk (0·98), West Hartlepool (1·15), and West Bromwich (1·13) have poor ratios (Cook and Walker, 1967).

The main reason for the maldistribution is variation in patterns of demand among the population, these patterns being affected by the factors previously discussed. In England there is evidence that more dentists tend to practise in areas where there are higher proportions of people of upper socio-economic status (Cook and Walker, 1967). This tendency explains the wide differences in urban and rural dentist: population ratios even in regions with good overall ratios. Thus in Ontario, Canada, where the dentist: population ratio was 1:2432 in 1961, some rural areas had a ratio of 1:20,892 (Royal Commission, 1964).

GROWTH TRENDS IN SUPPLY OF DENTAL MANPOWER

Because of the population growth the numbers of new dentists qualifying should continue to increase, if only to keep up with the increase in population. Add to that the manpower needed to cope with the increase in demand associated with improved education and economic status. There has been an increase in the total numbers of dentists but the increase is not keeping up with the world trend in population growth. In Canada, the rate of increase in population growth over the last four decades has been greater than the rate of increase in the number of dentists; since 1938 the population has increased by 65·1 per cent whereas dentists have increased by 39·9 per cent. Consequently, as shown in Table 13, the dentist: population ratio has become steadily worse (McFarlane, 1965).

TABLE 13

Population: dentist ratios, Canada 1881–1962 (McFarlane, 1965)

Year	*Ratio (to 1)*
1881	8480
1891	6419
1901	4100
1911	3301
1921	2783
1931	2569
1941	2733
1951	2791
1961	3047
1962	3108

PRODUCTIVITY OF DENTISTS

Perhaps the most important variable having an effect on the dentist component of the dentist: population ratio is productivity. Productivity is difficult to measure but it is known that the productivity will decrease with increasing age. Thus the older the members of the profession, the less productive they will be. This is due to reduction in manual dexterity and the physically exerting nature of dental practice which leads to a reduction of hours worked as physical vigour declines. The decrease in productivity is reflected by the drop in earnings although the reduction of hours worked may be gradual. Decreasing productivity with increasing age can lead to a manpower problem where the large segment of the dental manpower in a country or area with a high proportion of older dentists will be at a disadvantage in terms of productivity compared to another with a high proportion of younger dentists. In Canada, the percentage of dentists over 50 years of age varied from 58 per cent in Prince Edward Island to 15 per cent in Newfoundland (McFarlane, 1964). If the exact number of hours worked per week is computed for dentists over 60 years of age and converted into whole time equivalents of younger dentists then there will be a worsening of the dentist: population ratio for that region. For example Meskin and Martens (1970) estimated that if this was done for dentists in Minnesota the dentist:population ratio for the State would change from 1:1502 to 1:1826, and in one county of Minnesota it would drop from 1:2642 to 1:3230.

THE UTILIZATION OF DENTAL HEALTH MANPOWER

Analysis shows that the different patterns of utilization and the supply of dental health manpower are crucially linked. Areas with the greatest shortage of dental manpower have the poorest utilization of dental services, as reflected by under-employment, poor geographic distribution, emigration, early retirement, exaggerated trends towards specialization, poor staffing patterns, and the absence of or inappropriate task specifications. A clearer picture of the existing structure requires a scrutiny of the whole problem of productivity in the dental health care system in general, and of the pattern of dental health care and of dental manpower-utilization in particular. This overview of the provider side of dental care services must be related to social and demographic factors existing in the particular country.

Dental productivity is often related to quantity of work carried out and in dental terms to numbers of teeth filled, extracted, and replaced. These measures differ in principle from those used in estimating productivity of other health workers. There, productivity is measured by the reduction of infant mortality, increase in life expectancy, decrease in numbers of persons with specific infectious diseases as well as numbers of patients treated. A more rational measure of dental productivity, therefore, should include information on reduction of dental caries incidence and prevalence, reduction in numbers of extracted teeth and the increase in the percentage of the population with a complete natural dentition.

Manpower productivity takes into account not only the amount of disease prevented or treated but the level of training of the worker carrying out the procedures. Productivity is improved when functions are delegated from one level of performance to a lower one and by substitution of jobs. The higher skills are also more expensive and take longer to acquire. Ideally, therefore, each level of skill should be used only for tasks appropriate to it. The more highly skilled workers should not be burdened with tasks which can be done by those with less training (Brotherston, 1971). This involves the use of ancillaries for certain tasks carried out by professional personnel, a concept treated fully by Elderton in Chapter 9.

As stated earlier, the pattern of utilization of dental health manpower varies with certain social, economic, and demographic variables. Information on social trends must be collated and applied to known patterns of utilization. In the United Kingdom there are detailed data on social trends published by the Government Statistical Service (1970). This document outlines the sex and age structure of the population until the year 2001. In addition, birth and death rates, population changes, personal income and expenditure, trends, employment, and leisure are estimated. Many other countries publish similar sources of social data.

With these data, plus information on the dental health needs and demands of the population, and on the supply and utilization of dental health manpower, a policy for dental manpower can be formulated.

POLICY FORMULATION

DENTAL HEALTH MANPOWER PLANNING

The formulation of a manpower policy for a service such as dentistry cannot be developed without considering the national priorities for manpower. The medical services should have a high priority because the nation's health is of prime importance. The supply of dental manpower must be seen in the whole scheme of health services. The supply of more mental health workers, for example, may have to take precedence over that of dental health workers.

Dental health manpower planning is the process of estimating the quantity of manpower, plus their varying types of knowledge and skills, needed to bring about planned alterations in the dental health service system, so that the chances of improvements in the dental health of the population are optimal. Planning must specify who is going to do what, with whom, where and how—now and in the future. In general dental health manpower planning involves:

1. The analysis and projections of dental health needs and demands for services by the population. Such data are obtained by epidemiological surveys and from treatment records.
2. The assessment of present dental health manpower availability and the analysis of its pattern of utilization.
3. The formulation of policy.

4. The estimation of future manpower requirements and of relevant education and training needs in the light of the overall dental health plans.

Point (1) has been discussed earlier in this chapter, and is further touched on by Burt in Chapter 6. Points (2), (3), and (4) will now be considered in more detail:

2. Although considerable data are available on dental health manpower, very little objective analysis has been carried out on the patterns of utilization. One of the few detailed analyses which have been done was in Canada (Royal Commission, 1964) and the appraisal based upon that study can be readily applied to the dental services in the majority of countries. The appraisal was as follows:

> Information presented to the Royal Commission in Health Services revealed a grave shortage of dentists and dental schools, inadequate hospital dental facilities, and maldistribution of dentists. The cost of dental services is a deterrent to a sizeable proportion of the population. The cost of dental education discourages potential students from entering the profession. The contributions of auxiliary personnel have been barely exploited. This is some of the significant information on which the Commissioners based their dental recommendations. (McFarlane, 1964.)

3. The manpower requirements will depend not only upon the information regarding needs, demands, and available manpower, but upon the overall philosophy of dental health care. If the policy is based upon the commitment to maintain the dental well-being of the whole population in both the short and the long term, the manpower requirements both in numbers and types will differ significantly from the requirements of a system concerned chiefly with maintaining the status of the dental profession. This placing of professional interests ahead of community well-being, not unknown in the dental profession, has led Restrepo to say: 'The profession or its leadership rather than finding solutions often contributed additional barriers to existing obstacles' (Restrepo, 1968). These barriers can take the form of resistance to the introduction of operating ancillary personnel, and demanding unrealistic education programmes for ancillaries and specialists.

On the other hand if the commitment is to make good dental health care available to all, decisions can be made upon a comprehensive policy for a region or a nation. It is significant that where such a broad commitment has been made nations have been able to achieve some social change in the organization of their health services system. In such countries this change has been characterized by a greater role of the state in the financing and administration of dental health services. This has resulted in a concern for the adequacy, distribution, and costs of dental health manpower (Elling, 1968).

Depending upon the social philosophy towards dental health care the following models, or organizational patterns, may be applied in assessing manpower requirements:

SUPPLY AND DEMAND MODEL

This is the most commonly used method of assessing requirements and is often implemented for political reasons. When there is an expressed demand for health services, the politician will press for services to be created to satisfy that demand.

For this method, indices of demand are constructed based upon the utilization rates by age, sex, occupation, and race. On this basis the dentist:population ratio is projected at a given date. Then assumptions are made on the increase in numbers of dental visits to be made per year based upon reduction of financial barriers or increase in *per capita* income and education. The method of age-related utilization rates has been used to estimate projected medical manpower requirements in the United Kingdom (Royal Commission, 1968).

The supply-demand model of dental health manpower poses a number of methodological problems. First, the assumption is incorrectly made that there is not an underlying hypothesis regarding the nature of the overall services which are to be provided. Such a hypothesis must exist in order that decisions can be taken regarding which demands to satisfy and how to satisfy them. Secondly, the model does not analyse the changes which are occurring in the functions and the productivity of dental health personnel. They usually assume that the present staffing patterns are adequate and that changes in demand can be met by increasing the number of dentists. Thirdly, the users of the model assume that the supply of dentists will rise according to market demands or that the organization of the dental services system will remain constant. The impact of the system on society and the social changes in terms of expectations are neglected, thereby leading to gross miscalculations in manpower requirements.

FUNCTIONAL ANALYSIS MODEL

This method is based on the assumptions of supply-demand and on cost-benefit methods and is involved with matching qualifications of dental health personnel to the requirements of 'job performance'. There are numerous studies on the activities of dentists, hygienists, and dental auxiliaries but the relationship between the activities performed and the actual function of the particular worker has not been commented upon. Neither has there been any analysis of the extent to which dental care programmes have been redesigned as a result of these studies. Two examples of how functions have been transferred is found in the training and use of dental nurses in New Zealand (Leslie, 1961), and the use of corps men in the Royal Canadian Dental Corps (Baird et al., 1962). In both cases auxiliaries perform dental tasks which are usually carried out by dentists. Although such experiments have been widely publicized and in some cases tested (General Dental Council, 1966; Sutcliffe, 1969), there has been no major redesigning of dental care systems as a result of the studies.

TARGET SETTING APPROACH MODEL

The target setting model concentrates on identifying the deficiencies in the health service system which are identified by the desire to attain specified social priorities (Titmuss et al., 1964). This approach assumes that certain objectives, such as the eradication of certain infectious diseases, are social imperatives. Unfortunately, because few national health authorities recognize planning for dental services as priority need (Fendall, 1968), dental care is seldom included as a social priority in the large majority of countries, a problem touched on by Leatherman in Chapter 14. There are, however, some notable exceptions such as in Czechoslovakia and in the United Kingdom, where the service was described by Renson in the previous chapter. In Czechoslovakia (Poncova, 1969) the Ministry of Health have outlined the following objectives of dental care:

1. Provision of planned dental care on the largest possible scale, with priorities to age-groups under 18 years.
2. Effectuate all available preventive measures particularly against the development of caries.
3. Focus health education on a correct living regimen, hygiene, and on the importance of early treatment.

The target setting approach seeks to establish goals to be achieved, and its purpose is to influence the future course of development of the health services (Harbison and Myers, 1964). If the target of the profession is to '. . . make dental health care available to all citizens who need and want it so that the total health of the individual and of the nation is best served' (Federation Dentaire Internationale, 1968), a number of solutions are apparent. The first and most obvious solution is to reduce the need for dental care by prevention of dental disease, a subject comprehensively covered by McHugh in Chapter 2. In particular, fluoridation of the water supplies substantially reduces the prevalence of dental caries; this is discussed in detail by Burt in Chapter 3. Periodontal disease can be prevented and controlled by oral hygiene measures which are widely available (Sheiham, 1971), malocclusion can be prevented by interceptive measures and oral cancer can be treated effectively if the premalignant stages are diagnosed early.

Yet the dental profession displays a reluctance to act upon its own resolutions, as evidenced by the trivial amount of preventive dentistry which is taught and practised. In the main, the profession still clings to the traditional role of repairing diseased dental and oral tissues.

Water fluoridation reduces the manpower required to treat dental decay and, therefore, the cost of the dental services. Some examples of the effect of fluoridation on manpower requirements are given by Burt in Chapters 3 and 6. Others come from Striffler (1957), who estimated that in New Mexico areas with fluoride in the drinking water required 25 per cent fewer dentists than were required in non-fluoride areas, and from Gish (1968), who estimated that the cost-benefit of various preventive measures compared to restorative care. He estimated that given an expenditure of \$100,000 one could either prevent 666,666 cavities by spending the money on fluoridation of the water supply or 233,333 cavities prevented by topical fluoride professionally applied. On the other hand only 16,700 cavities would be restored for the same expenditure.

Dental health education is frequently stated to be a means towards achieving a high level of dental health. By this means individuals will be informed about disease prevention by oral hygiene and dietary control. Even in the highly developed welfare system in the United Kingdom dental health education is hardly practised although the need for it is frequently expressed.

These examples illustrate that although the dental profession gives the outward appearance of following a target setting approach, the actual method used is the supply-demand model. That model has not been successful in the past. This failure was summed up by Craig when he said:

> The sheer volume of dental disease, the shortage of trained manpower, the disappointing long-term results of conventional methods of dental health education and the slow progress to water fluoridation together create a situation in which the prospect of promoting the concept of positive dental health is remote. (Craig, 1970.)

4. The estimation of manpower requirements will depend on the method used as cited earlier. Whatever method is going to be used, the following information is required (World Health Organization, 1968):

Feature of national and regional profiles.

a. Essential profiles

- i. Population
  - —total
  - —rate of growth
  - —distribution: urban, rural, density
  - —school age population
- ii. Economics
  - —socio-economic status
  - —source of funds for health
- iii. Political factors
  - —government attitude towards and responsibility for health services
  - —level of authority of dental administrators
  - —prevalent status of dentistry, self or government employed
- iv. Communications
  - —transport
  - —distances between centres
- v. Demographic data
  - —ethnic groups
  - —educational levels
  - —cultural aspects
  - —religions

vi. Dental disease patterns
vii. Present manpower—availability
—distribution
—training facilities and capacity
—general education standard

b. Desirable profiles—features which any planner would desire, but which when unavailable do not stop planning.

i. Dental disease pattern. Estimates of malocclusion and tooth mortality. Detailed epidemiological data on dental caries and periodontal disease.
ii. Levels of oral hygiene.

c. Variable profiles—features which may be essential in some countries, desirable in some and of little importance in others.

i. General —geography
—climate
—economic factors
ii. Dietary pattern—customs, habits
—staple foods
—water supply
iii. Disease pattern—oral cancer
—orofacial defects
iv. Attitudes of dental personnel towards practice.

When this information is assembled the decision must be made regarding what manpower to use and how. Will there be all or some of existing categories permitted to delegate duties to operating auxiliaries (and if so under what degree of supervision) or will there be nonoperating auxiliaries who are allowed to become operating auxiliaries? Then priorities must be established and estimation of the manpower required to achieve the short, intermediate, and long-term goals of the plan.

The approach outlined above has been utilized in deciding on dental requirements for emerging countries, and plans have been formulated on the basis of the findings. The following three-phased programme has been suggested by Fendall (1968):

1. First Phase Training a minimal corps of superbly trained and dedicated dentists. They should know the wants of individual patients and the conservative care needs of children. The main task must be to act as a teacher, organizer, and supervisor to a team of auxiliaries. There must be a strengthening of departments of social medicine in medical schools and health departments of ministries of health by appointing health-minded dentists.

2. Second Phase Increase number of dentists but start training existing paramedical and auxiliary health personnel.

3. Third Phase Improve quality of service and train specific cadres of dental auxiliaries.

Fendall maintains, however, that in countries with underdeveloped dental services, e.g., Kenya, paramedical personnel with supplementary training of six weeks should be utilized. This situation is forced by the high cost of training professional dentists and in the basic demands of persons living in such countries for relatively simple treatment such as extractions to relieve pain, incision of abscesses, treatment of oral infections, and provision of simple dental prostheses.

If total outreach is to be achieved specific types of dental ancillaries must be trained. This training would emphasize preventive dental care and diagnosis of persons in more urgent need. The decision must be made whether to train single-skill or multiple-skill ancillaries. In the case of the single skill ancillary, one dental surgeon would diagnose and prescribe treatment, plan and perform advanced work and carry out oral surgery. One dental surgeon and six ancillaries would serve a population of 25,000 (Fendall, 1968). This system needs a large centre and is not mobile enough for countries with widely distributed populations. The alternative approach is to train two types of multiple-skill ancillaries, one orientated towards children and the other for adults.

INCENTIVE AND CONTROLS

The incentives offered by the types of work and the particular professional career, and the controls imposed upon dental health workers, together play an important role in achieving desired dental health objectives. Depending upon the state of the programme, either incentives, controls, or a variable blend of these two means of achieivng desired results can be used. Which alternative of the two means of effecting change comes to be used is largely determined by the social and political climate of the country.

Incentive policies cover such elements as mission-orientated education, satisfactory career structure, including the relevance of dental school curricula to the country's dental problems, an adequate salary or pay structure, opportunities for scientific growth and research promotions, suitable work schedules, special provisions for those working in rural areas, and job stability and prestige (Mejia, 1970).

A number of these incentives have been shown to be important in the recruitment of dentists. For example, the desire to work for people and to be of service to others is a frequently stated reason given by dental personnel to explain their liking for the dental professions (McFarlane, 1965). Income is another important incentive to join the profession. However, the method of remuneration is also very important for it should be considered by the dental worker to be fair. In the United Kingdom, the Tattersall Report on Methods of Remuneration concluded that there was widespread dissatisfaction with the item-of-service form of payment and concluded that: 'There is no future for the profession, or indeed general dental practice as an art or a science, in the system of remuneration as presently operated' (British Dental Association, 1964).

Other factors which are considered to be important incentives to joining the profession are the prestige of the occupation and the autonomy of the individual operator.

Many of the incentives relate to systems in countries based upon a free enterprise concept. Studies of incentives in welfare, socialist, and developing countries are required before generalizing these conclusions.

The types and the levels of controls are important in determining productivity and efficiency. Controls may be applied by the state, third-party agency, the profession and the consumer. The nature of these controls and their method of implementation may affect performance, but no worthwhile dental data are available of the relative impact of the effect of direct supervisory control, impersonal statistical control of performance, or professional peer judgement on dental personnel.

LEVELS OF DECISION-MAKING

Decisions must be made at all steps in the process of dental health and manpower planning. However, if these decisions are to be effectively implemented, those concerned in implementing the decisions should be represented during each stage in the planning, analysis and implementation processes. Efforts should be made to reach agreement at government, professional, dental public health, and the public level. At each of these levels of decision there should be informed technical and sociological personnel available to inform, and to communicate relevant information.

The implementation of dental health manpower plans requires political, financial, and administrative support and the administrative machinery for the formulation, preparation and implementation of the plans. It is very important that the dental profession recognizes that such an administrative structure exists and that a good liaison is developed between the dental manpower planning unit and those concerned with social, educational, and economic planning. Mejia (1970) has summarized the pattern of relationships which exists between social and economic planning bodies to national health manpower planning units:

1. A national body deals with social and economic plans: this body usually takes the form of a board made up of high government officials which formulates general manpower policies.

2. A national socio-economic planning secretariat with a general manpower division.

3. A manpower sub-committee of the board composed of senior officials of main government departments including representatives of the health sector, which provides recommendations to the board.

4. Reporting to the sub-committee there are working groups dealing with the collection and analysis of information, co-ordination with representatives of teaching institutions, projection of manpower, and improvement of utilization. The actual manpower planning may be the responsibility of the health planning unit of the department of health or

a joint working party including representatives of the department of health, other areas of national health administration and health teaching institutions. Some countries have created special commissions and/or manpower institutes either attached to the health planning unit of the department of health or set up a strong separate unit with greater autonomy.

The stimulus to the setting up of a dental manpower unit or commission may come from the department of health, from the professional association, or from the dental schools, but the final decision to implement the plans remains in the hands of the government whatever political system exists.

THE EVALUATION OF DENTAL SERVICES

Evaluation and criticism must be an integral part of a dental health service for without evaluation the administrator will have little objective information about the success and failings of his attempt at solving the dental problem.

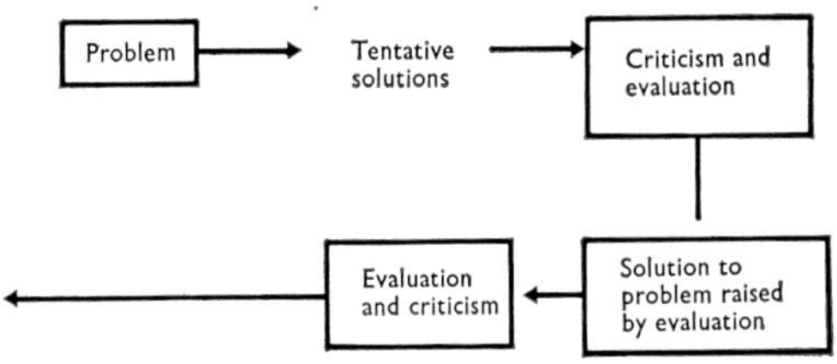

Fig. 2. Diagrammatic representation of the hypothetico-deductive method of evaluating health services.

The administrator has many reasons for evaluating his programme and these must be identified because aspects of the evaluation will hinge upon the reason. Knutson (1961) maintained that there were implicit and explicit reasons for evaluating a health programme and that these fell into two categories: reasons that are organization-oriented and reasons that are personally-oriented. The orientation will determine the selection of evaluation criteria. For example, if a dental administrator whose background is in restorative dentistry is called upon to evaluate a dental health programme he may measure the amount of restorative dental care carried out; he may pay less attention to measuring the severity of periodontal disease and malocclusion.

Various attempts have been made to develop models for evaluating health services. The following general approach known as the hypothetico-deductive method is suggested. This method can be diagrammatically illustrated (*Fig.* 2).

Once the problem is defined a series of tentative solutions to the problem are implemented. These solutions are criticized and evaluated and based upon the outcome of the evaluation the solution may be considered successful or not. If the evaluation indicates a failure to solve the problem, other solutions must be implemented. Evaluation of these solutions is carried out and thus we come closer to solving the problem. In order that the successful solutions may be identified, the criteria for success must be clearly stated at the outset of the programme. Quality of care, its availability, and its usage by the target population are essential considerations in developing criteria for measurement.

Schonfeld (1969) has suggested one approach to evaluation. He considers that the success and quality of dental care may be evaluated on four different levels: the dental procedure, the mouth, the person, and the community.

First Level The Restoration, Procedure, or Service: This level is the basis upon which all considerations are built.

Second Level The Mouth: Here the relationship of one dental procedure to another is evaluated.

Third Level The Person: Consideration of the patient's total health and the relationship of dental health care to it; in addition, the influence that the dental care given has had on the attitude to dentistry and future dental health behaviour.

Fourth Level The Family and Community: Evaluation of the dental services provided for groups and communities, and the number and social distribution of persons receiving adequate dental care.

These four levels of quality must be considered in conjunction with the settings for which the care was provided and those in turn must be evaluated.

Dimensions to be considered in evaluation are:

1. The Technical Dimensions which are concerned with the techniques, instruments, and materials used.

2. The Professional–Logistic Dimension. Technical perfection is not enough, quantity is also important. An evaluation of the kinds of dental services rendered, the sequences in which they were done, how many, how often, where, for whom, by whom, the number of visits required and the time spent at these visits must be carried out. In addition, the factors which may interfere with the provision and receipt of services must be assessed (Schonfeld, 1969).

3. The Organizational Dimension includes the broad organizational framework in which dental care is delivered. The effect that the type of organization has on the adequacy of dental care must be evaluated. The main type of practice, either solo or group and the qualification of operators may be important variables determining the outcome of dental care programmes.

4. The Financial Dimension. This is superimposed upon the other three dimensions and may affect the adequacy of dental care.

It is obvious that evaluation must be done at all levels in order that deficiencies or positive qualities may be identified. Evaluation is an ongoing process and requires well-defined criteria and objective methods of assessment. Failure to implement evaluation leads to a self-satisfied uncritical attitude under which no dental care programme can flourish.

REFERENCES

AKPABIO, S. P. (1966), 'Dentistry—A public health service in East and West Africa', *Dent. Practnr dent. Rec.*, **16,** 412.

ALDERMAN, A. J. (1965), *Volume of Dental Visits; United States, July 1963–June 1964.* Washington, DC: Public Health Service, National Centre for Health Statistics, Publication 1000, Series 10, No. 23.

ANDERSON, D. L. (1968), 'Oral cancer incidence in central and western Canada', *J. Can. dent. Ass.*, **34,** 180.

ANDERSON, O. W. (1957), 'Family dental costs and other personal health services: A nationwide survey', *J. Am. dent. Ass.*, **54,** 69.

ANDERSEN, R., and ANDERSON, O. (1967), *A Decade of Health Services.* Chicago: University of Chicago Press.

AST, D. B., CONS, N. C., CARLOS, J. P., and MAIWALD, A. (1965), 'Time and cost factors to provide regular, periodic dental care for children in a fluoridated and non-fluoridated area', *Am. J. Publ. Hlth*, **55,** 811.

— — — — POLLARD, S. T., jun., and GARFINKEL, J. (1970). 'Time and cost factors to provide regular, periodic dental care for children in a fluoridated and non-fluoridated area: Final report', *J. Am. dent. Ass.*, **80,** 770.

BAIRD, J. T., and KELLY, J. E. (1970), *Need for Dental Care among Adults; United States 1960–1962.* Washington, DC: Public Health Service, National Centre for Health Statistics, Publication 1000, Series 11, No. 36.

BAIRD, M. M., SHILLINGTON, G. B., and PROTHERO, D. H. (1962), 'Pilot study on the advanced training and employment of auxiliary dental personnel in the Royal Canadian Dental Corps: Preliminary report', *J. Can. dent. Ass.*, **28,** 633.

BALLARD, C. F., and WAYMAN, J. B. (1964), 'A report on the survey of orthodontic requirements of 310 army recruits', *Trans. Br. Soc. orthodont Study*, n.v. 81.

BARMES, D. E. (1969), 'The need for auxiliaries in developed as well as in developing countries', *Int. dent. J.*, **19,** 1.

BECK, D. J. (1968), *Dental Health Status of the New Zealand Population in Late Adolescence and Young Adulthood.* Wellington, NZ: Department of Health, National Health Statistics Centre, Special Report No. 29.

BINNIE, W. H., CAWSON, R. A., HILL, G. B., and SOAPER, A. E. (1972), *Oral Cancer in England and Wales. A National Study of Morbidity, Mortality, Curability and Related Factors.* Studies on Medical and Population Studies No. 23. London: HMSO.

BJÖRK, A., KREBS, A., and SOLOW, B. (1964), 'A method for epidemiological registration of malocclusion', *Acta odont. scand.*, **22,** 27.

BLANKEN, G. E. (1971), *Current Estimates from the Health Interview Survey, United States 1967.* Washington, DC: Public Health Service, National Centre for Health Statistics, Publication 1000, Series 10, No. 63.

BRITISH DENTAL ASSOCIATION (1964), 'Methods of remuneration; the report of the Ad Hoc Sub-Committee on methods of remuneration (Tattersall Report)', *Br. dent. J.*, **117,** 331.

BROTHERSTON, J. H. F. (1971), *Doctors in an Integrated Health Service; Report of a Joint Working Party appointed by the Secretary of State for Scotland.* Edinburgh: HMSO.

BROWN, W. A. B. (1967), 'Examiner variability', in *Proceedings of the Fourth Conference of Teachers of Orthodontics.* Cardiff: University of Wales Dental School.

BURKITT, D. (1964), 'A lymphoma syndrome dependent on environment', in *Lymphoreticular Tumors in Africa*, Paris, 1963. Basel and New York: Karger.

CARTER, C. O. (1967), 'Congenital malformations', *WHO Chron.*, **21,** 287.
CHATWIN, J. V. P., DELAQUIS, F. M., and WALKER, C. B. (1968), 'Accuracy of recall of dental care received during the preceding year', *J. Can. dent. Ass.*, **34,** 409.
CHULIS, G. S. (1966), *Dental Visits, Time Interval Since Last Visit, United States July 1963–June 1964.* Washington DC: Public Health Service, National Centre for Health Statistics, Publication 1000, Series 10, No. 29.
COOK, P. J., and WALKER, R. O. (1967), 'The geographical distribution of dental care in the United Kingdom', *Br. dent. J.*, **122,** 441, 494, 551.
CRAIG, J. W. (1970), 'Teamwork in dentistry', *Ibid.*, **128,** 198.
DRAKER, H. L. (1960), 'Handicapping labio-lingual deviations proposed for public health purposes', *Am. J. Orthodont.*, **46,** 296.
—— METZNER, C. A., and ALLAWAY, N. C. (1965), 'The dentists and the services they provided for two populations; comments on methodology of study', *J. Publ. Hlth Dent.*, **25,** 23.
ELLING, R. H. (1968), 'The design, institutionalization and evaluation of change in Colombian health services', in *Social Science and Health Planning* (ed. BADYLEY, R. F.). New York: Millbank Memorial Fund.
EMSLIE, R. D. (1963), 'Cancrum oris', *Dent. Practnr dent. Rec.*, **13,** 481.
FANNING, E. A., GOTTJAMANOS, T., and VOWLES, N. J. (1969), 'Dental health and treatment requirements of South Australian secondary schoolchildren', *Med. J. Aust.*, **2,** 899.
FEDERATION DENTAIRE INTERNATIONALE (1968), *Principles for Development of a Manpower Programme in Dentistry.* London.
——— (1970), *Basic Facts Sheets.*
FENDALL, N. R. E. (1968), 'Dental manpower requirements in emerging countries', *Publ. Hlth Rep.*, **83,** 777.
FU-TANG CHU, and CHUAN FAM (1963), 'Cancrum oris: A clinical study of 100 cases with special reference to prognosis', *Chin. med. J.*, **50,** 303.
GENERAL DENTAL COUNCIL (1966), *Final Report on the Experimental Scheme for the Training and Employment of Dental Auxiliaries.* London: General Dental Council.
GISH, C. H. (1968), State of Indiana; State Board of Health. ADA Newsletter vol. 21, No. 23; and personal communication.
GOVERNMENTAL STATISTICAL SERVICE (1970), *Social Trends No. 1.* London: HMSO.
GRAINGER, R. M. (1967), *Orthodontic Treatment Priority Index.* Washington DC: Public Health Service, National Centre for Health Statistics, Publication 1000, Series 2, No. 25.
GRAY, P. G., TODD, J. E., SLACK, G. L., and BULMAN, J. S. (1970), *Adult Dental Health in England and Wales, 1968.* London: HMSO.
GREENE, J. C. (1963), 'Epidemiology of congenital clefts of the lip and palate', *Publ. Hlth Rep.*, **78,** 589.
HARBISON, F., and MYERS, C. A. (1964), *Education, Manpower, and Economic Growth.* New York: McGraw-Hill.
HONIGSBAUM, F. (1970), *The Struggle for the Ministry of Health.* Occasional Paper and Social Administration No. 37. London: Bell.
HOUPT, M. I., ADU-ARYEE, S., and GRAINGER, R. M. (1967), 'Dental survey in the Brong Ahafo region of Ghana', *Archs oral Biol.*, **12,** 1337.
INTERNATIONAL LABOUR OFFICE (1969), *International Standard Classification of Occupation,* Revised ed. Geneva: ILO.
JAMISON, H. C. (1963), 'Prevalence of periodontal disease of the deciduous teeth', *J. Am. dent. Ass.*, **66,** 207.
JOHNSON, E. S., KELLY, J. E., and VAN KIRK, L. E. (1965), *Selected Dental Findings in Adults by Age, Race and Sex; United States 1960–1962.* Washington, DC: Public Health Service, National Centre for Health Statistics, Publication 1000, Series 11, No. 7.
JOLLY, R., and KING, M. (1970), 'The organization of health services', in *Medical Care in Developing Countries* (ed. KING, M.). London: Oxford University Press.

KAPRIO, L. J. E. (1967), 'Size and distribution of present world resources of doctors, specialists, nurses, midwives, medical technicians, sanatarians, and other health staff', *Health of Mankind* (ed. WALSTENHOLME, G., and O'CONNOR, M.). London: Churchill.

KEGELES, S. S. (1961), 'Why people seek dental care—a review of present knowledge', *Am. J. Publ. Hlth*, **51,** 1306.

KNUTSON, A. L. (1961), *Evaluation for What? Proceedings of a Conference on Neurologically Handicapping Conditions in Children.* Berkeley: University of California.

KOOS, E. L. (1954), *The Health of Regionville; What the People Thought and Did About It.* New York: Columbia University Press.

LEATHERWOOD, E. C., BURNETT, G. W., and CHANDRAVEJJSMARN, R. (1965), 'Dental caries and dental fluorosis in Thailand', *Am. J. Publ. Hlth*, **55,** 1792.

LESLIE, G. H. (1961), *Dental Health Planning at a National Level.* Manila: WHO Regional Office of Western Pacific, WP/RC12/TD5.

MALBERGER, E. (1967), 'Acute infectious oral necrosis among young children in Gambia, W. Africa', *J. periodont. Res.*, **2,** 154.

MCFARLANE, B. A. (1964), 'A sociologist's appraisal of the Report of the Royal Commission on Health Services', *J. Can. dent. Ass.*, **30,** 611.

— — (1965), *Dental Manpower in Canada.* Ottawa: Queen's Printer.

MEHTA, F. S., PINDBORG, J. J., and GUPTA, P. C. (1969), 'Epidemiologic and histologic study of oral cancer and leukoplakia among 50,915 villagers in India', *Cancer*, **24,** 832.

MESKIN, L. H., and MARTENS, L. V. (1970), 'Commentary on dental manpower; the dentist–population ratio', *J. Publ. Hlth Dent.*, **30,** 95.

MEJIA, A. (1970), *Introductory Note: Scientific Group on the Development of Studies in Health Manpower.* Geneva: WHO, Mimeograph, CHS/WP/70.3.

MILLS, L. F. (1966), 'Epidemiologic studies of malocclusion IV. The prevalence of malocclusion in a population of 1,455 schoolchildren', *J. dent. Res.*, **45,** 332.

MOORE, G. R. (1948), 'The orthodontic programme of the Michigan State Department of Health, with a new classification of occlusion for survey purposes', *Am. J. Orthodont.*, **34,** 355.

MOYERS, R. E. (1956), 'The basis for an index of malocclusion', in *The Practice of Dental Public Health* (ed. EASLICK, K. A.). Ann Arbor: University of Michigan School of Public Health.

NATIONAL ADVISORY COMMISSION ON HEALTH MANPOWER (1967), Report, volume 1. Washington, DC: US Government Printer.

NEWSHOLME, A. (1932), *Medicine and the State.* London: Allen & Unwin.

NIKIAS, M. K. (1968), 'Social class and the use of dental care under prepayment', *Med. Care*, **6,** 381.

O'LEARY, T. (1967), 'The periodontal screening examination', *J. Periodont.*, **38,** 617.

PELTON, W. J., DUNBAR, J. B., MCMILLAN, R. S., MOLLER, P., and WOLFF, A. C. (1969), *The Epidemiology of Oral Health.* Cambridge, Mass.: Harvard University Press, American Public Health Association Vital and Health Statistics Monographs.

PINDBORG, J. J., BHAT, M., DEVANATH, K. R., NARAYANA, H. R., and RAMACHANDRA, S. (1966), 'Occurrence of acute necrotizing gingivitis in South Indian children', *J. Periodont.*, **37,** 14.

PONCOVA, V. (1969), 'Dental health services in Czechoslovakia', Paper given at the WHO course in Dental Public Health, The London Hospital Medical College.

RAMFJORD, S. P. (1959), 'Indices for prevalence and incidence of periodontal disease', *J. Periodont.*, **30,** 51.

— — EMSLIE, R. D., GREENE, J. C., HELD, A. J., and WAERHAUG, J. (1968), 'Epidemiological studies of periodontal diseases', *Am. J. Publ. Hlth*, **58,** 1713.

RESTREPO, D. (1968), 'Some alternatives for national dental plans', in *Inter-regional Seminar on the Training and Utilization of Dental Personnel in Developing Countries, New Delhi, 1967.* Geneva: WHO DH/68.2.

ROSENSTOCK, I. M., HOCHBAUM, G. M., and KEGELES, S. S. (1960), 'Determinants of health behavior', Working paper prepared for the Golden Anniversary White House Conference on Children and Youth.

ROYAL COMMISSION (1964). *Report of the Royal Commission on Health Services: Dental Manpower in Canada.* Ottawa: Queen's Printer.

—— (1968), *Report of the Royal Commission on Medical Education* (*Todd Report*). London: HMSO.

RUDKO, V. (1970), *Consultation on Organisation and Planning of Dental Health Services.* Geneva: WHO, unpublished.

RUSSELL, A. L. (1956), 'A system of classification and scoring for prevalence surveys of periodontal disease', *J. dent. Res.*, **35,** 350.

—— (1967), 'Periodontal disease incidence in the United States', *The Periodontal Needs of the United States Population* (ed. O'LEARY, T.). Chicago: American Academy of Periodontology.

RUSSELL, S. L., LEATHERWOOD, E. C., LE VAN HIEN, and VAN REEN, R. (1965), 'Dental caries and nutrition in South Vietnam', *J. dent. Res.*, **44,** 102.

SALZMANN, J. A. (1968), 'Handicapping malocclusion assessment to establish treatment priority', *Am. J. Orthodont.*, **54,** 749.

SCHAMSCHULA, R. G., and BARMES, D. E. (1966), 'Dental education in Papua—New Guinea. Part I—The concept', *Aust. dent. J.*, **11,** 73.

SCHONFELD, H. K. (1969), *Peer Review of Quality of Dental Care.* Chicago: 20th National Dental Health Conference.

SHEIHAM, A. (1966), 'An epidemiological survey of acute ulcerative gingivitis in Nigerians', *Archs oral Biol.*, **11,** 937.

—— (1967), 'The prevalence of dental caries in Nigerian populations', *Br. dent. J.*, **123,** 144.

—— (1968), 'The epidemiology of periodontal disease: Studies in Nigerian and British populations', Ph.D. Thesis. University of London.

—— (1969), 'The prevalence and severity of periodontal disease in Surrey schoolchildren', *Dent. Practnr dent. Rec.*, **19,** 232.

—— (1971), 'The prevention and control of chronic periodontal disease', *Dent. Hlth*, **10,** 1.

—— and HOBDELL, M. H. (1969), 'Decayed, missing and filled teeth in British adult populations', *Br. dent. J.*, **126,** 401.

SKOUGAARD, M. R., PINCDORG, J. J., and ROED-PETERSEN, B. (1969), 'Periodontal conditions in 1,394 Ugandans', *Archs oral Biol.*, **14,** 707.

STRIFFLER, D. F. (1957), 'The relationship of endemic fluorides to the need and demand for dental services in New Mexico', *New Mex. dent. J.*, **8,** 13.

SUCHMAN, E. A. (1965), 'Social patterns of illness and medical care', *J. Hlth Human Behav.*, **6,** 2.

SUMMERS, C. J. (1971), 'The Occlusal Index: A system for identifying and scoring occlusal disorders', *Am. J. Orthodont.*, **59,** 552.

SUTCLIFFE, P. (1969), 'Dental auxiliaries: A method of measuring their clinical usefulness', *Br. dent. J.*, **126,** 418.

TAN, K. N. (1969), 'Oral cancer in Australia', *Aust. dent. J.*, **14,** 50.

TITMUSS, R., ABEL-SMITH, B., MACDONALD, G., WILLIAMS, A. W., and WOOD, C. H. (1964), *The Health Services of Tanganyika.* London: Pitman and African Medical Research Foundation.

VAN KIRK, L. E., and PENNELL, E. H. (1959), 'Assessment of malocclusion in population groups', *Am. J. Publ. Hlth*, **49,** 1157.

WORLD HEALTH ORGANIZATION (1965), *Organisation of Dental Public Health Services.* Geneva: WHO, Tech. Rep. Ser. No. 163.

——— (1968), *Inter-Regional Seminar on the Training and Utilization of Dental Personnel in Developing Countries, New Delhi, 1967.* Geneva: WHO, DH/68.2.

——— (1969), *Training in National Health Planning.* Geneva: WHO, Tech. Rep. Ser. No. 429.

World Health Organization (1970), '23rd World Health Assembly 1 and 2', *WHO* Chron., **24**, 289, 337.

——— (1971), *Oral Health Surveys; Basic Methods*. Geneva: WHO.

Young, M. A. C. (1967), *Review of Research and Studies Related to Health Education (1961–1966). What People Know, Believe, and Do about Health*. New York: Society of Public Health Educators Inc., Health Education Monographs, No. 25.

FURTHER READING

Fendall, N. R. E. (1970), 'The training and use of auxiliary personnel', in *Community Medicine* (ed. Latham, W., and Newbery, A.). New York: Appleton-Century-Crofts.

Grainger, R. M. (1961), *Indexing Malocclusion*. Geneva: WHO, Report WHO/DH/51.

Haefner, D. P., Kegeles, S. S., Kirscht, J., and Rosenstock, I. M. (1967), 'Preventive actions in dental disease, tuberculosis and cancer', *Publ. Hlth Rep.*, **82,** 451.

Hillenbrand, H. (1968), 'Problems of dental care in the United States', in *Oral Health; Fact, Figures, and Philosophy*. Harvard Dental Alumni Bulleting Special Supplement, Nov. 1968.

Russell, A. L. (1966), 'World epidemiology and oral health', in *Environmental Variables in Oral Disease* (ed. Kreshover, S. J., and McClure, F. J.). Washington: Am. Ass. Adv. Science.

Solow, B., and Helm, S. (1968), 'A method for tabulation and statistical evaluation of epidemiological malocclusion data', *Acta odont. scand.*, **26,** 63.

Chapter 9

Dental Ancillaries

Richard J. Elderton BDS (LOND), LDSRCS (ENG),
Research Fellow, Experimental Dental Care Project, The London Hospital Medical College

The necessity to develop the role of ancillaries in private practice and in public health programmes is no longer a question for debate. Social trends have forced the dental profession to move towards ever-greater utilization of ancillaries.

Several contributors to this book have already stressed the place of ancillaries in dental service programmes, and some specific examples of national programmes where they are employed have been given. In this chapter, Mr. Elderton looks at the different types of ancillaries which have developed around the world, and how they are utilized. He discusses some problems which still remain regarding the further development of ancillaries.

Anyone responsible for planning and organizing dental care services, whether he be a dentist, government official, or other interested person, is almost universally presented with one common problem. In the community that comes within his jurisdiction there is an abundance of untreated dental disease; he must seek to alter this situation.

Previous chapters have shown that programmes of dental treatment, without support from preventive dentistry, will not solve the problem of dental disease. On the other hand, even when prevention is well established, there will always be some reparative treatment required. There is, indeed, reason to believe that in an age when rapid population growth combines with increasing demands for health care, there will be considerably greater call on dental treatment services in the future than exists at present. If these services are to be adequately delivered, all countries are likely to require more dentists, or dental operators of some type, than they have at present.

Certainly if dentistry is to survive and stride forward as a profession there have to be dentists, but the nature and cost of their training puts an upper limit to their numbers. This being so, it seems reasonable that each should spend his professional life carrying out those duties that he alone is trained to undertake and that he alone is capable of undertaking. It will then be necessary for him to delegate the remaining functions to other individuals working under his direction.

DEFINITION OF DENTAL ANCILLARY

A dental ancillary is a person who is given responsibility by a dentist so that he or she can help the dentist render dental care, but who is not himself or herself qualified with a dental degree. The duties undertaken by dental ancillaries range from simple tasks, such as sorting instruments, to relatively complex procedures which form part of the treatment of patients.

CLASSIFICATION OF DENTAL ANCILLARIES

Dental ancillaries may be classified according to the training they have received, the tasks they are expected to undertake, and the legal restrictions placed upon them. While different titles have been given to groups of ancillaries classified in this way, terminology is not consistent from one country to another. At a conference conducted by the World Health Organization in New Delhi in 1967, the following titles and definitions were suggested (World Health Organization, 1968).

WORLD HEALTH ORGANIZATION CLASSIFICATION

NON-OPERATING AUXILIARIES

Clinical This is a person who assists the professional (dentist) in his clinical work but does not carry out any independent procedures in the oral cavity.

Laboratory This is a person who assists the professional by carrying out certain technical laboratory procedures.

OPERATING AUXILIARY

This is a person who, not being a professional, is permitted to carry out certain treatment procedures in the mouth under the direction and supervision of a professional.

This classification is particularly useful in that it draws a distinction between operating and non-operating ancillaries. However, the use of the term 'auxiliary' seems unnecessary and indeed confusing. This term is officially applied to a specific group of ancillaries in the United Kingdom though it has been used variously in the dental literature on many occasions when the more embracing term 'ancillary' has been implied. The classification could be made more meaningful by further subdivision of the categories as follows:

REVISED CLASSIFICATION

NON-OPERATING ANCILLARIES

Dental Surgery Assistant This is a person who assists the dentist with his clinical work but does not independently carry out any procedures in the mouth. (Other titles that are commonly used in some countries include dental assistant, chairside dental assistant, and dental nurse. The title 'dental technician' is used in some Armed Forces.)

Dental Secretary/Receptionist This is a person who assists the dentist with his secretarial work and patient reception duties.

Dental Laboratory Technician This is a person who assists the dentist by carrying out certain technical procedures in the laboratory. (The title 'dental mechanic' is also applied to this type of auxiliary.)

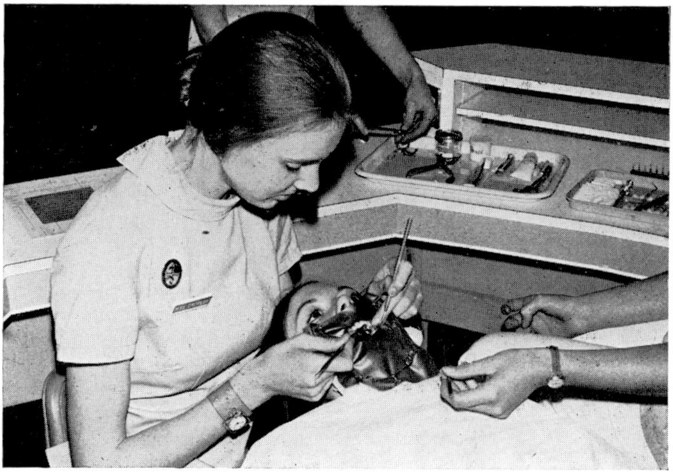

Fig. 1. The role of the dental auxiliary in the clinic.

OPERATING ANCILLARIES

School Dental Nurse (*New Zealand Type*) This is a person who is permitted to diagnose dental disease and to plan and carry out certain specified preventive and treatment measures, including some operative procedures in the treatment of dental caries and periodontal disease, in defined groups of people, usually schoolchildren. The school dental nurse has to work under the direction of a dentist and refer to him those patients requiring diagnosis or treatment that he or she is not able or legally entitled to carry out. Other titles that are used in some countries to refer to this type of ancillary include 'dental nurse' and 'dental auxiliary'; both are confusing.

Dental Auxiliary (United Kingdom) This is a person who is permitted to carry out *to the prescription of a supervising dentist*, certain specified preventive and treatment measures including some operative procedures in the treatment of dental caries and periodontal disease. In the United Kingdom the auxiliary has to work in the public health service, but in Western Australia, ancillaries with similar duties, and called dental therapists, may work under a dentist in private practice (Graebner, 1971). The United Kingdom dental auxiliary (Fig. 1) is sometimes referred to as a New Cross auxiliary. This is because the training school is located at New Cross General Hospital in south London.

Dental Hygienist This is a person who is permitted to carry out, *to the prescription of a supervising dentist*, certain specified preventive and treatment measures including some operative procedures in the treatment of periodontal disease. The dental hygienist is not permitted to carry out any operative procedures for the treatment of dental caries.

North American Expanded Function Operating Ancillary This is a person who is permitted to carry out certain specified preventive and treatment measures including parts of some operative procedures in the treatment of dental caries. The ancillary works in close co-ordination with a supervising dentist who is directly involved with each patient visit. These ancillaries are often referred to as expanded function auxiliaries, expanded duty dental auxiliaries or simply as auxiliaries. The title dental therapist is used by some sections of the Armed Forces in the United States of America and Canada. Some expanded function operating ancillaries have been trained first as hygienists and may therefore carry out the duties of both types of ancillary.

NUMBERS OF DENTAL ANCILLARIES

It is difficult to say precisely how many dental ancillaries there are in every country of the world, but in Table 1 are listed 1972 figures for representative countries (Federation Dentaire Internationale, 1972). It can be seen that the number of dental surgery assistants in each country corresponds roughly to the number of dentists but that otherwise there is little logic to the figures in the table.

NON-OPERATING ANCILLARIES

THE DENTAL SURGERY ASSISTANT

This type of ancillary, who in modern times is usually female, has probably been in existence since the time that dental treatment began. It is likely, however, that they only became numerous as itinerant dentists began to establish themselves into fixed practices. The function of the dental surgery assistant is to ensure general smooth running of the

TABLE 1

The numbers of dentists and dental ancillaries in representative countries (Federation Dentaire Internationale, 1972). Countries listed in order of increasing dentist to population ratio

Country	*Dentists*	*Ratio of dentists to population*	*Dental surgery assistants*	*Dental laboratory technicians*	*School dental nurses*	*Dental auxiliaries*	*Dental hygienists*	*Expanded functions operating ancillaries*
Sweden	7550	1072	8500*	2500	0	0	100	0
USA	104,000*	2001	112,000*	33,000*	0	0	24,000*	500†
Japan	38,055	2724*	31,858*	8215	0	0	7352	0
New Zealand	937	2980	1200*	306	1354	0	0	0
United Kingdom	15,900	3497	19,000*	7500*	0	280	495	0
Indonesia	1250*‡	96,000	1000	170	270*	0	0	0
Zambia	28	150,000	42	5	8	0	0	0
Burma	28*‡‡	893,000	150	153	3	0	3	0

* Estimated (FDI).
† Estimated by author.
‡ Also approximately 2000 unqualified dentists.
‡‡ Also approximately 320 unqualified dentists.

clinical area, and to help the dentist and other members of his staff so that they are able to spend more time providing actual dental care to patients. Traditionally she has been given responsibility for the management of instruments, equipment, and materials, including the cleansing, sterilizing, and recycling of these as necessary between patients. She supplies them to the dentist at the chairside as they are needed. She also has a duty to help look after the general well being of the patients. Some dental surgery assistants are also given patient reception and appointment-making duties, and general secretarial and clerical work. These jobs require little or no special dental knowledge and are more effectively undertaken by a secretary/receptionist who has had appropriate training.

In the past, dental surgery assistants received their training by apprenticeship in the employ of a dentist. While this situation still exists, formal training courses, usually of one to two years, have been introduced in a number of countries. In the United Kingdom, a dental surgery assistant, whether she has attended a course or not, may sit a national examination, the passing of which gives her official recognition as a qualified dental surgery assistant.

Klein (1944) showed that the addition of a dental surgery assistant to a dental practice was associated with a 33 per cent increase in the number of patients treated. Findings of this type have been confirmed on many occasions since, and are probably a prime factor in the increase in utilization of these ancillaries by the dental profession since Klein first published his findings. However, not only has the number increased, and indeed also the number of locations at which they are employed, but as well there have been changes in the way in which dental surgery assistants are utilized, so that they are more efficient. Following appropriate training, they are being increasingly employed to give more direct and constant assistance to the dentist. The dentist and dental surgery assistant sit closely beside the supine patient, the assistant anticipating the instruments and materials that are required, and passing them to the dentist in such a way that he may not have even to take his eyes momentarily away from the field of operation when changing to another instrument. The term 'four-handed dentistry' has been coined to describe this somewhat more sophisticated method of working. The dental surgery assistant must work in a close and co-ordinated manner with the dentist and it will be clear that the operating area must be well organized and contain equipment of suitable design.

THE DENTAL LABORATORY TECHNICIAN

This ancillary, who is usually male, works in a laboratory constructing dental appliances to the prescription of the dentist. He undertakes mechanical tasks, many of which are time consuming and some of which the dentist has not himself been trained to carry out. Most of his time is spent working to models of the patients' teeth and supporting tissues. His specific duties, in addition to the casting of these models from impressions made by the dentist, include the fabrication of dentures, splints, orthodontic appliances, inlays, crowns, and sundry items such as special trays for the topical application of fluoride agents to the teeth.

In the past the dentist himself undertook all his own laboratory work; indeed in some countries before the establishment of dentistry as a profession, some dentists probably spent more time carrying out laboratory procedures in the patients' absence than clinical procedures in their presence. In the United Kingdom the dental laboratory technician became distinguishable from the dentist in 1921 after the Dentists Act of that year had been passed as law. Since that time only qualified dentists have been permitted to work directly with patients. This is in line with the recommendation of the World Health Organization Expert Committee on Auxiliary Dental Personnel (World Health Organization, 1959). It is, however, interesting to note that in Tasmania, a state of Australia, laboratory technicians are legally permitted to work directly with the public to provide a prosthetic service (Department of Labour and National Service, 1970).

Dental laboratory technicians receive their training through apprenticeship which is sometimes associated with formal training in academic and practical subjects at a dental school or technical college. In the United Kingdom such formal training lasts from three to five years on a part time basis (British Dental Association, 1968).

Dental laboratory technicians may be employed by dentists in private or public health practice, they may be self-employed and accept work from dentists in the area or they may be employed by commercial laboratories established by other dental technicians.

OPERATING ANCILLARIES

THE SCHOOL DENTAL NURSE (NEW ZEALAND TYPE)

This type of ancillary was established in New Zealand in 1923 (training began in 1921) to deal with the large amount of dental disease present among the schoolchildren. The government made provision for training of young women, to be known as school dental nurses, who would provide the bulk of the treatment in the school dental service which was introduced at the same time.

It should be realized that operating ancillaries with functions similar to those of the New Zealand school dental nurse are also employed in a number of other countries, many of which have started their own training schemes. There are 26 countries apart from New Zealand with school dental nurses; they are: Australia, Brunei, Burma, Central Africa, Ceylon, Costa Rica, Cuba, Ghana, Haiti, Hong Kong, Indonesia, Italy, Jamaica, Kenya, Malaysia, Nigeria, Papua-New Guinea, Paraguay, Senegal, Sierra Leone, Singapore, South Vietnam, Taiwan,

Thailand, Uganda, and Zambia (Federation Dentaire Internationale, 1972). Most of these countries are employing under one hundred school dental nurses, though in 1971 in New Zealand there were 1354 and in Malaysia, 403. Cuba and Indonesia were each employing between two and four hundred school dental nurses. Length of training, conditions of employment and specific duties vary slightly from country to country. (Federation Dentaire Internationale, 1972).

THE NEW ZEALAND SCHOOL DENTAL NURSE

Interest in an organized plan to improve dental conditions among children in New Zealand first became evident in 1905 (Gruebbel, 1950). Treatment of these children was particularly difficult on account of the distances which often separated quite small communities. Also there were insufficient dentists to provide an adequate dental service on their own, and very few dentists were being trained at that time.

The duties of the New Zealand school dental nurse, which are essentially the same today as when they began treatment in 1923, are the examination of the children and the diagnosis and treatment of the most prevalent dental diseases, dental caries and periodontal disease. She prepares cavities and restores teeth with amalgam and silicate cement, extracts deciduous teeth, scales and polishes teeth, applies topical fluoride solutions, provides dental health education singly and on a group basis, and refers more complex cases to a dentist in the area. She is permitted to use local infiltration anaesthesia, but not block anaesthesia.

A supervising dentist of the school dental service has overall responsibility for the dental care of the children, but he does not have to be on the premises where the ancillary works. However, he is expected to make periodic visits to ensure that she is providing an effective service.

Approximately two hundred young women are trained as school dental nurses each year under the auspices of the Department of Health. Training takes place over a two-year period at one of three specially designed training schools (which are separate from those involved with undergraduate dental student education). Upon completion of training, each school dental nurse is assigned to a school where she is employed by the government to provide regular dental care of between 450 and 700 children (Leslie, 1971). The lower figure applies to areas without fluoridated water supplies and the higher figure to areas that have had fluoridation for a considerable length of time. Leslie (1971) has also stated that in some places with fluoridation, the school dental nurses are able to provide regular care for 1000 children.

It is of special interest to note that each school which takes more than 100 children has its own dental clinic. This may be part of the structure of the rest of the school or it may be housed in a separate building.

When a school dental nurse is assigned to a school, she is accepted as a member of the staff of that school in the same way as are the teachers; she is responsible to the principal of her school for matters which effect the running of the school such as the scheduling of group dental health instruction sessions.

A number of aspects of the New Zealand scheme warrant discussion. Here is a well-developed country with a dental service for its children which has been acclaimed on numerous occasions to be providing good and effective dental care (United Kingdom Dental Mission, 1950; Fulton, 1951; World Health Organization, 1959). Criticism of the overall service has been far less common (Gruebbel, 1950).

The overall effect of the service has been dramatic. In 1923, 78·6 teeth were extracted for every 100 fillings placed. This ratio has changed to just 2·9 extractions to every 100 fillings in 1969 (Leslie, 1971). Undoubtedly the school dental nurse has played a major part in bringing about this success.

In 1970, approximately 95 per cent of all schoolchildren up to the age of 13 were receiving regular dental care by school dental nurses (Leslie, 1971). In addition, 60 per cent of all preschool children between $2\frac{1}{2}$ and 5 years of age were also receiving regular care. These are undoubtedly impressive figures, especially when one realizes that, in addition, some children receive dental care from private dental practitioners. However, the service has been in operation for almost 50 years and it should be pointed out that only during the last decade has the number of children enrolled with the service approached the maximum possible. In 1955, only about 60 per cent of schoolchildren up to the age of 13 were receiving care in the service, even though the total schoolchild population was then about 40 per cent lower than in 1970 (Leslie, 1971).

With most children now receiving regular dental care and with the effects of fluoridation reaching more than half the population, the dental profession and government may well be faced shortly with a manpower problem that is unusual in any health field; there may be an excess number of school dental nurses. At the same time it is highly likely that preventive measures will be adopted more and more in the future, thereby further reducing the demands placed upon the school dental nurses. This situation could be dealt with by reducing their numbers or expanding their roles to provide care for a larger segment of the population.

The school dental nurses appear to be fully accepted by the dentists, there being about equal numbers of each in the country. The nurses themselves find the job acceptable and satisfying, they have a good rapport with their patients and the *esprit de corps* is very high (Davies, 1971). It should be appreciated, however, that New Zealand is a small country and one with advanced social services. Because the system described above works well in New Zealand this does not necessarily mean that a similar system would work well, or even at all, in every other country. The role of the school dental nurse in the overall pattern of dental treatment services in New Zealand has been discussed by Burt in Chapter 6.

THE DENTAL AUXILIARY (UNITED KINGDOM)

This type of ancillary began operating in the United Kingdom in 1962. Training began in 1960, following a revision of the Dentists Act in 1957 (British Dental Association, 1968). They have been likened to New Zealand-type school dental nurses but their role is quite different as they are not permitted to diagnose and plan dental care. They are permitted to work to written treatment plans devised by the supervising dentists, though the operative procedures they are entitled to carry out are similar to those of the New Zealand school dental nurses, including the administration of local infiltration anaesthesia. The supervising dentists give nerve-block anaesthesia when it is required.

Dental auxiliaries may only work in the local authority and hospital services (described by Renson in Chapter 7) and they are required to carry out their duties under the direction of a registered dentist. 'Direction' does not imply 'personal supervision' though before a change in the Ancillary Dental Workers Regulations in 1968 this was the case (British Dental Association, 1969). The directing dentist is responsible for determining the degree of supervision required in each individual case, according to the capacity and experience of the auxiliary concerned.

Compared to the New Zealand school dental nurse, it is clear that the dental auxiliary functions much less independently and consequently accepts less responsibility. She does not have to learn clinic management in anything like the same detail. However, both types of ancillary undergo a training course of two years' duration; perhaps a case could be made for reducing that of the auxiliary.

It is interesting to note that the school dental nurses in Malaysia are required to have direct supervision. While they have been classified as school dental nurses, this is only partially correct as in a way they are more akin to the United Kingdom dental auxiliaries. However, as there is an inadequate number of dentists in that country, the supervision becomes impracticable (Berman, 1966). The principle that supervision should be 'as close as possible' is adopted, so that every completed case is checked by a dentist (Berman, 1964). Malaysian dental services are described in detail by Burt in Chapter 6.

THE DENTAL HYGIENIST

This type of ancillary was first employed in 1906 in a private dental practice in the United States of America, and in 1913 the first formal training course for hygienists was established (Fones, 1926).

The duties of the dental hygienist are essentially the scaling and polishing of teeth, the topical application of fluoride and the provision of dental health education. In some countries dental hygienists are permitted to take radiographs, make impressions for study models, and polish restorations. In Denmark and the Netherlands they are allowed to make a preliminary examination and charting of the teeth, while in Manitoba they are permitted to take impressions, record jaw relationships, and repair some broken dentures (Federation Dentaire Internationale, 1970).

Dental hygienists usually work with adults, though in many countries there is no legal restriction for this to be the case. They are employed both in private dental practice and in public dental services.

Dental hygienist training is usually of 1–2 years' duration though one year training was thought appropriate by an expert committee of the World Health Organization for countries wishing to train hygienists to enter their governmental health services (World Health Organization, 1959). In the United Kingdom training is from nine months to one year, while a number of schools in the United States of America offer a four-year degree programme in dental hygiene as well as the two-year certificate programme which is standard in that country. Training may or may not take place in an undergraduate dental school (US Department of Health, Education and Welfare, 1968).

There are dental hygienists in many countries, that with the largest number being the United States of America where there are over 20,000 (Federation Dentaire Internationale, 1970). Most are employed in private practices and, in 1964, 19 per cent of practising dentists employed one on a full or part-time basis. Eleven per cent employed a hygienist full time (American Dental Association, 1966).

Young and Striffler (1969) have pointed out that in America a peculiar relation exists between the supply of hygienists and the demand for their services by the dentists. In states with relatively large numbers of hygienists the demand exceeds the supply, whereas in areas with few hygienists this is not the case. The former areas have had hygienists for many more years than the latter. This seems to demonstrate, perhaps without surprise, that as dentists become more accustomed to employing hygienists, so they realize the advantages of so doing and consequently increase their demand for them. This is a different mechanism from that which operates for school dental nurses and dental auxiliaries in other countries; these ancillaries can not be employed by a dentist in private practice, and therefore can not directly influence him. In other words while it is the dental needs of the community that map the way for school dental nurses and dental auxiliaries, this same situation appears not to have existed with regard to some dental hygienists. After a number of years in the field it will be interesting to examine the pattern of employment of the Western Australian dental therapists who are employed by private practitioners (Graebner, 1971).

THE EXPANDED-FUNCTION OPERATING ANCILLARY

In North America ancillaries are being trained to carry out certain restricted restorative procedures on patients. In particular they are taught to undertake such procedures as placing rubber dams and restoring with amalgam and other plastic filling materials teeth that have had cavities prepared by a dentist. The taking of radiographs and making of certain impressions are also undertaken by some of these expanded-function ancillaries.

The procedures delegated to the expanded-function ancillaries exclude diagnosis, treatment planning, the cutting of hard or soft tissues, and the prescription of drugs. This leaves those parts of the dental procedures that have been described as 'reversible' to be carried out by the ancillaries, who must necessarily work with dentists to provide a treatment service. Being reversible, it is considered that parts undertaken by the ancillary could be repeated by the dentist without excessive 'harm' to the patient, in the event of the ancillary's work being of unacceptable quality. This is in keeping with a policy statement by the American Dental Association regarding experimentation in training and utilization of ancillary personnel (American Dental Association, 1962).

Most of the ancillaries who have been instructed in these duties have been trained previously as dental surgery assistants or dental hygienists, and hence the term 'expanded function' has arisen. The first report of this use of dental ancillaries concerned an original piece of research that was undertaken by the Royal Canadian Dental Corps (Baird et al., 1962; Baird et al., 1963). Male dental hygienists were given training to enable them to undertake clinical duties of the type mentioned above.

In the pilot study, one hygienist who had been given four weeks of special additional training was employed. He participated in 75 per cent of 332 dental operations. It was found that he performed dental treatment equivalent to nearly four dentist-hours per six and a half hour working day. This means in effect that the dentist increased his productivity by 61·5 per cent by utilizing this ancillary.

In the main study, three hygienists were provided with sixteen weeks of additional training and then employed in clinics in different parts of the country. It was found that productivity rose on average by 62 per cent when an operating ancillary and a clerical assistant were added to a team consisting of one dentist and two dental surgery assistants. The team operated in three surgeries instead of two. This increase in the size of the team added 34 per cent to the total salary costs.

In 1966 a similar type of study was reported by the United States Navy Dental Corps at Great Lakes, Illinois (Ludwick et al., 1966). However, in this case it was dental surgery assistants whose duties were expanded. They were given an additional seven weeks training course to enable them to undertake the extra duties. Five dentists worked with twelve of the special operating ancillaries in various combinations and with varying numbers of dental chairs. One finding was that a dentist operating with three chairs and delegating the procedures mentioned, could treat twice the number of patients compared to his operating upon just one patient at a time. The quality of the restorations was shown to be similar to that undertaken by control groups of dentists. Quality assessment was carried out by means of peer review by dentists not otherwise connected with the project.

A further study along the same lines was conducted by the Division of Indian Health of the Public Health Service (Abramowitz, 1966). Again, dental surgery assistants were trained to carry out restricted operative procedures and a peer assessment of quality confirmed the findings of the Great Lakes study.

Quality of operative procedures was examined rather more carefully, though in a manner which is still open to criticism, in a project initiated at the University of Alabama in 1963 (Hammons and Jamison, 1967). In this study, five selected young women, none of whom had received any previous dental training, were given a special two-year course of instruction in the 'reversible' operative procedures that were to be studied. The quality of their work was compared to that of senior dental students. Evaluation was made in a double blind manner and according to specific written criteria. For the various aspects evaluated, the proportions of the clinical procedures judged excellent were consistently greater for the operating ancillaries than for the dental students, though overall gradings were comparable. Further work at the University of Alabama (Hammons et al., 1971), confirmed that operating ancillaries carrying out 'reversible' clinical procedures produced work of similar quality to practising dentists and dental school clinical instructors.

A rather more complex study was conducted by the Division of Dental Health, National Institutes of Health, in Louisville, Kentucky (Lotzkar et al., 1971a, 1971b). This study extended over five and a half years and provided dental treatment for 6400 patients. During the course of the project dental surgery assistants were given a one-year training in 'reversible' clinical procedures to enable them to assist dentists who worked in teams with varying numbers of the operating ancillaries. The dentists delegated about two-fifths of their work to the ancillaries. It was found that a dentist's productivity rose about 75 per cent when he worked in a team with three operating ancillaries, and by about 120 per cent when he worked with four of them. Peer assessment of the quality of the work performed by the ancillaries and the dentists showed that both were comparable. It is worth noting, however, that of 27 dental surgery assistants who completed their additional one-year training to become operating ancillaries, 6 failed to achievc sufficiently high quality to be allowed to join the clinical experiment.

As a result of these experimental studies, it is current practice in some parts of North America for dental surgery assistants and hygienists to undertake additional duties to those traditionally assigned to them. In the United States of America state legislation concerning the utilization of dental ancillary personnel is undergoing constant change towards more liberal practice acts (United States Public Health Service, 1970).

The Indian Health Service, which is responsible for the dental health of 403,500 American Indians and Alaska natives, is increasingly teaching its 146 dental surgery assistants to undertake additional 'reversible' operative clinical procedures and the topical application of fluoride (Lathrop, 1971).

In Canada the Armed Forces in some areas train experienced dental hygienists and expand their duties even further than described above. The title dental therapist has been adopted. In addition to the 'reversible' operative procedures described above, these ancillaries are permitted to organize and conduct dental inspections and categorize patients into priority order (Federation Dentaire Internationale, 1972).

In Prince Edward Island, hygienists who have received $2\frac{1}{2}$ months of special training in expanded duties at Dalhousie University, are being employed in six private dental practices in a study conducted by the Island's Department of Health (Canadian Dental Association, 1971). Productivity, cost-benefits, and patient acceptance are being studied.

Expanded function operating ancillaries are not confined to North America. In Costa Rica dental surgery assistants receive one year's training at the University at San José which permits them to place rubber dams, polish in the mouth, and apply fluoride topically (Federation Dentaire Internationale, 1972). They are also instructed in certain laboratory duties including the production of study models, impression trays, and the moulding, casting and polishing of inlays and dentures.

In a much more limited way, Sweden has expanded the functions of some dental surgery assistants by providing two additional weeks of training and allowing them to conduct fluoride mouthrinsing programmes to groups of schoolchildren. These ancillaries are called Dental Health Educators (Federation Dentaire Internationale, 1972). It is interesting to note that in the United Kingdom, Dental Health Education Officers are employed by a number of local authorities to educate in matters of prevention. They are not, however, allowed to undertake any intra-oral procedures and cannot therefore be classified as operating ancillaries. Their training is minimal (British Dental Association, 1968).

EFFECT OF ANCILLARIES ON DENTAL EDUCATION

As dental ancillaries come to be accepted more and more by the dental profession, so their numbers increase and individual dentists have to carry a greater responsibility for them. Accordingly it has been realized in some countries that dental students should be trained to work with ancillaries and begin to accept responsibility for them at an early stage in their undergraduate careers.

With this in mind, in 1961 the United States Public Health Service established the Dental Auxiliary Utilization (DAU) programme (American Dental Association, 1968). Under this scheme, Congress made available until recently sums of money to American dental schools to initiate programmes for training dental students in modern methods of working with dental surgery assistants, including the practice of four-handed dentistry. The scheme was popular and all the dental schools in the country became recipients of grants enabling each to set up a modern (DAU) teaching clinic and to employ trained full-time dental surgery assistants under the guidance of a specially appointed member of the teaching staff. Every dental student in each school spent a minimum of several weeks during his dental training receiving instruction in the DAU clinic. Such teaching is also taking place in undergraduate dental schools in other countries (Purdy, 1966; Nixon and Rowbotham, 1970).

Interest is being shown in some quarters in the need to train dental students to become the leaders of teams which include operating as well as non-operating ancillaries. The student would learn to direct a team so that he could eventually accept the responsibility for working in the field in a similar manner. In Britain, the London Hospital Medical College Dental School has put forward the hypothesis that:

> In the future, dental care will be the responsibility of specifically designed teams whose members will be trained together to combat dental disease on the community scale. The size and composition of each team will be determined by the needs of the community it will serve. The teams will be led by one or more dentists who will have been educated and trained to exercise overall control of patients' care, to diagnose; to prescribe treatment; to check and supervise simple procedures and to carry out only the more complex operations demanding their unique skill and training. (Allred et al., 1972.)

This dental school has already begun to experiment into methods of delivery of dental care with special reference to the role of ancillary personnel as a preliminary to testing this hypothesis (Allred et al., 1973). This project is discussed by Allred in an appendix to this volume.

In the United States of America the Public Health Service has announced a plan to make funds available for teaching dental students to work with, manage and supervise dental health teams comprising both operating and non-operating ancillaries. It is called the Training in Expanded Auxiliary Management (TEAM) programme (United States Public Health Service, 1970). Each dental school in the country is eligible to apply for a TEAM grant. Included in the programme is the facility for training the appropriate dental school supervisory staff in the utilization of expanded function operating ancillaries. Such training takes place at the Dental Manpower Development Center at Louisville, Kentucky.

In describing the TEAM programme, the Public Health Service has stated the following:

> That the practice of four-handed dentistry alone would not increase dentists' productivity sufficiently to keep pace with projected need and demand for dental care has become increasingly evident. Consequently many states have reviewed their dental practice acts for the purpose of redefining the duties of dental auxiliaries [ancillaries]. Such review has led to the expansion of the roles of auxiliaries [ancillaries] in several states. . . . In order to keep pace with these changes within the dental profession, . . . and to encourage further improvements in the use of manpower to provide dental services, the TEAM programme has been established. (United States Public Health Service, 1970.)

On a smaller scale, a project is underway in Colombia at the University of Antioquia to provide ten young women with an eighteen-month course of instruction to enable them to carry out simple operative procedures in children and adults. They will undertake these procedures in patients being cared for by dental students to enable the students to devote more time to other skills (Federation Dentaire Internationale, 1972).

QUESTIONS UNANSWERED

The dental ancillary scene has been described above and certain conclusions concerning ancillaries may be reached after a study of the facts. It should be realized, however, that there are many questions still to be answered before the ultimate role of ancillaries in the delivery of dental care is established.

One of these questions concerns the ancillaries themselves. Are they happy and satisfied workers? Suitable people to train as dental ancillaries are not always easy to find and indeed once trained they do not necessarily function as dental ancillaries for lengthy periods. For example in 1970, of the 423 United Kingdom dental auxiliaries who have graduated from New Cross General Hospital since 1962, only 205 were registered with the General Dental Council (Federation Dentaire Internationale, 1970). While some of the others have married and ceased to work for this reason, many others have failed to find suitable employment as auxiliaries and taken other work. Manning (1971) has stated that heavy resistance from the dental profession is the main reason. If true, then perhaps the role of the dental auxiliary should be redefined or her training and conditions of employment changed. While these remarks have been made specifically about United Kingdom dental auxiliaries, they may also apply to other types of ancillary dental worker.

Another question involves the patients themselves. This important factor has received very little attention and yet must be of great importance. What are their reactions to dental care when ancillary personnel are involved? Do they like it? Do they prefer one type of ancillary or dental team to another? Do they feel that they are being looked after competently? Do the answers to these questions affect the response of the patient to dental care? Each of these questions requires an answer before firm decisions regarding ancillary personnel can be made.

Another fundamental issue about which little is known concerns quality of dental care. This has only received minimal attention to date and the role of the ancillary in quality control has not been defined. While most of the experiments in ancillary personnel utilization have been concerned to some extent with the quality of the care being provided, much more thorough investigation is required. It is not sufficient simply to make peer assessments of technical excellence for this is only a small part of the whole picture that has to be built up.

It is clear that much sound research is required in the broad field of dental care delivery. First though, it will be necessary to define the tasks that have to be undertaken in order to deliver total dental care on a community scale, and then to define the precise roles that ancillary personnel should play in this delivery. These definitions are likely to differ from country to country, and will therefore need to be reached within the social and cultural context of each individual society.

LOOKING TO THE FUTURE

With the problems and unknowns that have been discussed, it is difficult to predict how dental ancillaries will be employed in the future. As more experimental results come forth and more experience is gained, it seems likely that ideas will clarify and that ancillaries will come to be utilized in a less haphazard manner than is currently the case. As advances are made in aspects of prevention and control of dental disease, so ancillary utilization will have to change to keep pace with the developments. The recipients of dental care will have to decide how important they feel this care to be, in terms of how much they are prepared to pay for it. If political pressures to provide care are not accompanied by adequate financial support, then there is the danger that decisions will be made that allow premature development of dental services without proper control by those responsible, ultimately the dental profession.

Whatever events take place, it is essential that those people who plan and organize dental care services should be aware of the problems that exist, and are able to relate them to their own particular situations. Only if this is the case will wise decisions be made regarding the utilization of dental ancillary personnel and real dental care be available, eventually, to all communities in the world.

REFERENCES

ABRAMOWITZ, J. (1966), 'Expanded functions for dental assistants: a preliminary study', *J. Am. dent. Ass.*, **72,** 386.

ALLRED, H., DUCKWORTH, R., JOHNSON, N. W., and SLACK, G. L. (1972), 'Proposals for planned change in dental education and practice', *Br. dent. J.*, **133,** 1.

—— HOBDELL, M. H., and ELDERTON, R. J. (1973), 'The establishment of an experimental dental care project', *Ibid.*, **135,** 205.

AMERICAN DENTAL ASSOCIATION (1962), *Increasing the Efficiency of Dental Practice: Proceedings of the Workshop on the Future Requirements of Dental Manpower and the Training and Utilization of Auxiliary Personnel.* Ann Arbor: University of Michigan.

——— (1966), 'Bureau of Economic Research and Statistics. Survey of dental practice; IV. Professional expenses, auxiliary personnel', *J. Am. dent. Ass.*, **72,** 1181.

——— COUNCIL ON DENTAL EDUCATION, THE DIVISION OF DENTAL HEALTH, UNITED STATES PUBLIC HEALTH SERVICE (1968), 'The Dental Auxiliary Utilization Program', *Ibid.*, **76,** 953.

BAIRD, K. M., PURDY, E. C., and PROTHEROE, D. H. (1963), 'Pilot study on advanced training and employment of auxiliary dental personnel in the Royal Canadian Dental Corps: Final Report', *J. Can. dent. Ass.*, **29,** 778.

—— SHILLINGTON, G. B., and PROTHEROE, D. H. (1962), 'Pilot study on advanced training and employment of auxiliary dental personnel in the Royal Canadian Dental Corps: Preliminary Report', *Ibid.*, **28,** 627.

BERMAN, D. S. (1964), 'Dental auxiliaries: New Zealand—Federation of Malaya—United Kingdom', *Br. dent. J.*, **117,** 95.

—— (1966), 'The role of dental auxiliaries in child dental health', *Dent. Practnr dent. Rec.*, **16,** 360.

BRITISH DENTAL ASSOCIATION (1968), 'Dental ancillary personnel: Report of the Ancillary Personnel Committee of the British Dental Association', *Br. dent. J.*, supplement, **124,** 1.

——— (1969), 'Advice to dental surgeons directing dental auxiliaries', *Ibid.*, **126,** 41.

CANADIAN DENTAL ASSOCIATION (1971), 'Prince Edward Island dental manpower study', *J. Can. dent. Ass.*, **37,** 50.

DAVIES, G. N. (1971), personal communication.

DEPARTMENT OF LABOUR AND NATIONAL SERVICE (1970), *Dentists: Professional and Technical Manpower Study No. 1.* Melbourne: Department of Labour and National Service.

FEDERATION DENTAIRE INTERNATIONALE (1970), *Basic Fact Sheets.*

——— (1972), *Basic Fact Sheets.*

FONES, A. C. (1926), *The Origin and History of the Dental Hygienist Movement.* Philadelphia: Proceedings of the Seventh International Dental Congress.

FULTON, J. T. (1951), *Experiment in Dental Care.* Geneva: WHO. Monograph Series No. 4.

GRAEBNER, A. (1971), 'Dental therapists. Australian Dental Association, W.A. Branch', *Dent. Bull.*, **13,** 3.

GRUEBBEL, A. O. (1950), *A Study of Dental Public Health Services in New Zealand.* Chicago: American Dental Association.

HAMMONS, P. E., and JAMISON, H. C. (1967), 'Expanded functions for dental auxiliaries', *J. Am. dent. Ass.*, **75,** 658.

—— —— and WILSON, L. L. (1971), 'Quality of service provided by dental therapists in an experimental program at the University of Alabama', *Ibid.*, **82,** 1060.

KLEIN, H. (1944), 'Civilian dentistry in wartime', *J. Am. dent. Ass.*, **31,** 648.

LATHROP, R. L. (1971), 'Expanded functions from the perspective of dental assistants of the Indian Health Service', *Ibid.*, **82,** 591.

LESLIE, G. H. (1971), *School Dental Service; New Zealand 1921–1971.* Wellington: Shearer.

LOTZKAR, S., JOHNSON, D. W., and THOMPSON, M. B. (1971a), 'Experimental program in expanded functions for dental assistants: Phase 1; base line, and phase 2; training', *J. Am. dent. Ass.*, **82,** 101.

——————(1971b), 'Experimental program in expanded functions for dental assistants: phase 3; experiment with dental teams', *Ibid.*, **82,** 1067.

LUDWICK, W. E., SCHNOEBELEN, E. O., and KNOEDLER, D. J. (1966), 'Greater utilization of dental technicians', Presented before the 17th National Dental Health Conference, American Dental Association.

MANNING, J. E. (1971), 'Dental ancillaries for the 70's; A personal view', *Br. dent. J.*, **131,** 413.

NIXON, G. S., and ROWBOTHAM, T. C. (1970), 'Student teaching with chairside assistance', *Ibid.*, **129,** 214.

PURDY, C. E. (1966), *Student Training in the Utilization of Dental Assistants at the Faculty of Dentistry.* University of Toronto: Summer report.

UNITED KINGDOM DENTAL MISSION (1950), *New Zealand School Dental Nurses.* London: HMSO.

UNITED STATES DEPARTMENT OF HEALTH, EDUCATION AND WELFARE: PUBLIC HEALTH SERVICE (1968), *Health Resources Statistics, 1968.* Washington, DC: Public Health Service Publication No. 1509.

————————————(1970), *Objectives and Guidelines for the TEAM Program.* Bethesda. Mimeograph.

WORLD HEALTH ORGANIZATION (1959), *Expert Committee on Auxiliary Dental Personnel.* Geneva: WHO Tech. Rep. Ser. No. 163.

——— (1968), *Inter-Regional Seminar on the Training and Utilization of Dental Personnel in Developing Countries.* New Delhi, Dec. 1967. Geneva: WHO. Mimeograph.

YOUNG, W. O., and STRIFFLER, D. F. (1969), *The Dentist, his Practice, and his Community*, 2nd ed. Philadelphia: Saunders.

Chapter 10

Statistical Principles in the Analysis of Dental Data

John Osborn PHD
Lecturer in Medical Demography, The London School of Hygiene and Tropical Medicine

Epidemiology has been established as a fundamental aspect of the delivery of dental services and correct interpretation of epidemiological data requires some knowledge of statistical procedures.

In this chapter, Dr. Osborn discusses the place of statistics in epidemiological research. He then presents a number of principles and methods used in the conversion of field observations into data which can be applied to dental service administration.

INTRODUCTION

Statistics is a relatively new branch of mathematics which is finding increasing application in the study of community health. Statistical principles have been used in the design and execution of medical research projects for many years, but workers in dental public health have, perhaps, only more recently recognized the benefits to be derived from their use.

The subject, statistics, involves the quantitative study of aggregates. Its principles and methodology should be considered throughout an investigation from the design of the experiment or survey, the recording of observations, the sorting and the presentation of the data, the calculation of descriptive characteristics such as averages and proportions, to the inferences made from the results.

For example, suppose it is required to investigate the cariostatic action of a new dentifrice. Should the children on whom the dentifrice is to be tested be of a given age, sex, race, and social class, or should the test group be matched to a control group as closely as possible? How are the children to be chosen for inclusion in the survey? How is cariostatic action of the dentifrice to be measured? If by DMFS scores, how precisely are these to be defined? What checks will be kept on examiner error and examiner consistency? When the record cards for each child are complete, the observations must be classified, tables constructed, and graphs and histograms drawn in order to reduce the bulk of the data to a summary form.

Perhaps most important is the use of statistical reasoning to provide objective methods for drawing conclusions from observations. For example, if the experimental dentifrice is supplied to a sample of 20 children and their average annual DMFS increment is smaller than that of a control group, can it be concluded that the dentifrice will have a beneficial effect on all children? With a sample of only 20 children the conclusions must be doubtful but what is a reasonable sample size: 100, 1000, or 10,000 children? What can be concluded from the magnitude of the reduction of increment? DMFS increments vary considerably between children and thus sample means will differ irrespective of the dentifrice used. Is the increment for the test group within the range that could be expected merely as a result of sampling fluctuations? If it is, little can be said of the beneficial effect of the new dentifrice.

Thus the subject biostatistics has a very wide field of application, the whole of which cannot be covered here. This chapter is, of necessity, only a brief introduction to the subject and will only consider some of the basic principles. For discussion of topics not included here and for greater detail, reference can be made to other textbooks on biostatistics. some of which are listed at the end of the chapter.

The subject will be discussed under these headings:

1. Histograms and graphs.
2. Descriptive statistics.
3. Sample means and proportions.
4. Pairs of observations.
5. Sample survey design.
6. Summary.

HISTOGRAMS AND GRAPHS

The subject, statistics, is essentially concerned with the study of variability and the diagram most often used to display variability is the histogram. For example, the age at which edentulous people lost their last tooth varies from person to person. This conclusion is reached by observing the frequency distribution of the ages at which a sample of edentulous persons lost their last teeth, such as that in Table 1.

A frequency distribution is a statement of the number of observations counted in each class, where in this example the classes are the age groups 11–15, 16–19, 20–24, and so on.

At first sight, to draw a histogram of these data presents no problem if the observed frequency is plotted vertically and age horizontally, as in *Fig.* 1A. However, this diagram is misleading. It implies that the

TABLE 1

The age at which respondents to a survey of an edentulous population lost their last tooth

Age	*No. of respondents*	*Class width (yr.)*	*Average no. per year of age*
11–15	1	5	0·20
16–19	7	4	1·75
20–24	21	5	4·20
25-29	35	5	7·00
30–34	40	5	8·00
35–44	58	10	5·80
45–54	28	10	2·80
55–74	10	20	0·50

most likely age for an edentulous person to have lost his last tooth is around 40 years, even though this column is tallest merely because this class width (age range) is ten years while others are only 5 years.

When the class widths of the frequency distribution are not all equal, if the histogram is to describe the distribution of ages realistically the

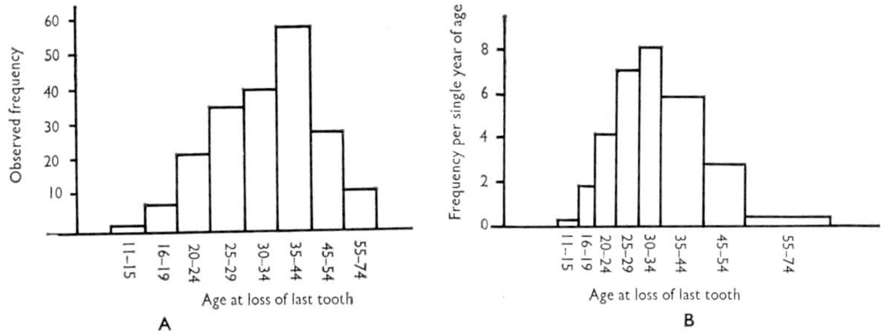

Fig. 1. Histogram showing age at loss of last tooth, of respondents in a survey of an edentulous population. A, Wrong method. B, Correct method.

observed frequencies must be adjusted. Thus, in Table 1, the final two columns show the class widths (in years) and the average frequency per single year of age. If these values are used to draw the histogram as in *Fig.* 1B, it can be seen that, in fact, the most likely age for an edentulous person to have lost his last tooth is between 30 and 34 years not 35–44 years.

The histogram in *Fig*. 1B has been drawn with the number of persons per single year of age plotted vertically. It is not essential that the average per *single* year is taken. Indeed, in this example to plot the average number per 5-year interval would involve less calculation. Thus for each 5-year interval the observed frequency could be plotted but frequencies in the 10-year and 20-year intervals would be halved and quartered respectively. In the 4-year interval, the observed frequency would be increased by a factor 5/4. The base for the average, or as it is commonly called, the unit class width, can take any value, one year as plotted, 5 years, or whatever is considered convenient, always provided that all the averages are calculated using the same unit class width.

It can be seen, therefore, that when histograms with unequal class widths are drawn, the *frequency per unit class interval* must be plotted

TABLE 2

The decline of two imaginary incidence rates A and B 1961–70

Year	*Rate A per 1000*	*Absolute decrease*	*Rate B per 1000*	*Absolute decrease*	*Percentage decrease*
1961	92	—	100·0	—	—
1962	82	10	80·0	20·0	20
1963	72	10	64·0	16·0	20
1964	62	10	51·2	12·8	20
1965	52	10	40·6	10·6	20
1966	42	10	32·5	8·1	20
1967	32	10	26·0	6·5	20
1968	22	10	20·8	5·2	20
1969	12	10	16·6	4·2	20
1970	2	10	13·3	3·3	20

vertically, rather than just the observed frequency. This gives the histogram an important property: the observed frequency in each class is proportional to the area of the column, not the height. There are several reasons why this is important, but since the eye associates frequency with the size of the blocks rather than just the height, the histogram will not give a misleading impression.

Graphs Two kinds of graphs are commonly used to display trends in observed data; the first, in which both axes of the graph have simple arithmetic scales is the most usual and needs little introduction. The second kind has its vertical axis calibrated with a logarithmic scale.

A graph drawn on ordinary arithmetic graph paper will be a straight line if the absolute change per unit interval is constant. Thus the first column of Table 2 shows a series of incidence rates A, decreasing each year by 10 per 1000. It is often the case that it is of greater importance to consider proportionate changes, and the incidence rates B in Table 2 decline by 20 per cent every year.

If these rates are plotted on arithmetic graph paper as in *Fig*. 2, the graph for rate A is a straight line whereas that for B is curved.

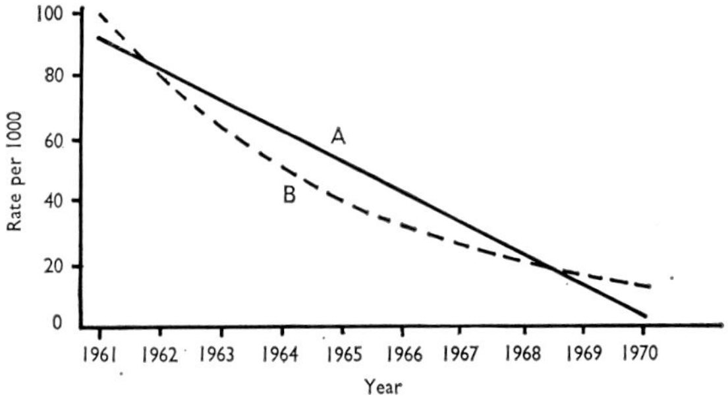

Fig. 2. Incidence rates A and B plotted on an arithmetic grid.

If it is of particular interest to study proportionate changes, it is useful to plot the rates in such a way that for a constant proportional change a straight line is obtained. This is achieved by the use of semi-logarithmic graph paper which has its vertical axis marked with a logarithmic scale. Some examples of logarithmic scales are shown in *Fig*. 3 and it should be noted that a logarithmic scale can never reach zero.

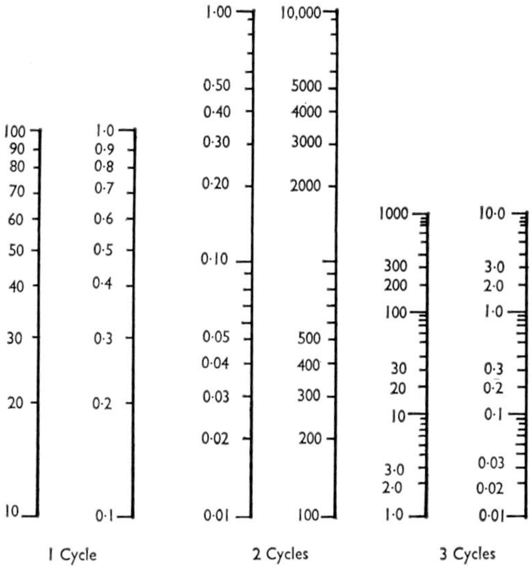

Fig. 3. Some examples of logarithmic scales.

Thus, if rate B (from Table 2) is plotted on a semi-logarithmic grid as in *Fig*. 4, a straight line is obtained.

Plotting graphs on semi-logarithmic graph paper is particularly useful for comparing the proportionate change in two or more series of observations since the slopes of the graphs show which series has the greater proportionate change. If the proportionate changes are equal the graphs will be parallel.

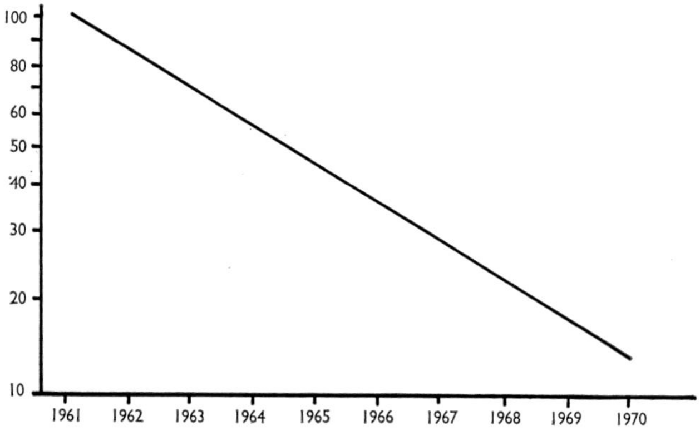

Fig. 4. Incidence rate B plotted with a logarithmic vertical scale.

For example, suppose it is required to compare graphically the expenditure by the central government on general medical services with that on general dental services, during the financial years 1963–4 to 1969–70. The expenditure on these two Services for these years is shown in Table 3.

TABLE 3

Expenditure (*£millions*) *by central government on National Health Service for general medical services and general dental services 1963–4 to 1969–70* (*Annual Abstract of Statistics No. 107 1970, Central Statistical Office, HMSO 1970*)

	1963–4	*1964–5*	*1965–6*	*1966–7*	*1967–8*	*1968–9*	*1969–70*
General medical services	93·5	94·5	104·4	111·8	130·1	137·7	147·7
General dental services	54·0	56·3	57·9	66·8	68·9	69·9	76·3

If these expenditures are plotted on arithmetic graph paper as in *Fig.* 5A, the absolute increase in expenditure is seen to be greater for the general medical services. This is not surprising since the expenditure on general medical services is higher than that on general dental services and the absolute change of the larger expenditure will be naturally greater than the absolute change of the smaller. If, however, the expenditure is plotted on a logarithmic scale as in *Fig.* 5B, it can be seen that, since the two graphs are roughly parallel, the proportionate increases in expenditure on the services are approximately equal.

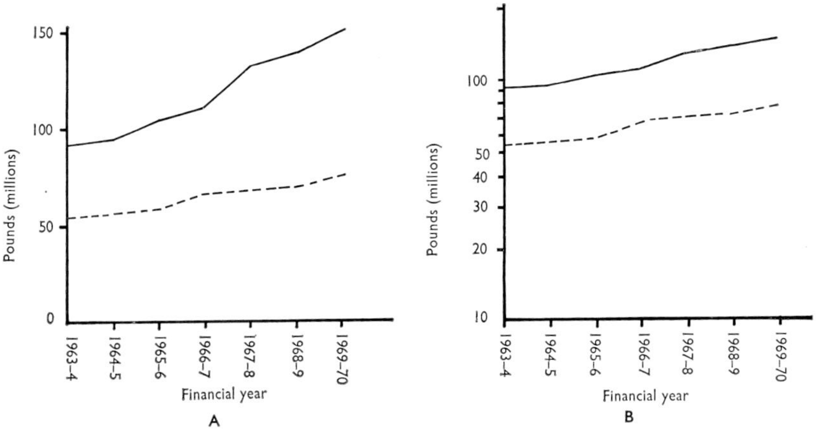

Fig. 5. The expenditure by the central government on the National Health Service for general medical services and general dental services 1963–4 to 1969–70. A, Arithmetic vertical scale. B, Logarithmic vertical scale.

Misleading Diagrams Most statistical diagrams can be misleading if they are constructed incorrectly. Table 4 shows the number of patients treated each year at a dental clinic between 1960 and 1969.

TABLE 4

Number of patients treated per year at a dental clinic

Year	1960	1961	1962	1963	1964
Number of patients	20,000	20,000	20,200	20,500	20,900
Year	1965	1966	1967	1968	1969
Number of patients	21,500	22,200	23,000	24,200	26,000

Figs. 6 and 7 show graphs of these data. However, *Fig.* 6 grossly exaggerates the increase in patients treated because the vertical scale starts at 18,000 patients. If the vertical scale includes zero, the gradual increase in the number of patients treated each year is apparent.

Sometimes pressure of space precludes the use of the complete vertical scale. In such situations it is possible to exclude part of the scale but when the graph is drawn in this way it is essential to draw the attention of the reader to the omitted part of the scale by drawing a zig-zag on the axis.

A graph can also become distorted if the scale on one axis is over-expanded or contracted compared with the other. *Figs.* 8 and 9 show graphs of the same data of patients attending a clinic given in Table 4.

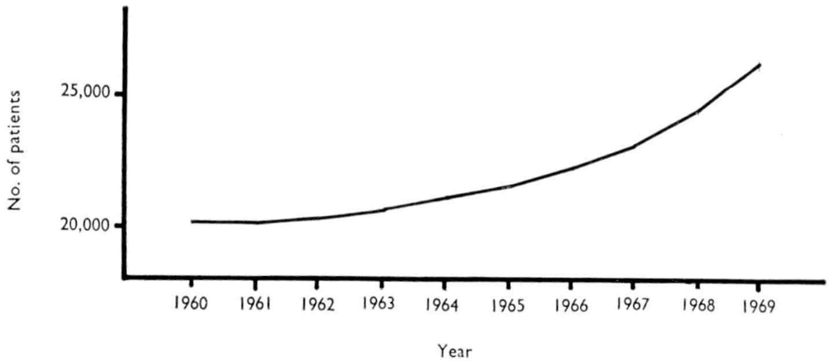

Fig. 6. The number of patients treated per year at a dental clinic 1960–9.

In *Fig.* 8, the vertical scale has been exaggerated and the zero point is omitted, while the horizontal time scale is compressed. The resulting graph implies a rapidly increasing annual number of patients. On the other hand, *Fig.* 9 shows the same data but in this case the vertical scale

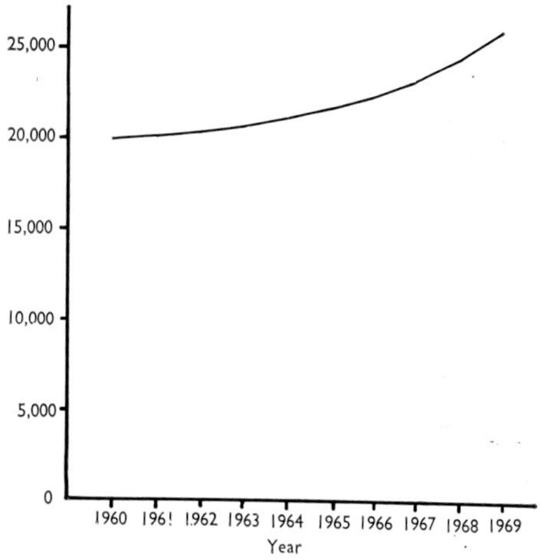

Fig. 7. The number of patients treated per year at a dental clinic 1960–9.

is compressed and the horizontal time scale is expanded, giving the impression that the trend is negligible. The graphs shown in *Figs.* 8 and 9 are both misleading and while it is difficult to give a rule of thumb about scales which is applicable to all graphs, in general they should occupy an area which is approximately square.

When constructing or interpreting graphs and histograms the following points should be considered:

1. A graph or histogram is a pictorial aid to the presentation of observed data. All detailed information is lost and hence a graph cannot be a substitute for a full analysis.

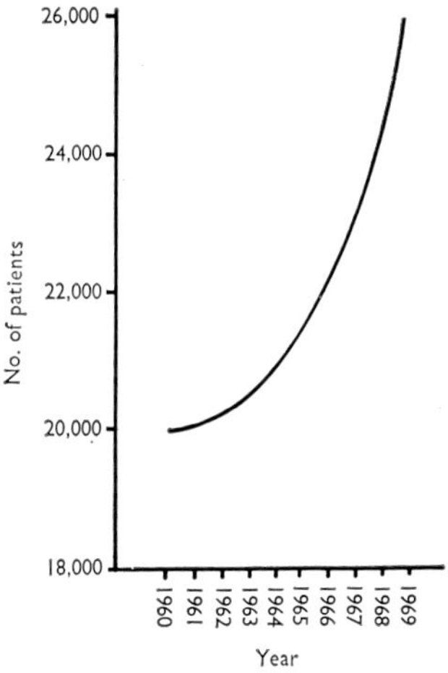

Fig. 8. The number of patients treated per year at a dental clinic 1960–9.

2. Graphs and histograms can be misleading especially if an arithmetic vertical scale does not start at zero or if one scale is very over-expanded compared to the other.

3. When interpreting graphs it is advisable to calculate the approximate magnitude of any trend before drawing conclusions.

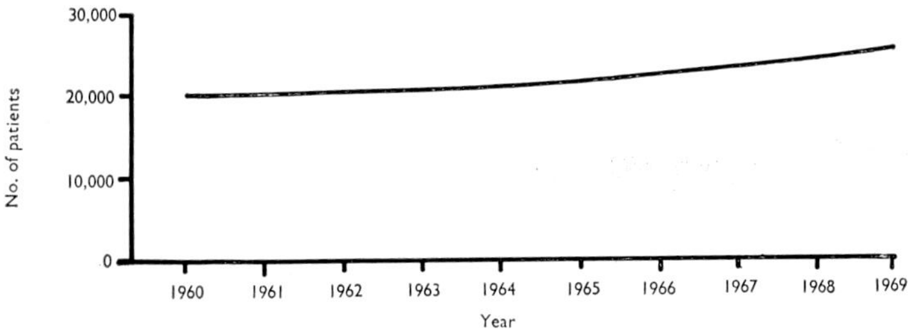

Fig. 9. The number of patients treated per year.

4. The axes of a graph should be clearly labelled and the scales should be marked.

5. A graph can only describe situations which occur within the range of the observations. Extrapolating a graph and using it to predict values

outside the range of the observations can at worst be grossly misleading, and at best little more than a reasonable guess.

DESCRIPTIVE STATISTICS

The use of sampling is not confined to estimating averages. If the sample is randomly selected, it should resemble the parent population in other respects, for example, in the variability of the measurements. Descriptive statistics are calculated and used to measure attributes of distributions, particularly the magnitude of the observations and their variability. If the distribution is plotted as a histogram, the position or location of the distribution on the scale of the horizontal axis determines the general magnitude of the observations and the dispersion of the observations within the distribution indicates their variability.

THE ARITHMETIC MEAN AND THE MEDIAN

The most useful measures of position or location are the arithmetic mean, or ordinary average value of the observations and the median. The *arithmetic mean* of a series of observations is calculated by adding up the values of the observations and dividing this total by the number of observations. The median is defined to be the middle observation when the values are listed in ascending order of magnitude. When the number of observations is even, there is strictly no middle observation and the median is defined as the average of the two middle values.

The arithmetic mean is the most commonly used measure of position but in some circumstances, particularly where a few observations are very much larger, or very much smaller, than the rest, it can give a result which is not typical of the observations. For example, the following observations represent the waiting time (in minutes) of 10 patients at a surgery: 2, 0, 0, 3, 3, 2, 0, 5, 55, 60. The sum of the waiting time is 130 minutes and hence the mean waiting time is 13 minutes. This mean waiting time is not typical of the observations because the two large values give much weight to the total sum of the observations. On the other hand, if the observations are arranged in order of magnitude—0, 0, 0, 2, 2, 3, 3, 5, 55, 60—the median (since the number of observations, 10, is even) is the average of the fifth and sixth value, that is $\frac{2+3}{2} = 2\frac{1}{2}$.

Thus the median, in this extreme example, gives a more typical value than the mean. In general, however, the mean is the preferable measure of position because it uses all the information from the observations. The median only considers the middle of the distribution and takes no account of the precise values of the rest of the observations.

THE RANGE, VARIANCE, AND STANDARD DEVIATION

The range is the difference between the largest and smallest observation in a sample, but because most of the information contained in the sample is ignored it is seldom used analytically as a measure of variability.

A more efficient approach to the measurement of dispersion is to consider the difference between each observation and the arithmetic mean. These deviations from the mean will tend to be large if the observations are very spread out and small if they are not, but it is of no help to consider the average value of the deviations, since the differences less than zero obtained from observations smaller than the mean cancel out the positive differences. If the deviations are squared this problem does not arise and the mean of the squared deviations is called the *variance*. Theoretical considerations show that in fact a better estimate of the population variance is obtained if, instead of dividing the sum of squared deviations by the number of observations, say n, it is divided by $n-1$. Algebraically, if there are n observations:

$x_1, x_2, x_3, \ldots x_n$ and the mean of these is $\bar{x}$, the sample variance, s^2 is

$$s^2 = \frac{(x_1 - \bar{x})^2 + (x_2 - \bar{x})^2 + (x_3 - \bar{x})^2 + \ldots + (x_n - \bar{x})^2}{n-1}$$

$$= \frac{\Sigma(x - \bar{x})^2}{n-1} = \frac{\Sigma x^2 - n\,\bar{x}^2}{n-1}.$$

The divisor, $n - 1$, in the estimate of variance is called the 'degrees of freedom', and is the number of independent items of information which exist in the observations. In this example if the mean is known, all the information is contained in $n - 1$ of the observations since the final observation can be calculated from the others.

The units of variance are the square of the units of the observations. It is useful to have a measure of the spread of a distribution which has the same units as the original observations and the square root of the variance is usually calculated. The square root of the variance is called the *standard deviation*. Some idea of the practical meaning of the standard deviation can be obtained by consideration of the *normal distribution*. The normal distribution is a mathematical ideal which is used as a model for distributions found in practice; it is symmetrical about the mean and is bell-shaped.

For example, the distribution of respondent's age at loss of last tooth, whose histogram is shown in *Fig.* 1, is reproduced in *Fig.* 10 with a normal distribution curve drawn around it. The observed distribution does not fit the mathematical ideal exactly, but for descriptive purposes at least, the distribution of respondent's age at loss of last tooth is said to be approximately normal.

This mathematical ideal, the normal distribution, also has the following very important properties, while for the observed distributions which approach this ideal these properties are approximate:

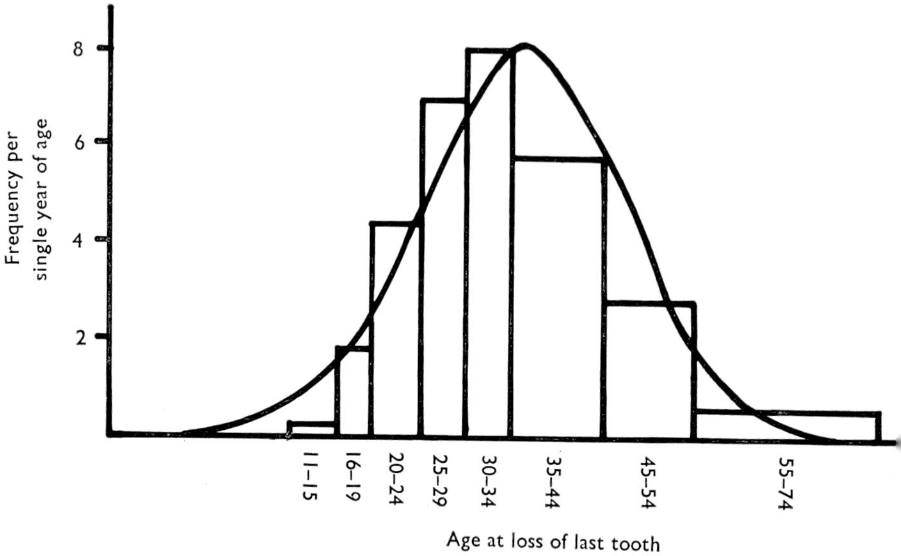

Fig. 10. Histogram showing age at loss of last tooth of respondents to a survey of an edentulous population with the normal distribution superimposed.

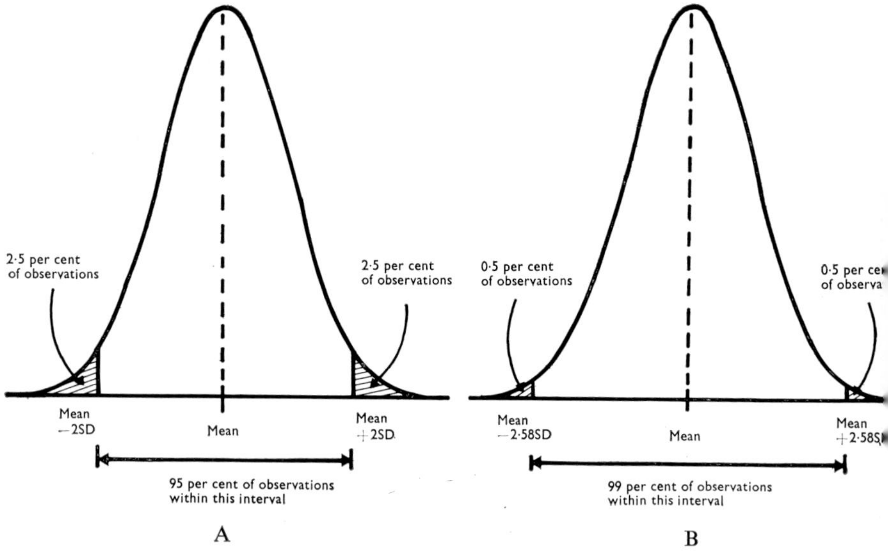

Fig. 11. The normal distribution. A, Five per cent of observations are more than 2 standard deviations from the mean. B, One per cent of observations are more than 2·58 standard deviations from the mean.

1. About 95 per cent of the observations lie within the interval: mean ± 2 standard deviations (more precisely, mean $\pm 1{\cdot}96$ standard deviations).

2. About 99 per cent of the observations lie within the interval: mean $\pm 2\frac{1}{2}$ standard deviations (more precisely, mean $\pm 2{\cdot}58$ standard deviations).

These intervals with a normal distribution are shown in *Fig.* 11 A, B. Distributions with larger standard deviations are flatter and more spread out, while distributions with smaller standard deviations are taller and more narrow.

SAMPLE MEANS AND PROPORTIONS

Suppose a sample of n observations is taken from a population whose values (e.g., DMFS scores) form a distribution with mean μ and variance σ^2 (i.e., the standard deviation is σ). It is unlikely that the sample mean $\bar{x}$ will equal μ exactly and if a second sample of n observations is taken a slightly different value of the sample mean may be obtained. If this procedure of taking samples of n observations were continued a series of sample means would result. What can be said about the distribution of sample means? Statistical theory can prove the following:

1. The sample means tend to be normally distributed even if the original observations, here the DMFS scores, are not normally distributed.

2. The mean of the distribution of sample means is μ the mean of the population of original observations.

3. The variance of the sample means is σ^2/n and hence the standard deviation of the sample means is $\sigma/\sqrt{n}$. To avoid confusion with the standard deviation of the original observations (DMFS scores), the standard deviation of the sample means is called the *standard error of the mean* and is written as $\mathrm{SE}(\bar{x})$.

Since the distribution of the sample means tends to follow the normal distribution, 95 per cent of the observations of $\bar{x}$ lie within the interval $\mu \pm 1{\cdot}96\ \mathrm{SE}(\bar{x})$ and 99 per cent within $\mu \pm 2{\cdot}58\ \mathrm{SE}(\bar{x})$. In practice only one sample of n observations is taken and one value of $\bar{x}$ is found and it can be argued that there is a 95 per cent chance that this sample mean will lie within the interval $\mu \pm 1{\cdot}96\ \mathrm{SE}(\bar{x})$. Alternatively, there is 95 per cent confidence that the interval $\bar{x} \pm 1{\cdot}96\ \mathrm{SE}(\bar{x})$ will include the true mean μ. Similarly there is 99 per cent confidence that the interval $\bar{x} \pm 2{\cdot}58\ \mathrm{SE}(\bar{x})$ will include μ. These intervals are called 95 per cent and 99 per cent confidence intervals for the true mean and are statements of the maximum likely error of the sample estimate, $\bar{x}$, of the population mean. The chance that the error in the sample estimate will exceed $\pm 1{\cdot}96\ \mathrm{SE}(\bar{x})$ is 5 per cent and $\pm 2{\cdot}58\ \mathrm{SE}(\bar{x})$ is 1 per cent.

TESTING HYPOTHESES

The first problem of importance when considering the results of a survey is the accuracy of the sample estimates. For example, how close is the sample mean $\bar{x}$ to the population mean μ? This question is answered, at least in terms of the maximum *likely* error by consideration of confidence intervals.

A second problem is that of *comparison* of the sample estimate with previously obtained results. For example, previous experience may suggest that the population mean should be some particular value, say μ_0. Are the results of a sample survey, with sample mean $\bar{x}$, consistent with this prior information? Or is the observed difference between $\bar{x}$ and μ_0 so great as to suggest that the sample was *not* taken from a population with mean μ_0 but some other population with unknown mean μ?

This problem of comparison of results is investigated by consideration of a *null hypothesis*. In the above example the null hypothesis would be that the difference between μ_0 and μ is zero and the observed difference between $\bar{x}$ and μ_0 is merely the result of taking a sample.

Thus, suppose it is required to investigate the hypothesis that the mean value, μ, of a population is some particular value say μ_0. If a sample of n observations is taken from the population and the sample mean $\bar{x}$ is calculated 95 per cent confidence limits for the true mean are $\bar{x} \pm 1{\cdot}96$ SE($\bar{x}$). If the hypothesis that the population mean, μ, is μ_0 is true, there is a 95 per cent chance that this confidence interval will include μ_0.

If μ_0 is not included in the confidence interval, either (1) the hypothesis that the population mean is μ_0 is true and the sample mean has an error which is exceeded rarely, i.e., in one sample out of 20, or (2), the hypothesis is false; the population mean is not μ_0.

Of these alternatives, it is concluded that (2) probably occurred since the chance of (1) occurring is small (5 per cent). If (2) is accepted, the difference between $\bar{x}$ and μ_0 is said to be significantly different to zero. Equivalently, the normal deviate, which is the ratio of a difference to its error is calculated. Thus if $(\bar{x} - \mu_0)/\mathrm{SE}(\bar{x})$ is greater than 1·96 or less than −1·96 the difference is significant at the 5 per cent level. Similarly if the normal deviate exceeds 2·58 or is less than −2·58 the difference is significant at the 1 per cent level.

THE *t* TEST

The t test is a refinement of the normal deviate test. To calculate the normal deviate it is necessary to know the population standard deviation, σ, since the $\mathrm{SE}(\bar{x}) = \sigma/\sqrt{n}$. In general σ is not known and s, the standard deviation of the sampled observations is used in its place. When the sample size is large, s will approximate closely to σ and the test will not be affected, but if the sample is small, this substitution may make the normal deviate test unreliable. If σ is replaced by s in the normal deviate formula another value, say t, is obtained. Thus:

$$t = \frac{\bar{x} - \mu_0}{s/\sqrt{n}}.$$

Now the normal deviate is compared with the critical values 1·96 and 2·58 for the 5 per cent and 1 per cent levels of significance respectively. The critical values for t depend on the number of observations, or more precisely the degrees of freedom, used to estimate σ by s. Here s is estimated with $n - 1$ degrees of freedom.

Thus to test the hypothesis that the population mean is a particular value μ_0, t is calculated from the above formula and if this exceeds the critical value at the 5 per cent or 1 per cent level given in Table 5, the hypothesis is rejected at that level.

TABLE 5

Critical values of t at the 5 per cent and 1 per cent levels of significance

Degrees of freedom	*Critical values of t at 5 per cent level*	*Critical values of t at 1 per cent level*	*Degrees of freedom*	*Critical values of t at 5 per cent level*	*Critical values of t at 1 per cent level*
1	12·71	63·66	10	2·23	3·17
2	4·30	9·92	12	2·18	3·05
3	3·18	5·84	15	2·13	2·95
4	2·78	4·60	20	2·09	2·85
5	2·57	4·03	24	2·06	2·80
6	2·45	3·71	30	2·04	2·75
7	2·36	3·50	40	2·02	2·70
8	2·31	3·36	60	2·00	2·66
9	2·26	3·25	120	1·98	2·62
			∞	1·96	2·58

The normal deviate test is a particular case of the t test. As the degrees of freedom increase, so the critical values of t get closer to those of the normal deviate. With infinite degrees of freedom (that is where σ is known exactly) the critical values of t are equal to those of the normal deviate.

When σ is unknown, confidence intervals for the true mean are calculated using the critical values of t in place of the normal deviate values 1·96 and 2·58. Thus writing the critical values of t with $n - 1$ degrees of freedom as t (5 per cent, $n - 1$) and t (1 per cent, $n - 1$) for the 5 per cent and 1 per cent levels respectively, confidence intervals for the true mean are

$$\bar{x} \pm t(5 \text{ per cent}, n - 1)\ \mathrm{SE}(\bar{x})$$

and

$$\bar{x} \pm t(1 \text{ per cent}, n - 1)\ \mathrm{SE}(\bar{x})$$

for 95 per cent and 99 per cent confidence respectively.

COMPARISON OF TWO SAMPLE MEANS

A common problem which arises in research projects is the consideration of the mean responses to two different treatments. Here, the word treatment does not necessarily mean that of a dentist to his patient, but it is used in its broadest sense. Thus any specific procedure applied to experimental units may be called a treatment. For example, it may be required to compare the mean DMFS increments after a period of time in two groups of children who have been using different dentifrices. In an experiment to compare the abrasiveness of two denture cleaners, the mean weight loss in samples of dentures which have been cleaned may be compared.

Sample means are compared by considering the difference between them and investigating the hypothesis that the difference between the population means is zero. Thus if the hypothesis is true the observed difference between the sample means is merely the result of random sampling fluctuations. On the other hand if the difference is large the validity of the hypothesis may be doubted.

The normal deviate test or t test can be applied to test this hypothesis. Where before, $\bar{x}$, the sample mean was compared with a hypothetical value μ_0, here $\bar{x}$ is replaced by the difference between two sample means say $\bar{x}_1 - \bar{x}_2$ and μ_0, the hypothetical difference is zero. Thus the ratio of the difference to its standard error is

$$\frac{(\bar{x}_1 - \bar{x}_2) - 0}{\mathrm{SE}(\bar{x}_1 - \bar{x}_2)}.$$

Some difficulty is experienced here since the standard error of a difference is required. Statistical theory can show that the *variance* of a difference is equal to the *sum* of the individual variances. Thus

$$\text{variance } (\bar{x}_1 - \bar{x}_2) = \text{variance } (\bar{x}_1) + \text{variance } (\bar{x}_2).$$

If the variance of the population values in group 1 is $\sigma_1{}^2$, and group 2 is $\sigma_2{}^2$ then the variances of the sample means $\bar{x}_1$ and $\bar{x}_2$ are $\frac{\sigma_1{}^2}{n_1}$ and $\frac{\sigma_2{}^2}{n_2}$, where n_1 and n_2 are the two samples sizes. Thus

$$\text{variance } (\bar{x}_1 - \bar{x}_2) = \frac{\sigma_1{}^2}{n_1} + \frac{\sigma_2{}^2}{n_2}$$

and hence the standard error is

$$\mathrm{SE}(\bar{x}_1 - \bar{x}_2) = \sqrt{\frac{\sigma_1{}^2}{n_1} + \frac{\sigma_2{}^2}{n_2}}.$$

Thus the normal deviate is

$$\frac{(\bar{x}_1 - \bar{x}_2)}{\sqrt{\dfrac{\sigma_1{}^2}{n_1} + \dfrac{\sigma_2{}^2}{n_2}}}.$$

In general σ_1 and σ_2, the population standard deviations in samples 1 and 2, are unknown, and they are replaced by the sample estimates s_1 and s_2. Clearly, if the sample sizes are large s_1 and s_2 will be close to

σ_1 and σ_2 and the normal deviate can be compared with 1·96 or 2·58. On the other hand, if the sample sizes are small this substitution may make the test unreliable.

If the population variances $\sigma_1{}^2$ and $\sigma_2{}^2$ are equal, $s_1{}^2$ and $s_2{}^2$ are two sample estimates of the same quantity. This statement could be part of the hypothesis to be tested. For example, the hypothesis: 'The population from which the samples were taken are identical' includes the equality of the variances. Then, $s_1{}^2$ and $s_2{}^2$ can be combined to give a more accurate single estimate, say, s^2, where

$$s^2 = \frac{\Sigma(x_1 - \bar{x}_1)^2 + \Sigma(x_2 - \bar{x}_2)^2}{(n_1 - 1) + (n_2 - 1)}$$

and so

$$t = \frac{(\bar{x}_1 - \bar{x}_2)}{\sqrt{\dfrac{s^2}{n_1} + \dfrac{s^2}{n_2}}} = \frac{\bar{x}_1 - \bar{x}_2}{s\sqrt{\dfrac{1}{n_1} + \dfrac{1}{n_2}}}.$$

This value of t is calculated and referred to the table of critical values of t with $(n_1 - 1) + (n_2 - 1) = n_1 + n_2 - 2$ degrees of freedom. If the calculated value is greater than the critical value at the 5 per cent level of significance it is concluded that a difference between sample means as large as that observed is unlikely (i.e., there is only a 1 in 20 chance) to occur if the hypothesis is true. That is, the hypothesis is probably false; there is some evidence of a real difference between the means and it is said that the difference is significant at the 5 per cent level.

PROPORTIONS AND PERCENTAGES

Qualitative observations, such as whether a person is edentulous, are usually measured by estimating their prevalence as a proportion or percentage. Suppose in a population a proportion μ_p or percentage 100 μ_p have a characteristic, such as that they are edentulous. If a sample of n observations is taken and, p, the proportion in the sample with the characteristic is calculated, what can be said about the accuracy of p as an estimate of μ_p?

The distribution of p is binomial with mean μ_p and variance $\mu_p(1 - \mu_p)/n$ but when the sample size is large and μ_p is neither very small or nearly 1, use can be made of the normal approximation to the binomial distribution. In this case the proportion can be treated as though it were a mean and thus 95 per cent confidence limits for μ_p are

$$p \pm 1{\cdot}96\sqrt{\frac{p(1-p)}{n}}.$$

The significance of the difference between two sample proportions p_1

and p_2 is tested by calculating the ratio of the difference to its standard error, that is,

$$\frac{p_1 - p_2}{\sqrt{\frac{p_1(1 - p_1)}{n_1} + \frac{p_2(1 - p_2)}{n_2}}}$$

where n_1 and n_2 are the sample sizes and comparing it with 1·96 or 2·58.

When the sample size is small, the normal approximation to the binomial distribution can be improved by introducing a continuity correction. Alternatively the binomial probabilities can be calculated exactly. Further details of these calculations are given by Armitage in the textbook listed at the end of the chapter.

LEVELS OF SIGNIFICANCE

The use of 5 per cent and 1 per cent as standard levels of significance is purely arbitrary. If lower levels of significance, say 10 per cent, are accepted more differences treated as significant will, in fact, be the result of sampling fluctuations; while if only higher levels, say 0·1 per cent, are accepted, small but real differences may not be detected.

Hypotheses cannot be proved correct by these tests. If the normal deviate or t is smaller than the critical value it is concluded that, at this level of significance, there is no evidence to disprove the hypothesis. On the other hand a normal deviate or t value very much greater than the critical values may lead to the rejection of the hypothesis with a high degree of confidence.

PAIRS OF OBSERVATIONS

In most sample surveys more than one measurement is made on each sampled unit. For example, in a survey of children's DMF scores several other observations may be made, such as age, sex, social class, weekly sugar consumption, state of oral hygiene, and type of dentifrice used. The association between these concomitant observations and the response measurement, the DMF score, may be important since it may, for example, provide information about the aetiology of dental caries.

In the simplest case, in which only one other observation is taken, the association between the two measurements can be displayed by a scatter diagram. A scatter diagram is a plot of points such that the position of each point is determined by the two measurements. The response variable, conventionally denoted by y and measured on the vertical axis is called the 'dependent variable' since its value is believed to be in some way dependent on the concomitant variable x which is called the 'independent variable'. The pattern of points gives an indication of the form and closeness of the association between the two variables. If the pattern is such that there is a tendency for the points to be scattered about a straight line there is said to be a linear association between the two measurements.

How closely the points lie around a straight line can be measured by the product moment correlation coefficient. This coefficient can take values from -1 through zero to $+1$. Consider the scatter diagrams in *Fig.* 12.

In *Fig.* 12A the points lie exactly on a straight line and there is a perfect linear relationship between x and y in which as x increases y increases. In this situation, which rarely, if ever, occurs with biological measurements, the correlation coefficient is $+1$. *Fig.* 12B shows another perfect linear relationship, but here, as x increases y decreases, and the correlation coefficient is -1. *Figs.* 12C, D, E show the type of association most commonly encountered in practice. In *Fig.* 12C there is some tendency for y to increase as x increases and the correlation coefficient is greater than zero but less than 1. In *Fig.* 12D the tendency is for y to decrease as x increases and the correlation coefficient is between -1 and zero. *Fig.* 12E shows no tendency for y to increase or decrease as x increases. There is no association between x and y and the correlation coefficient is zero.

However, a correlation coefficient of zero does not necessarily imply that there is no association between x and y. *Fig.* 12F is a scatter diagram showing an array such that there is no overall tendency for y to increase or decrease as x increases and the correlation coefficient is zero but there is a strong association between x and y. A correlation coefficient of zero means that the association, if any, between x and y is not linear.

It is sometimes of interest to draw a straight line through the points of a scatter diagram. If the points are closely linear, fitting the line by eye may be satisfactory. Techniques of *linear regression* provide an objective method of fitting the line. The *regression coefficient* is the slope of the fitted line and therefore measures the average increase in y per unit increase in x. For example, if the dependent variable y is DMF score and the independent variable x is weekly consumption of sugar then the regression coefficient measures the average increase in the DMF score per unit (say 100 g.) increase in weekly sugar consumption.

If all points lie exactly on the straight line y increases by the regression coefficient for each unit increase in x. In practice this is not so and y can take a range of values for any fixed value of x. Thus for each level of weekly sugar consumption a distribution of DMF scores is observed. The mean DMF score for each value of x can be calculated but the DMF score for an individual child cannot be predicted exactly since factors other than sugar consumption affect the DMF score. Thus, the regression coefficient only measures the average increase in y per unit increase in x and is not affected by how closely the points are scattered about the line. The closeness of the linear relationship is measured by the correlation coefficient.

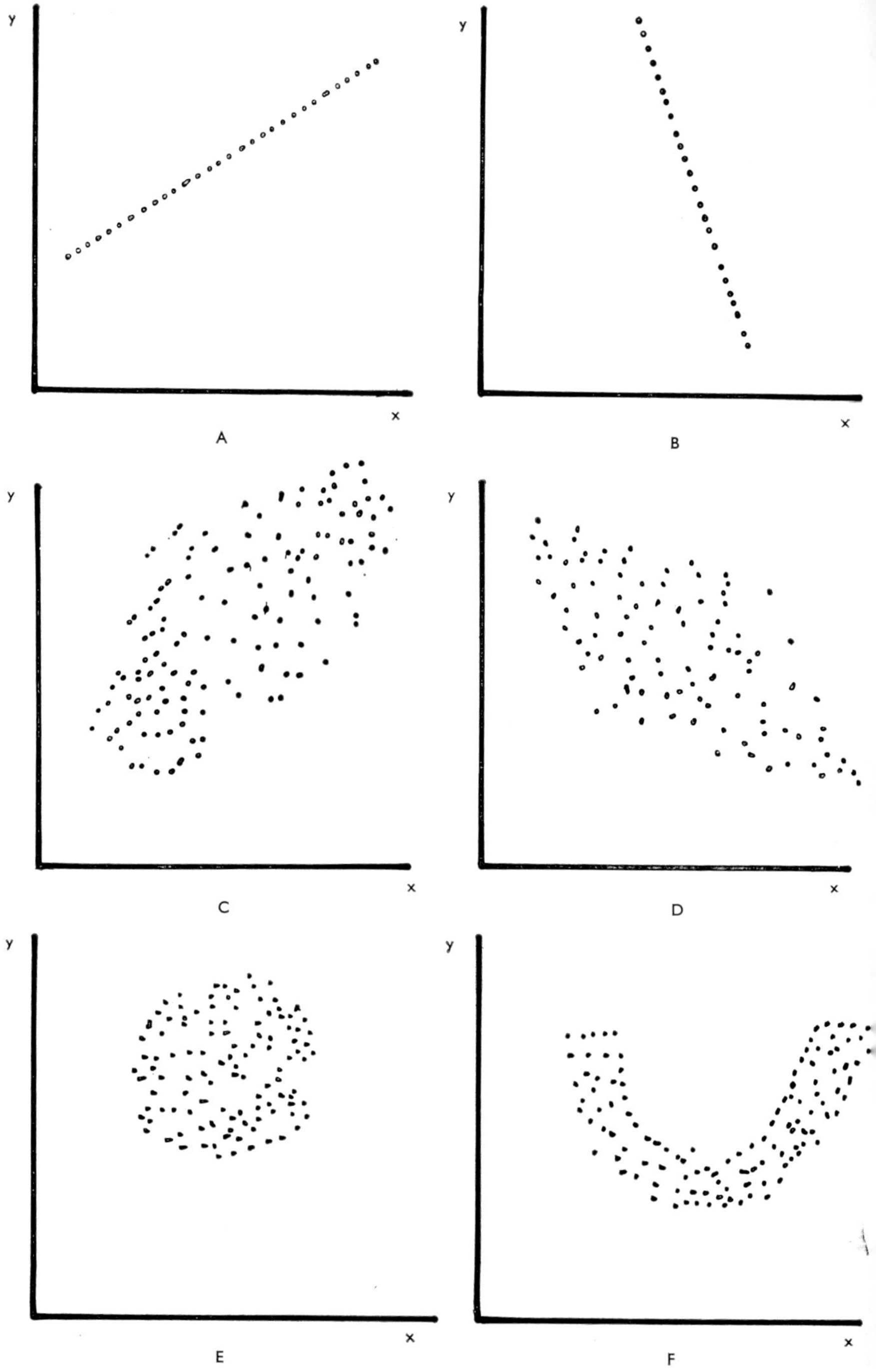

Fig. 12. Scatter diagrams. A, Perfect postive correlation. Correlation coefficient is 1. B, Perfect negative correlation. Correlation coefficient is −1. C, Some degree of positive correlation. D, Some degree of negative correlation. E, Correlation coefficient is zero. F, Correlation coefficient is zero.

Scatter diagrams, correlation, and regression cannot, of themselves, prove cause and effect relationships. For example, two variables may appear to be closely associated from the scatter diagram but this could merely be a reflection of the association of each with a third variable. If in a survey of schoolchildren, DMF score and head circumference are measured and the results plotted in a scatter diagram a tendency for DMF score to increase as head circumference increases would be apparent. However, this would not mean that decaying teeth cause the head to grow larger nor would it mean that teeth decay more easily in a large head. The apparent association between DMF score and head circumference would merely reflect that both measurements are associated with the age of the child.

SAMPLE SURVEY DESIGN

A sample survey is undertaken to obtain information about a population which is too large to be investigated completely. The characteristics of the sample are used as estimates of the characteristics of the population, but estimates, such as means and proportions, are liable to sampling error. However, this disadvantage is offset by the saving of the labour, time and expense of a complete survey of the population.

The population to be sampled must consist of a set of non-overlapping elementary units upon which an observation is made. Thus in a survey of the DMF scores of the children in a particular district, the individual child is the elementary unit and the group of all children in the district constitutes the population. The list of all elementary units in a population is called the sampling frame.

A sample may be selected according to some predetermined scheme or it may be randomly selected. If for example the sample is chosen to consist of 'typical' elementary units it will not be a random sample. A random sample is defined as one in which each unit in the sampling frame has a known chance of selection. When the selection is not random the sample may be biased and hence not representative of the population. In some circumstances it may provide more accurate estimates than a random sample but it is difficult if not impossible to assess the likely error of the estimates. Random sampling is always assumed in this discussion of biostatistics.

A random sample is called *simple* if each of the elementary units in the sample are selected independently and all units in the population have an equal chance of inclusion. The standard errors of estimates of the population mean and proportion are calculated from the formulae given on page 236, and there is a 5 per cent chance that the sampling error exceeds two standard errors. The maximum likely error which can be tolerated by an investigator should be decided before the sample survey is undertaken since this can be used to help determine the smallest sample size required. If the investigator will take a 5 per cent chance that the error in an estimated mean will exceed E, say, then by considering the 95 per cent confidence interval for the true mean, E can be expressed by

$$E = 2\sigma/\sqrt{n}$$

where $\sigma/\sqrt{n}$ is the standard error of the estimate of the mean. Algebraic manipulation of this expression shows that

$$n = \frac{4\sigma^2}{E^2}.$$

Thus if, from a pilot or some other source, an estimate of the variance of the observations is obtained the above formula gives the sample size required for a given maximum likely error E.

STRATIFICATION

If the population to be sampled can be classified into groups, or strata, in such a way that the units in each group are more homogeneous than those of the population as a whole, the accuracy of an estimate for a given sample size may be improved by taking separate simple random samples from each of the strata. The reduction in the standard error of an estimate from a stratified random sample is dependent on the allocation of the total number of units in the sample to the separate simple random samples. If the allocation is such that the simple random sample size for a stratum is proportional to the number of elementary units in the stratum and their standard deviation, the standard error of the estimate is the minimum possible for the given total sample size. Such an allocation of the total sample to separate simple random samples of the strata is called the *optimum allocation.*

Stratification can either reduce the total sample size (and hence costs) to achieve a given level of accuracy in the estimate or, alternatively, the most accurate estimate for a given sample size is obtained.

MULTI-STAGE SAMPLING

To construct a sampling frame of a large and scattered population may prove difficult or even impossible in certain situations. If it were constructed, and a simple random sample selected, the elementary units to be examined may be scattered thinly over a wide area. This would usually make the cost of the sample survey excessively high. Costs and administrative difficulties can sometimes be reduced by sampling in two or more stages. For example, suppose it were required to investigate the dental health of children of a particular age in a large city. If a sampling frame of all children of the required age were constructed, and a simple random sample taken, the children selected would be scattered all over the city. If on the other hand a sampling frame of schools were constructed and a random sample of schools were selected, a second stage sample of children could be taken from the selected schools. Such a sampling scheme as this has the advantages that it is not necessary to construct a sampling frame of all children, only those attending the schools selected, and secondly, the cost of examining each child is reduced because the children would be seen in batches at each school. For a given sample size such as the children examined in the above example, a multi-stage sample does not give so accurate estimates as a simple random sample. On the other hand, for a given fixed financial or labour budget it may be possible to examine more elementary units than if they were a scattered simple random sample.

Cluster Sampling is a special case of two stage sampling in which *all* the elementary units of each selected first stage unit are examined. Thus in the above example the schools are sampled in the first stage but every child in the selected schools is examined.

SUMMARY

Statistical principles and methods have an important part to play in almost all objective biological investigations. Thus the design of a trial or experiment should be planned in such a way that the analysis of the results can be anticipated. For example, experimental units (patients or teeth are the most common units in dental research) should, in general, be allocated to treatments randomly. The bias which could be introduced by non-random allocation cannot usually be assessed quantitatively and consequently the results of such work must be interpreted with caution. Only with random allocation can the errors in estimated parameters such as means and proportions be assessed, and then only in the form of a probability statement, the confidence intervals. It is unlikely that even very complicated statistical techniques can compensate for a badly planned and/or executed investigation.

Statistical techniques in detail appear many and varied, but, together, they provide a systematic and objective approach to the problems that abound in the study of measurements whose values are influenced by random fluctuation. The use of statistical parameters such as means, proportions and correlation coefficients, together with the construction of appropriate diagrams, graphs and charts gives a basis for description, but the statistical method goes further and provides positive, logical techniques of analysis which enable decisions to be made and rational action to be taken. The principles of statistical inference, which include the simple procedures of hypothesis testing herein described, are themselves part of the whole system of scientific inference by which knowledge is advanced.

However, although the basic principles are not in themselves difficult to understand and apply, there are pits into which the unwary can fall, and the advice of persons experienced in the application of statistical methods could prevent the collection of biased data which may be impossible to interpret satisfactorily.

FURTHER READING

ARMITAGE, P. (1971), *Statistical Methods in Medical Research.* Oxford and Edinburgh: Blackwell. [This is a very comprehensive account of the concepts and methods of statistics applied to medical research. Very little mathematical experience is assumed and algebraic proofs are kept to a minimum. This and the author's clear literary style make this not only a useful reference book but also a lucid text for students.]

BOURKE, G. J., and MCGILVRAY, J. (1969), *Interpretation and Uses of Medical Statistics.* Oxford and Edinburgh: Blackwell. [This is not a text of statistical methods but the emphasis is almost always on the meaning of statistical results. This elementary and very readable book will probably be of most interest to those workers who already have some knowledge of medical statistics.]

HILL, A. B. (1971), *Principles of Medical Statistics*, 9th ed. London: The Lancet. [This is the standard text of medical statistics. Emphasis is on the application of statistical methods to medical problems. No knowledge of mathematics is assumed. The sections on mortality may not have direct application to dental problems.]

Chapter 11

The Use of Computers in the Analysis of Dental Data

R. J. Anderson BSC, BDS, PHD
Senior Lecturer, Department of Dental Health, University of Birmingham, Honorary Consultant in Dental Health, United Birmingham Hospitals

Computers are rapidly becoming a part of everyday life. Their use as an administrative aid is increasing as the machines become more compact and easy to operate, and many dental administrators are now employing computers for a variety of purposes.

Dr. Anderson here describes the various kinds of computers and the uses to which they may be put. He effectively removes the mystique which still surrounds computers in many minds and he explains the principles of programming in a simple, step-by-step manner.

DEVELOPMENT OF COMPUTERS

There can be little doubt that one of the technical developments for which the past two decades will be remembered is that of the computer.

Prior to 1946, the only machines available for data processing were desk calculators, originally conceived by Pascall and Leibnitz in the seventeenth century but not commercially available until the nineteenth century, and the punch card system designed by Hollerith in the last part of the nineteenth century. Operations of the latter system are limited to sorting, counting, and some limited mathematical operations.

In 1946, Eckert and Mauchly working at the Moore School of Engineering in Pennsylvania developed a machine known as ENIAC. It had the facilities to perform the operations described above, but in addition it had one other most important attribute. This was the facility to assist the human brain in judgements and decisions which previously had been the exclusive function of the cerebral cortex; in addition it was able to perform all its operations about 1000 times faster than was possible by manual means. This machine contained 18,000 valves and was very unreliable. Apparently it had to be nursed by a team of engineers for occasional brief but phenomenal bursts of activity.

Following this, steps were taken to reduce the number of valves required and in the early 1950s the manufacturers produced the so-called 'first generation' computer. These were large, expensive, and unreliable but were used for some prodigious feats of calculation and provided valuable experience for all concerned.

Development would probably have been slow from this stage, as the machines were so unreliable and difficult to use that they were not really a commercial proposition, had it not been for the advent of the transistor. These replaced the conventional valves and enabled the size and the amount of heat produced to be considerably reduced. Early in 1960 the manufacturers took advantage of this development to produce the so-called 'second-generation' computers. These machines were much more reliable, easy to operate and worked at a speed 100 times faster than ENIAC.

These changes meant that it was now more economically possible to use computers in areas other than that of calculation. As more people learned to use them so the applications and demand grew and the industry was able to develop 'third generation' machines, which were first produced in 1965. These are basically the same as their predecessors but are 1000 times faster than ENIAC and have facilities for working on many different jobs at the same time.

Finally, techniques developed in 1966 have enabled several thousand transformers to be manufactured on a piece of silica one inch in diameter and only a few thousandths of an inch thick. Thus complicated systems can be reduced in size and it is now possible to produce compact computers (*Fig.* 1) no bigger than electric calculators.

The present situation is that computer techniques have advanced to such a stage where these machines can be used to assist with any project. The problem now, however, is the education of those who could benefit from their effective use.

One fact which tends to dissuade people from developing an interest in computers is the very fact that makes them so useful. Their ability to assist with judgements and decisions is taken to mean that they can think for themselves. The early machines were referred to as giant brains and anthropological terms such as this are still applied to present day machines. They should be regarded as inanimate machines whose function is to help in the processing of data and making judgements with regard to that data, just as the motor car assists us with our travel.

It is important to realize that however advanced and sophisticated the machine, it can only make a decision of the simplest style. That is one in which the answer is either yes or no. All other apparent abilities of the machine depend on the facilities of the particular unit and the skills of the user.

It is possible to understand the principles of computers, and to use them, without an expert knowledge of how they work. This may also be likened to the car where a lack of detailed knowledge of how the engine functions does not prevent many from driving most efficiently.

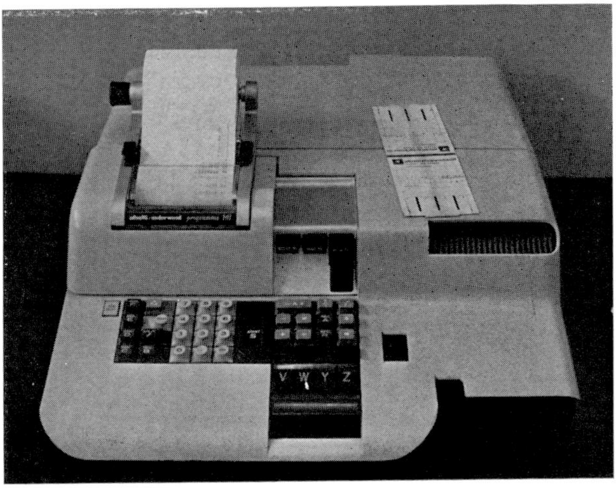

Fig. 1. A desk top computer.

BASIC PRINCIPLES OF COMPUTING

The basic principles of the computer are simple and can be understood by describing them in terms of analagous situations which are familiar to all.

All computers consist of three basic parts. The input unit, the central processing unit, and an output unit. The input unit is that part of the machine which accepts the data, the central processing unit (CPU) is the region where the appropriate operations are performed and the output is the unit where the results of the processes are presented to the user. *Fig.* 1 shows a desk top computer. Here the input unit is represented by the keyboard, the output is the unit which prints the results on the tally toll and the remainder of the machine is the central processing unit. *Fig.* 2 shows an electric calculator which also has input and output units and a processing unit where the calculations are performed.

The essential differences between the two machines is the way in which they operate. Examination of the keyboard of the calculator (*Fig.* 2) shows that the keyboard comprises of two types of key. There are rows identified by numerals, which are used for entering the data and the remainder which are identified by mathematical symbols which are the instruction keys. Keys in the latter group have to be depressed to enable the machine to perform the appropriate mathematical operation. Every time a calculation is required the operator has to enter the data and depress the appropriate instruction button for each step of the calculations.

When using a calculator it is normal for the operator to determine which operating instruction button is required next as the calculation proceeds. However, it is possible to write down a list of instructions giving the order in which the buttons are to be depressed. If this is done, the calculations can be performed by anyone, even if they have no

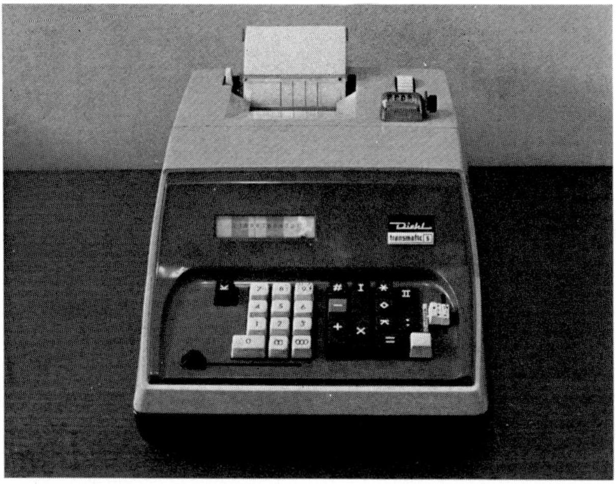

Fig. 2. An electric calculator.

knowledge of the formulae and procedures being used. Provided that they adhere rigidly to the instructions they would produce the correct answer. The computer shown in *Fig.* 1 also has instruction keys and it can be used in exactly the same way as a calculator. However, if a list of instructions has been prepared, then with this machine it is possible to use the instruction keys to feed the instructions into the machine before a calculation is started. When a calculation is required, the operator enters the data and the machine is able to act on the instructions stored within it to produce the result without any further operator intervention. If further calculations are required of a similar nature, these can be performed with the same set of instructions. In addition, the computer is able to store data once it has been entered and so the results of intermediate calculations can be retained for further use. It is unusual for electric calculators to be able to store more than one intermediate result so these have to be printed out and re-entered when appropriate.

This list of instructions used by the computer is known as a program (this form of spelling is universally adopted, British Standards

Institution, 1962), and it is stored together with the data in the central processing unit.

PRINCIPLES OF PROGRAMMING

We may imagine the central processing unit as consisting of a room in which we have the facility to store data, containing also a clerk who is unable to think for himself but who can carry out procedures in accordance with a set of instructions. To make the unit work we have to give the clerk the necessary program and data by way of the input unit, and he will then communicate the results by way of the output unit. Thus using such a machine depends not on the knowledge of how it performs its operations but on being able to provide it with a suitable program.

If it is imagined that the storage space within our computer consists of a series of pigeon holes similar to those used for sorting letters, it is first necessary to be able to identify each separate location. This may be done by giving each position an identifying name. In the following example three storage locations will be required which for the sake of convenience will be called A, B, and C. To use the computer for the simple task of adding two figures together the instructions could be as follows:

1. Read the first number on the input unit, copy this number onto a piece of paper, place this piece of paper in Box A. If there happens to be a piece of paper already in Box A destroy it first.
2. Read the second number on the input unit, copy this number onto a piece of paper, place this piece of paper in Box B. If there happens to be a piece of paper already in Box B destroy it first.
3. Look at the number written on the paper stored in Box A. Look at the number written on the paper stored in Box B. Add these two numbers together, write the total on a piece of paper and place it in Box C. If there is a piece of paper already in Box C destroy it first.
4. Look at the number written on the piece of paper stored in Box C, and transfer it to the output unit.

With these instructions the operation would be performed. The instructions may seem unnecessarily lengthy and detailed but the clerk can only follow a set of instructions implicitly in the order in which they are given. If any part of the above instructions were missing he could not perform the procedure correctly.

With the above instructions the procedure could be completed only once. However, with the addition of a fifth instruction:

5. Return to instruction number 1.

the program could now be used to repeat the process over and over again.

Instructions in this form are very clumsy and may be expressed in a form of shorthand. If for convenience the input and the output unit are represented by codes 1 and 3 respectively, the above instructions could be shortened as follows:

1. READ (1) A
2. READ (1) B
3. C = A + B
4. WRITE (3) C
5. GO TO 1

The meaning of each of these statements is exactly the same as described before and is now in a form acceptable to many computers.

A critical inspection of these instructions reveals that they go round and round indefinitely and our clerk could never stop. To overcome this we may insert a further statement between statements 1 and 2 and this might be as follows:

Look at the number written on the piece of paper in Box A and if it is equal to 99 continue with instruction number 7, if it is not equal to 99 continue with the next instruction.

This type of instruction takes advantage of the ability of the computer to make decisions. In addition it demonstrates that it is possible to alter the order in which the remaining instructions are carried out as a result of a decision. In shorthand it would be:

IF (A.EQ.99) GO TO 7

Instruction number 7 could be:

7. STOP

The completed program would now be as follows:

1. READ (1) A
2. IF (A.EQ.99) GO TO 7
3. READ (1) B
4. C = A + B
5. WRITE (3) C
6. GO TO 1
7. STOP

It is now necessary to add the value 99 to the end of the data on which we wish the computation to be undertaken. The program will now run and the machine will add together pairs of values (first and second, third and fourth, etc.) until the value 99 was sensed and then it would stop.

The complete program illustrates the precise way in which a program will act. It can be seen that if any one of the values which is to be summed to a second is 99, the machine will stop when it detects this value even if there is more data to be processed. Thus the program cannot process the value 99; if it is to do so, instruction number 2 of the program must be modified so that A is tested against a value which would never be found as one of the values for computation. Secondly, the arrangement of the data values is important as the 99 value must be the last, and the total number of values must be odd; if this is not so the 99 value will be read into Box B which is not tested. In this way the stop signal will be missed and the machine will attempt to read more values even though they are not present.

The program in this example was run on a computer and the print-out is shown in *Fig.* 3. It can be seen that apart from some additional statements it is very similar to the example.

```
                                        FORTRAN     RUN
FORTRAN COMPILATION    VER 2 MOD 2
              INTEGER     A,B,C
          100 FORMAT (I2)
          200 FORMAT (1H0,15X,I4)


            1 READ (1,100)   A
            2 IF (A.EQ.99) GO TO 7
            3 READ (1,100)   B
            4 C = A + B
            5 WRITE (3,200)   C
            6 GO TO 1
            7 STOP


              END
```

Fig. 3. The printout of a program written in FORTRAN.

Learning to program consists very simply of learning the instructions which the computer will accept and knowing the correct shorthand for these instructions. It is then just a matter of arranging these instructions so that the computer performs the operation required. There is no correct way to write a program, provided it produces the correct answers, the method used is unimportant.

PROGRAMMING LANGUAGES

Computers work by possessing many thousands of small electric circuits. The usual form of arithmetic suitable for these circuits is binary arithmetic. This is based on a unit of two, which can be represented in the circuits by the fact of whether they are carrying an electrical current or not. Thus basically all information fed into a computer has to be numerical information in a binary form. This means that all programs have to be coded into numerical form, translated into binary. For example, the code for addition might be 3 which in binary is 0011, and the code for subtraction might be 4, 0100 in binary. Programming in binary machine language was a very specialized art and one which few attempted to master. When the 'second generation' machines were introduced the manufacturers realized that if they were to make them available to the widest possible field they must make the programming easier. Much time and effort were spent by the manufacturers in developing systems which would enable the users to write their programs in forms which were easier to master, the computer itself could then be used to translate these 'higher level' programs, known as human orientated programs, into machine language. These translating programs known as compiler programs, some of which are reputed to have taken 100 man years to produce, are provided by the manufacturers and are available on computer systems for use when required.

Initially each manufacturer tended to develop his own individual human orientated programs, but recently they have become more standardized and the main ones are FORTRAN, ALGOL, and COBOL. The first two are basically for scientific applications and the latter is for business applications.

If potential users are going to learn a language then their choice must be governed by the languages available on the system they are going to use. However, if several are available, then the author would recommend FORTRAN, as most computing systems possess this compiler and it can be used almost universally. It has two main versions, FORTRAN II and FORTRAN IV. These differ in some of the details as to the particular statements which may be used, FORTRAN II being slightly less sophisticated than FORTRAN IV. The program shown in *Fig*. 3 is written in FORTRAN IV.

FORTRAN was devised by one particular manufacturer and often computer systems manufactured by others possess this compiler which is similar except for minor details. However, often it is given a different name. EGTRAN is such an example.

To anyone who wishes to study this language the books by McCracken (1961, 1965) are particularly recommended. However, this author uses problems from the physical sciences as his examples, and the book by James et al. (1970), although not so comprehensive, is a good primer as many of the examples are from the medical field, and some are very similar to the problems encountered in dental epidemiology.

Once a language has been mastered the user now requires the programming manual supplied by the manufacturer for the particular machine he intends to use. This gives all the details of the language as applied to the particular machine. It is not recommended, however, that anyone attempts to learn a programming language from these detailed manuals.

From the foregoing description of languages, it can be seen that when a job is run it consists of two separate stages. The first step is the compilation of the human orientated language into basic machine language and the second step, known as execution, is the processing of the data using the translated program.

THE COMPUTER

As previously described a computer consists basically of an input unit, an output unit, and a central processing unit. The outward appearance of the latter is most uninteresting as it comprises a series of metal cabinets. The other units are more interesting and may be in a variety of forms.

INPUT UNITS

The units for receiving the program and data are basically of two types. One type reads the punch card which was designed originally for the Hollerith system. This card has 80 vertical columns, in each of which there are 12 positions which may be punched out and using a code of single, double and treble punching any numeral, alphabetical character or certain special characters may be represented in each column (*Fig*. 4).

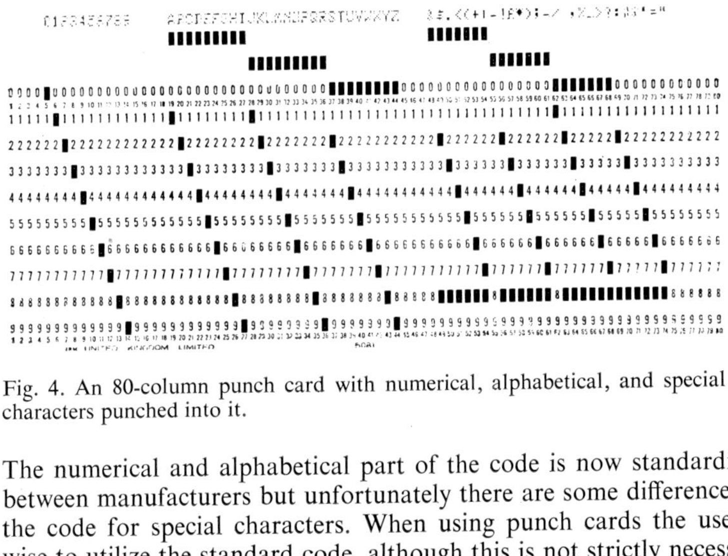

Fig. 4. An 80-column punch card with numerical, alphabetical, and special characters punched into it.

The numerical and alphabetical part of the code is now standardized between manufacturers but unfortunately there are some differences in the code for special characters. When using punch cards the user is wise to utilize the standard code, although this is not strictly necessary if the card is to be used on the Hollerith system only; many applications end up on the computer even if at the outset there seemed little chance of doing so. If the information is not in standard code it cannot be analysed by a computer.

The card read unit of a computer (*Fig*. 5) allows these cards to be placed in stacks and read one at a time as required.

Another type of reader is the paper tape reader (*Fig*. 6). For this, information is punched in a continuous strip of paper, each character being represented by a group of one or more punchings in one of seven positions, or channels, across the tape (*Fig*. 7). There is a range of

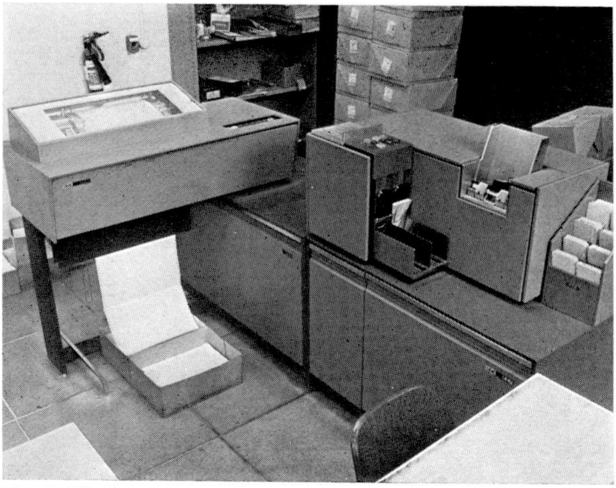

Fig. 5. The input and output units of an IBM 1440 computer unit, showing the card reader on the right and the line printer on the left.

paper tape coding systems which vary in the code used and the number of channels available for the coding.

THE OUTPUT UNIT

The most usual form of output is the line printer (*Fig.* 5) which prints the output a line at a time onto a continuous sheet of stationery. The arrangements of the layout of the results are decided by the programmer and are written into the program.

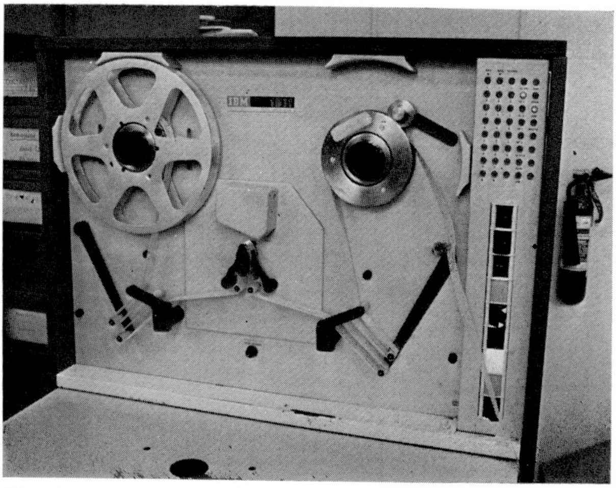

Fig. 6. A paper tape reader.

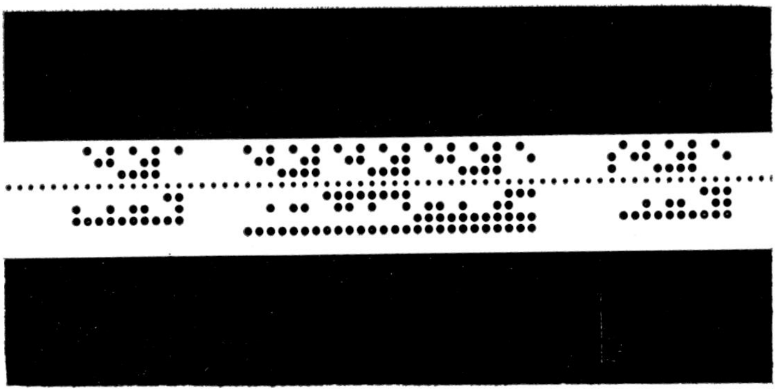

Fig. 7. A section of seven track punched paper tape showing from left to right numerical, alphabetical and special characters.

Output can also be put onto punch cards using a card punch, or onto a paper tape using a paper tape punch.

INPUT AND OUTPUT UNITS

In addition to the units described above which can only be used for the transfer of data in one direction as described, there are two other units which may be used for input and output. One of these is the magnetic

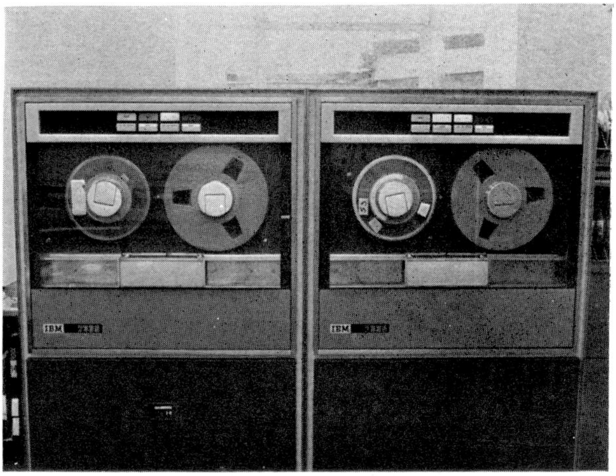

Fig. 8. Magnetic tape input/output units.

tape unit. This enables the computer to store information onto and read back from magnetic tape, in the same way a sound can be recorded onto and played back from magnetic tape from a tape recorder (*Fig.* 8).

The other input/output unit is the magnetic disc unit. Basically this unit consists of a flat rotating disc, the surfaces of which are covered with a sensitive magnetic coating. Information can be stored upon or retrieved from these discs in a manner analagous to the recording and playing back of a gramophone record. Larger disc units may have five or more of these discs arranged vertically above one another and spinning on the same axis (*Fig*. 9). The advantage of this disc unit is that any item of information is almost immediately accessible whereas with a tape unit the information is stored sequentially and it may be necessary for the computer to search to the end of the tape for the particular item of information it requires. The analagous situation is that the pick up of a record player may be placed directly on a particular track of a record but with a tape recording it is necessary to search through the tape to find the particular sequence required.

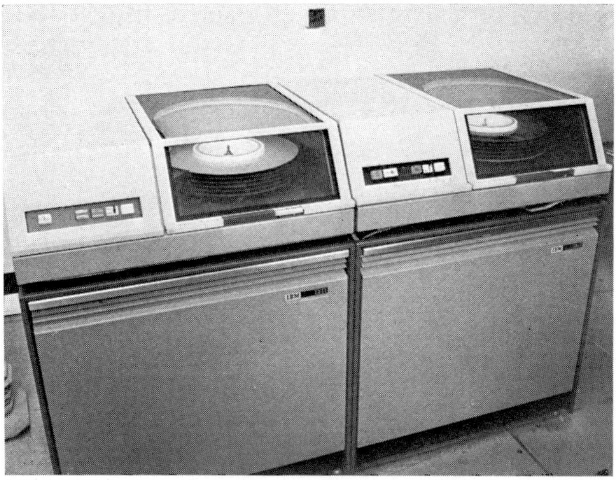

Fig. 9. Magnetic disc input/output units.

All magnetic tapes and many of the magnetic discs are removable from their units so they may be stored for use at a later date. For long term storage, tape is the most convenient as these cost considerably less than discs.

THE APPLICATION OF COMPUTERS TO DENTAL EPIDEMIOLOGICAL DATA

The computer has now been used in almost all fields of medicine. These applications form the basis of a series of articles in the *British Medical Journal* (1968) and books edited by Rose (1969) and McLachlan and Shegog (1968).

In dentistry the computer is being used to an ever increasing extent. Christopher (1967) and Moore (1969) give details of the role of computers in dentistry in North America where they are used in hospital administration, laboratory and radiological investigations, the storage of patients' records, dental education, and dental research. In some centres these machines are also used for planning the treatment of patients (Glass et al., 1969), for recording students' clinical achievements (Glass et al., 1965; Ehrlich et al., 1969) and for students' examinations. James et al. (1968) describe how a computer has been used in Britain to assess the efficacy of an oral hygiene campaign and also for investigation into a hospital's record system.

The use of two different ways in which punch card systems could be used for analysing dental data was described by Klein and Palmer (1940) and Klein and Kramer (1948). Marthaler (1963) described the use of the computer to analyse dental epidemiological data and Solow (1964) used one for the examination of epidemiological malocclusion data.

The problem of analysis of dental epidemiological data is the amount of data which has to be collected to make any study worthwhile. Having assembled this data the observer often wishes to look at it in several ways and compare it with the results of previous studies. After examination of some of the results additional interesting ways in which the data may be analysed may become apparent.

If such a study is to be undertaken by hand, several months of hard work are required to obtain the interim results and often any further analysis is abandoned simply because of the time factor. Until recently, epidemiological data from all parts of the world was extremely scarce, not because there was any difficulty in its collection but because of the tedious nature of its analysis. In the last few years, the dental epidemiologist has begun to use the computer to assist in this task and more epidemiological data are becoming available.

THE PREPARATION OF EPIDEMIOLOGICAL DATA FOR THE COMPUTER

The use of punch cards and paper tape as computer input have been described, and it has been shown that alphabetical and numerical characters can be punched onto these. Unfortunately, the data collected in a dental survey is not in the form of simple alphabetical or numerical characters so it is necessary to decide how the information should be recorded. For example, when recording the sex of an individual we could punch MALE or FEMALE into the card. This method is perfectly satisfactory but the character M or F would be sufficient. Alternatively, this information could be coded so that the males were represented by 0 and the females by 1. In the last two examples there would be a considerable saving of space as only one column of the card would be used instead of six. In a similar way, dental cleanliness which may have been classified as 'good', 'fair' or 'poor' could be coded G, F, or P, or 1, 2, 3. As a general rule it is easier to write programs for data which has been coded numerically and this is the method of preference. All qualitative information to be collected in a survey has to be coded in this way. Quantitative data is already numerical so does not need to be coded.

In addition to the coding it is necessary to decide the position at which each item of information is to be punched onto the card. Some items will require only a single column, sex is an example, some such as DMF or DMFS values will require more than one. The total number of columns designated for each item is known as a 'field'.

The precise manner in which a computer works makes it necessary that each field is always in the same position in every card and great care must be taken during the preparation of the data to ensure that this rule is obeyed. Once the position and code for each field have been determined details should be fully documented, as they are easily

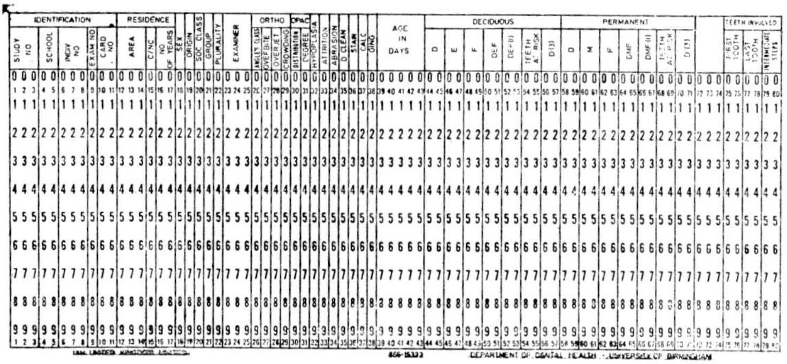

Fig. 10. A punch card with the fields printed upon it.

forgotten and processing of the information is impossible without them.

It is possible to have punch cards prepared with the fields printed on them (*Fig.* 10), and this can be of enormous benefit during the data processing. However, this is only a financial proposition if many thousands of cards with a similar layout are to be used.

If a user is designing a system, the field length and the details of the coding should be arranged to suit the user's requirements and the computer programmed accordingly. It is wise, however, to bear the programming in mind at this stage in the design, as often simple rearrangement of the data can lead to considerable simplification of the programming details. If the user is to collect data for analysis using programs which have already been written then the field layout and coding must be exactly as required by the program.

Once the details of the coding have been settled the preparation of the data consists of three phases: the collection, coding, and the punching.

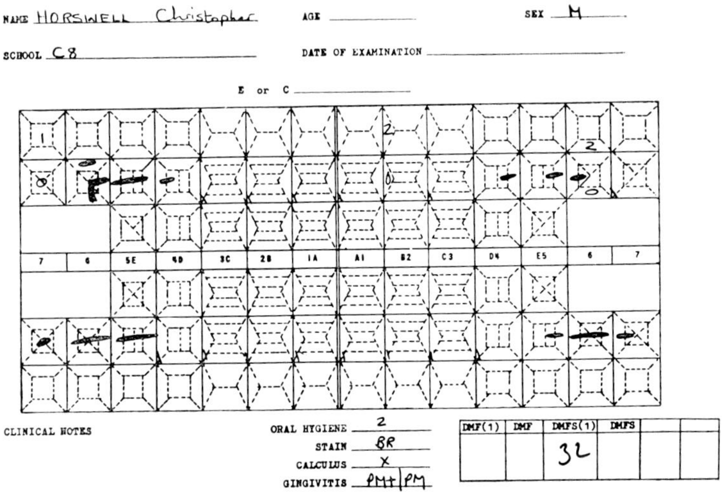

Fig. 11. A conventional dental survey chart.

Dental data is normally recorded on a chart in a diagrammatic form (*Fig.* 11). This information then has to be coded and to ensure accuracy at the punching stage this coding is usually recorded on a second form.

The basic design of this abstract document comprises a series of boxes, each box represents one column of the punch card and has two

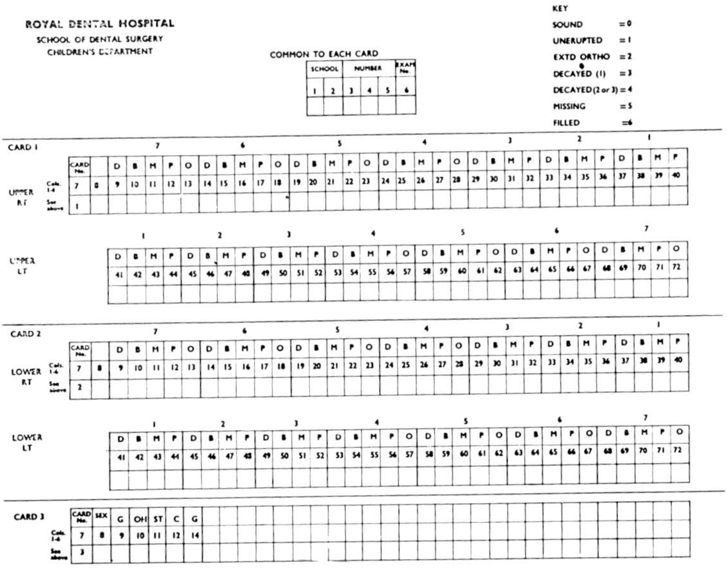

Fig. 12. An abstract sheet suitable for coded dental information.

distinct labels. One identifies it to a particular column of the card and the second gives details of the information which is to be recorded into it. The document shown in *Fig*. 12 has a space into which details of each surface of every tooth may be recorded and some additional boxes for recording the details of sex, status of oral hygiene and so on. In this particular application three punch cards were necessary to record all the information.

Once the abstract document has been completed it is a simple matter to punch the cards from it. The operator uses a machine as shown in *Fig*. 13 and enters the data by way of the typewriter keyboard. During the punching the operator simply transfers the figures recorded in the boxes into the appropriate columns of the card and

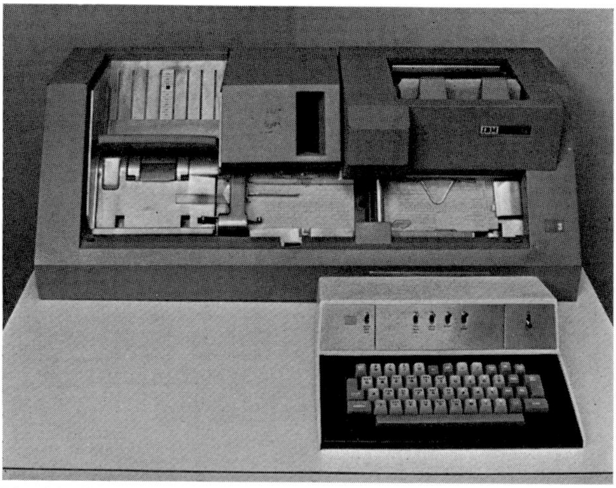

Fig. 13. An automatic card punch.

usually will have no knowledge as to the meaning of this data. The punch operator, therefore, cannot be expected to check the accuracy of the coding.

If dental data is collected in this manner it soon becomes apparent that the bottle neck in this procedure is the coding of the data from the dental record onto the abstract sheet. In an attempt to overcome this problem and speed up this part of the processing, a special set of punch cards was designed specially for dental data (Anderson, 1968; Anderson and Beal, 1971).

These sets combine the features of the dental chart, abstract sheet, and punch card. For convenience the first card is used for recording personal details about the individual such as their name, date of birth, sex, area of residence, and each of the four remaining cards is for recording details of one quadrant of the mouth. The basic form of each of the cards for the clinical part of the data is shown in *Fig*. 14. It has the relevant portion of the clinical chart and a series of boxes for the coded information similar in design to those of the abstract sheet previously described. The various possibilities as to the state of each surface of the teeth was coded and this code was printed on the cards (*Fig.* 14).

At the clinical examination, the examiner calls out his findings in code rather than in the usual manner. Thus a call of, upper right six, occlusal seven, means that this tooth has an occlusal filling. Details of each surface of each tooth and details of any other conditions examined are called out in this way. If at any time the examiner cannot remember the details of the coding he would call it in the usual way and the recorder who has the details in front of her would do the coding.

It may seem that this method of coding at the time of recording is too complex to work satisfactorily and it was for this reason that the dental chart was included on each card so that it could be used as a standby

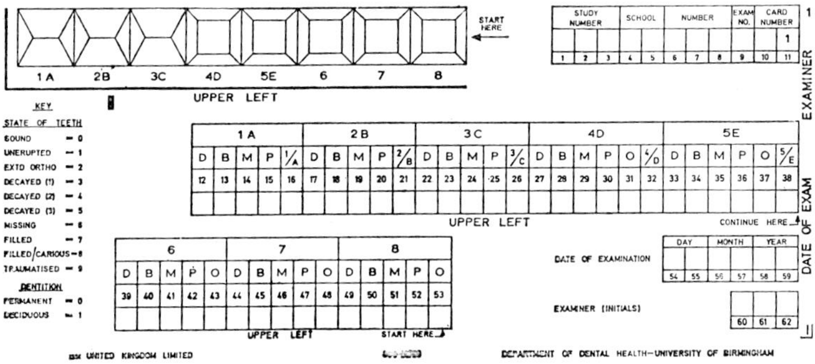

Fig. 14. A punch card designed for recording data from the upper left quadrant.

in the event of failure of the other system. In practice the system of coding the information as it is collected works extremely well and has been used by many examiners and recorders, several of whom have had no knowledge of the data processing principle involved. In all cases it was only necessary for a few minutes' familiarization before the system could be used with ease. Several examiners reported that they preferred this method of recording. Checks on the accuracy of the recorder using this method were undertaken using a tape-recorder. It was found that there was no loss of accuracy when this method was compared with the conventional methods.

After the collection of the data these cards are designed so that they may be fed into an IBM 029 card punch and the details recorded on the cards can be punched into the same cards (*Fig.* 13). After punching the cards are passed through a verifier in which a similar sequence of events takes place but instead of punching the cards this machine checks to ensure that the holes are in the correct place. This must be undertaken by a different operator to ensure that the same mistakes are not made twice, and to give a second opinion on any badly written figures. Any errors detected are corrected before the analysis begins.

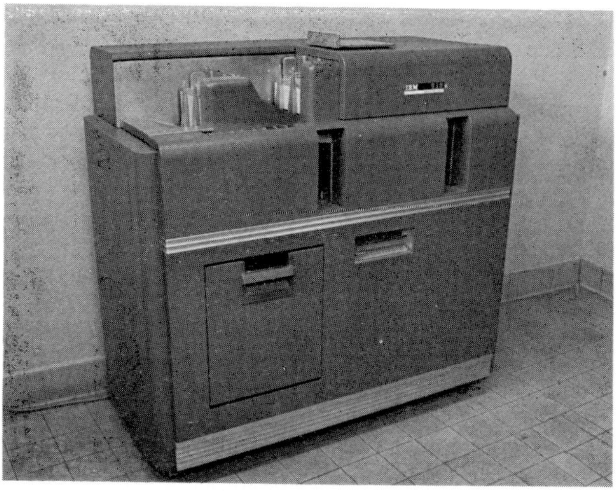

Fig. 15. A mark sense punch.

Using this method of collecting data it is possible for a skilled punch operator to prepare the data for computation at about the same rate as it is collected.

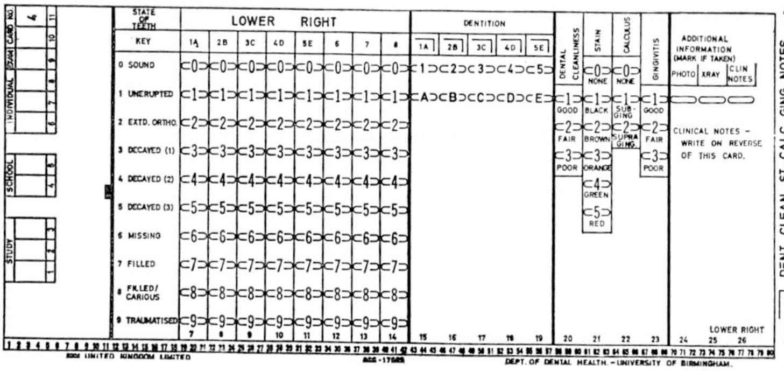

Fig. 16. A punch card designed for recording dental data in a form suitable for mark sensing.

It is also possible to punch the information automatically if it is collected in a different way. A mark sense punch (*Fig.* 15) can sense pencil marks electronically. By redesigning the card sets this system can also be used. The layout of one of the cards is shown in *Fig.* 16.

The only difference is that for each tooth there is a series of alternative positions for recording a mark. Each of the positions corresponds

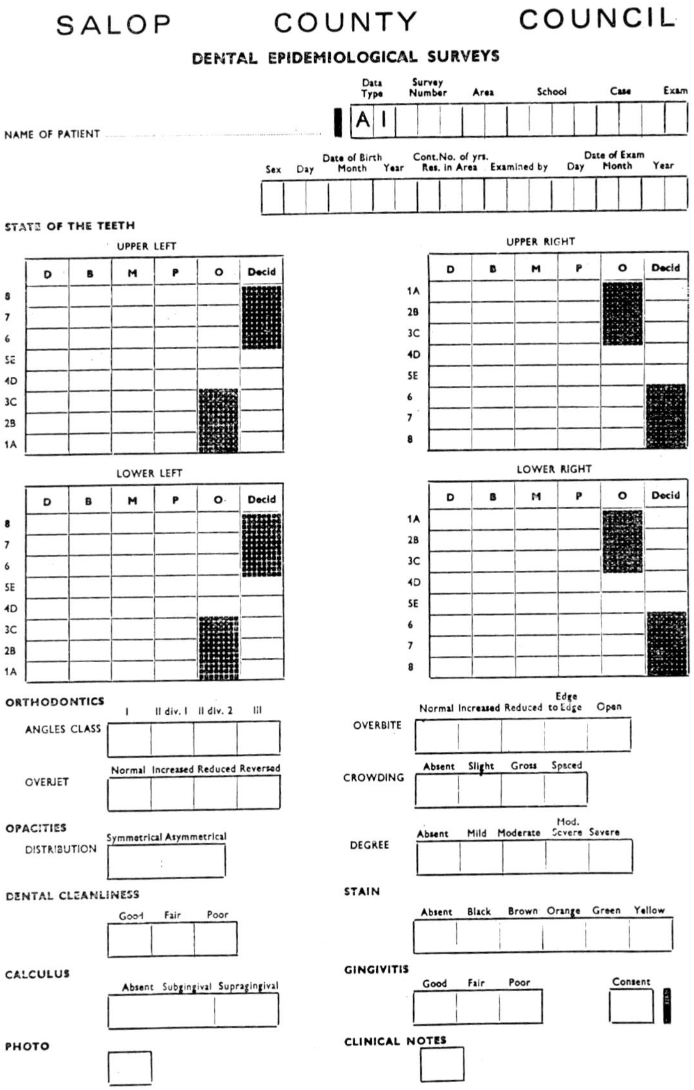

SALOP COUNTY COUNCIL

DENTAL EPIDEMIOLOGICAL SURVEYS

Data Type | Survey Number | Area | School | Case | Exam

A I

NAME OF PATIENT ....

Sex | Date of Birth: Day, Month, Year | Cont. No. of yrs. Res. in Area | Examined by | Date of Exam: Day, Month, Year

STATE OF THE TEETH

UPPER LEFT

	D	B	M	P	O	Decid
8						
7						
6						
5E						
4D						
3C						
2B						
1A						

UPPER RIGHT

	D	B	M	P	O	Decid
1A						
2B						
3C						
4D						
5E						
6						
7						
8						

LOWER LEFT

	D	B	M	P	O	Decid
8						
7						
6						
5E						
4D						
3C						
2B						
1A						

LOWER RIGHT

	D	B	M	P	O	Decid
1A						
2B						
3C						
4D						
5E						
6						
7						
8						

ORTHODONTICS

ANGLES CLASS: I | II div. I | II div. 2 | III

OVERBITE: Normal | Increased | Reduced | Edge to Edge | Open

OVERJET: Normal | Increased | Reduced | Reversed

CROWDING: Absent | Slight | Gross | Spaced

OPACITIES

DISTRIBUTION: Symmetrical | Asymmetrical

DEGREE: Absent | Mild | Moderate | Mod. Severe | Severe

DENTAL CLEANLINESS: Good | Fair | Poor

STAIN: Absent | Black | Brown | Orange | Green | Yellow

CALCULUS: Absent | Subgingival | Supragingival

GINGIVITIS: Good | Fair | Poor

Consent

PHOTO

CLINICAL NOTES

Fig. 17. A document designed for collecting dental data in a form suitable for punching on paper tape.

to a possible state of the tooth. During the clinical examination the recorder makes the appropriate marks on the card which can then be punched and verified automatically at a speed of 100 cards per minute.

This is considerably faster than when processing by hand but has some disadvantages. One is that only 26 vertical columns are available when using this system instead of 80, which means a considerable reduction in the amount of detail which can be recorded. Thus the card sets which have been designed to utilize this system can only be used for recording details of each tooth instead of details of each surface. As it seems that in prevalence studies analyses utilizing surface indices add little information to that gained from the analyses of tooth indices (Jackson et al., 1963, Anderson, 1967) this disadvantage is small when compared to the speed of the data preparation. The other disadvantages are that if the cards are not filled in correctly many problems can arise during their preparation. These may be overcome by ensuring that the recorder understands that the cards are to be processed by machine and insisting that the rules laid down for the completion of these cards are always obeyed.

The method of collection and preparation of dental data described above was specifically designed for punch card input. If paper tape is the input facility available then a modified form for data collection is necessary. An example of such a form is shown in *Fig*. 17, and this replaces the card sets but is used in exactly the same way for recording the clinical information directly in code (Clarke, Maycock, and Price, 1973). The punched paper tape can be prepared and verified directly from this form.

ANALYSIS OF DENTAL DATA

The dental data collected on punch cards as described above is analysed in two steps. First, the abstraction of the data according to the various epidemiological indices and secondly the analysis of the results of groups of individuals using these indices.

It is necessary to store the results of the abstraction stage in some way, either on magnetic tape or disc or on punch cards. The records then have to be sorted into groups for analysis. If the abstracted information is stored on magnetic tape or disc then the sorting may be done by the computer. If the information is on cards it can be done away from the unit.

The computer unit upon which the card sets are analysed at present is an early second generation machine and the time taken for sorting the abstracted information is ridiculously long when related to the time for the rest of the analyses so it was decided that the best method of storage of the abstracted information in this case was on cards. For this output a special card design is used (*Fig*. 10). The abstract programs are arranged so that they may abstract details from the full mouth, or from any named quadrant or quadrants, teeth or tooth groups. In this way the programs are very flexible and can be used for partial as well as complete analysis.

To prepare the cards for the analyses they are sorted into groups using a counter sorter (*Fig.* 18). The appropriate heading cards are added and the cards resubmitted to the computer.

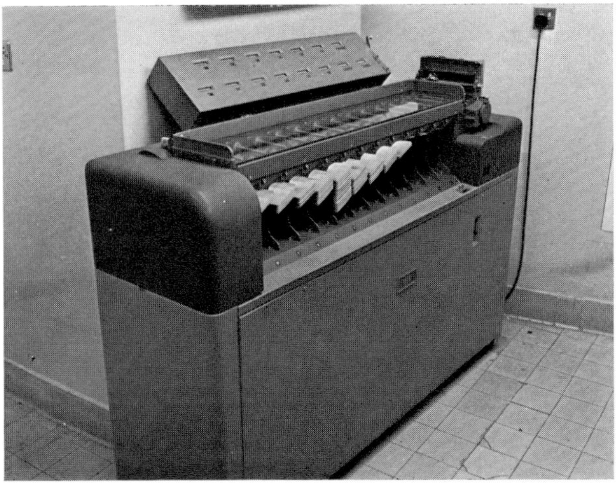

Fig. 18. A counter sorter.

The output of the analyses are usually in the form of tables (*Figs.* 19 and 20) giving detailed results for each group. When required the necessary statistical test between groups can be undertaken. It is also

	NUMBER	AVERAGE	SUM	SUMSQ	S.D.	S.E.
AGE(YEARS)	52.	5.00	259.96	1299.64	0.00	0.00
DECIDUOUS DECAYED	52.	1.23	64.00	296.00	2.06	0.29
DECIDUOUS MISSING	52.	0.33	17.00	39.00	0.81	0.11
DECIDUOUS FILLED	52.	0.44	23.00	55.00	0.94	0.13
DECIDUOUS DMF	52.	2.00	104.00	644.00	2.92	0.41
DECIDUOUS DMF(1)	52.	2.06	107.00	669.00	2.97	0.41
DECIDUOUS NO AT RISK	52.	19.23	1000.00	19308.00	1.23	0.17
DECIDUOUS DECAYED(3)	52.	0.13	7.00	11.00	0.44	0.06
DECIDUOUS DECAYED(2)	52.	1.10	57.00	219.00	1.75	0.24
DECIDUOUS DMF 100 TH	52.	10.57	549.53	17872.54	15.38	2.13
PERMANENT DECAYED	23.	0.00	0.00	0.00	0.00	0.00
PERMANENT MISSING	23.	0.00	0.00	0.00	0.00	0.00
PERMANENT FILLED	23.	0.00	0.00	0.00	0.00	0.00
PERMANENT DMF	23.	0.00	0.00	0.00	0.00	0.00
PERMANENT DMF(1)	23.	0.00	0.00	0.00	0.00	0.00
PERMANENT NO AT RISK	23.	3.26	75.00	329.00	1.96	0.41
PERMANENT DECAYED(3)	23.	0.00	0.00	0.00	0.00	0.00
PERMANENT DECAYED(2)	23.	0.00	0.00	0.00	0.00	0.00
PERMANENT DMF 100 TH	23.	0.00	0.00	0.00	0.00	0.00

EAST ANGLIAN STUDY
WEST MERSEA CHILDREN AGED 5 EXAMINED 1969

Fig. 19. An example of the output of results showing quantitative data in tabular form.

possible to produce bar charts giving details of the DMF of each group (*Fig*. 21). Further analyses are undertaken by rearranging the groups of cards on the sorter and re-submitting them for analysis using the same programs.

ATTRITION	ABSENT	MILD	SEVERE			
NUMBER	52.	0.	0.			
PERCENT	100.00	0.00	0.00			
ABRASION	ABSENT	MILD	SEVERE			
NUMBER	52.	0.	0.			
PERCENT	100.00	0.00	0.00			
DENT CLEAN	GOOD	AVERAGE	POOR			
NUMBER	24.	24.	4.			
PERCENT	46.15	46.15	7.69			
STAIN	ABSENT	BLACK	BROWN	ORANGE	GREEN	RED
NUMBER	39.	0.	7.	2.	4.	0.
PERCENT	75.00	0.00	13.46	3.85	7.69	0.00
CALCULUS	ABSENT	SUBGING	SUPRAGING			
NUMBER	51.	0.	1.			
PERCENT	98.08	0.00	1.92			
GINGIVITIS	GOOD	AVERAGE	POOR			
NUMBER	42.	8.	2.			
PERCENT	80.77	15.38	3.85			

EAST ANGLIAN STUDY
WEST MERSEA CHILDREN AGED 5 EXAMINED 1969

Fig. 20. An example of the output of results showing qualitative data in tabular form.

This system has been found to be very flexible and no reprogramming has been necessary in order to undertake any analysis desired, by any of the users.

The system described has now been in use for several years and has been used by many examiners, the large majority of whom were public

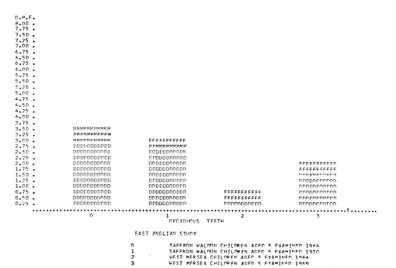

Fig. 21. An example of the output of results in diagrammatic form.

dental officers conducting surveys in their areas. All have reported that the system was easy to use and many have indicated that in the absence of the computer they would not have considered starting their surveys.

To date, over 50,000 records have been processed in this manner so there can be little doubt that the application of computers in the field of dental epidemiology is now firmly established.

WHEN SHOULD A COMPUTER BE USED FOR EPIDEMIOLOGICAL DATA?

The public health dentist who conducts a survey must decide early in the planning stages whether or not the data will be processed by computer. What are the factors which influence this decision?

There are several important considerations each, of which is dependent on the others. The major points are the amount of processing involved, access to a computer, a decision as to who is going to supervise the planning, programming and processing involved, and the cost.

The amount of analysis required depends on the number of subjects involved, the quantity of data collected for each subject, and the amount and complexity of the analyses involved. If the survey is relatively simple and is only to be undertaken once, then it is possible that it could be more easily and cheaply processed by hand. If the study is to be repeated a number of times, however, it is often worthwhile using a program and the computer. Some surveys have so much data or require so much complex analyses that the required results can only be produced by a computer.

The availability of a computer may not be as large a problem as it at first appears. Most local authorities in this country have a unit or have access to one, and several are already being used for dental work. All the universities have computers and are often prepared to help, and there are several commercial bureaux who can provide a service. Burt has described in chapter 6 the system developed by WHO, and they are prepared to help in areas where access to a computer is difficult (World Health Organization, 1971).

Possibly more difficult than obtaining access to the machine is the development of the processing system. Frequently a computer unit is prepared to run work but is unable to provide any assistance with the programming other than in an advisory capacity. It is possible to use a system which has been developed elsewhere. This has the advantage that all the development and testing of the program has been completed but has the disadvantage that the data has to be collected according to the criteria laid down for that system, and this may mean restricting the scope of the study. It is usual to use such a system on the unit for which it was intended, as with the WHO system. In theory, it is possible to use a program written for one computer on another, but in practice this may mean a lot of modifications and often it is quicker to write a new program.

The alternative is to devise a new system for the available unit, but for this it is necessary to have someone who is conversant with the system and the programming language. This may be one of the unit's programmers.

If there is a programmer available to help, this is a very satisfactory arrangement but it must be remembered that they are usually employed to undertake specific jobs and the dental work is an extra load, so often it is necessary to wait before help is available. Obviously two experts from such different fields working together on a program make it necessary for at least one of them to learn a certain amount about the other's discipline. Often it is the programmer who is expected to master the techniques of dental epidemiology in order to be able to write the program. This means additional delays. It is also possible that the programmer may tackle the problem as he understands it and not as it really is. This can give rise to errors, which if the dental researcher has no knowledge of the processing, may pass undetected. There is also an unfortunate tendency among some researchers to assume that because the results have been produced by a computer, they must be correct.

One solution to these difficulties is for someone in the dental team to be responsible for the programming and supervising of the processing, using the professional programmer as a consultant adviser. It is not difficult to learn to program. A course of approximately 50 hours should be sufficient to enable someone to tackle most of the programming problems associated with the dental data, provided professional assistance is available if required.

Cost is a factor which must be considered early in the study. Many beginners are surprised by the costs involved. This is not only the costs of the processing but also of the preparation of the data and for the services of the programmer.

The importance of early consultation with the computer personnel cannot be over stressed. It allows for the necessary understanding of mutual problems to be sorted out. Failure to communicate at this stage has cost some surveys dearly in time, money and effort wasted when the data comes to be processed.

THE FUTURE OF COMPUTERS IN DENTAL EPIDEMIOLOGY AND DENTAL PUBLIC HEALTH

It is not possible to say in which direction the next developments will be made in the field of dental epidemiology, but there are two large areas which are beginning to receive consideration.

The first is that the speed of the collection and preparation of data is still the slowest part of the whole process and it is possible that in the future this will be considerably increased. Some steps have already

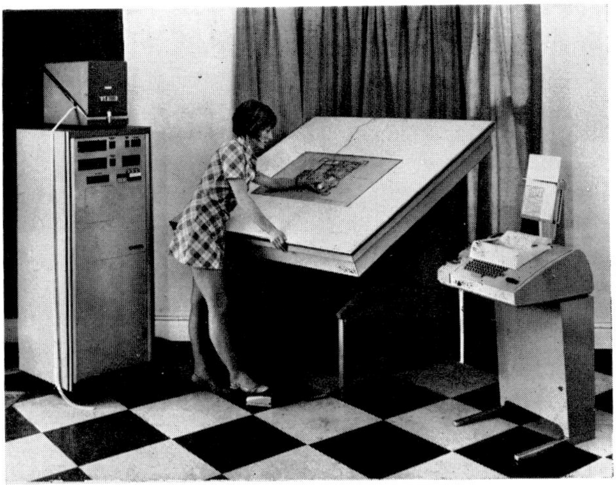

Fig. 22. A tracing table being used to record information, which is in diagrammatic form, onto paper tape. The paper tape punch is situated on the top of the left hand cabinet and the typewriter keyboard on the right hand side may be used to insert additional information onto the paper tape.

been made in this direction. The use of the mark sense punch has already been described and it was noted that a disadvantage of this system in the dental application was that it was necessary to reduce the amount of data recorded. It is now possible, however, to obtain readers which scan marks optically instead of electronically. They enable much larger amounts of information to be read at any one time and operate

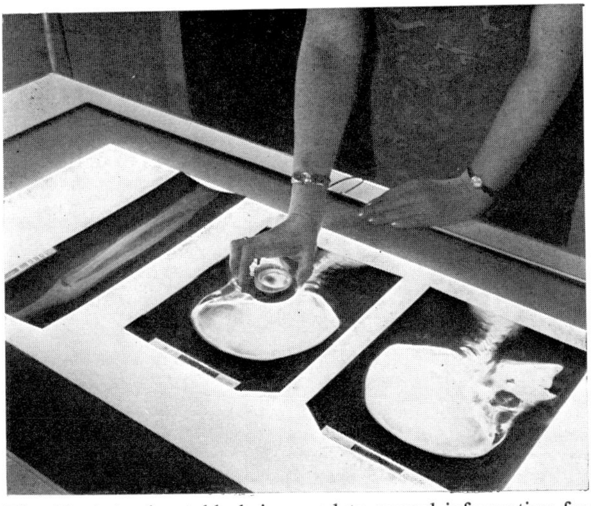

Fig. 23. A tracing table being used to record information from lateral skull X-rays.

at a much faster speed. These optical readers can be used to produce punch cards, store the information onto magnetic tape, or for direct input to the computers.

There are also available tracing tables which automatically record the co-ordinates of any information which is in diagrammatic form (*Fig.* 22). It enables data in the form of photographs, X-rays (*Fig.* 23), maps, or graphs to be directly coded, stored on magnetic or paper tape, or input directly to a computer. In the dental field this table has already been used successfully for measuring photographs and radiographs (Houston, 1970). Using such a table, large-scale orthodontic surveys become a practical possibility and it is also conceivable that

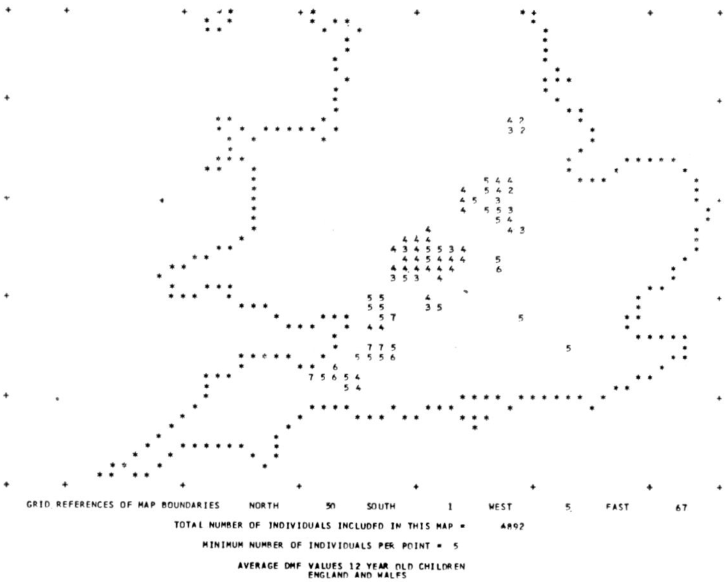
GRID REFERENCES OF MAP BOUNDARIES NORTH 50 SOUTH 1 WEST 5 EAST 67
TOTAL NUMBER OF INDIVIDUALS INCLUDED IN THIS MAP = 4892
MINIMUM NUMBER OF INDIVIDUALS PER POINT = 5
AVERAGE DMF VALUES 12 YEAR OLD CHILDREN
ENGLAND AND WALES

Fig. 24. An example of computer output showing the mapping of dental information.

such a unit could be used for recording the results of a dental examination directly onto magnetic tape.

The second area of development is that new methods of analysis for the data will now become available. In all fields in which the computer is used new methods of analysis are now being introduced which because of their complexity could never have been considered previously. Some of the methods now in use in the fields of medicine and biology have direct applications to dental epidemiology. One example is the mapping of dental epidemiological data. If an individual's place of residence, in the form of a map reference, is added to the dental information then the computer can be used to map the prevalence of dental disease (*Fig.* 24). However, many of these maps are not easy to interpret so it is necessary to use statistical methods to calculate the position of 'contour lines' joining areas of equal disease prevalence. These trend surface analyses are complex and could not possibly be undertaken by hand. The results that they produce mean that the dental data will be directly comparable with the results of other environmental studies, analysed in the same way, and should make any association between dental disease and the natural environment much easier to detect.

In the wider field of dental public health the computer is playing an increasingly important role. Apart from the epidemiological aspects which may also be used to gain information about the future development, how the service is running, and where it is most needed at present;

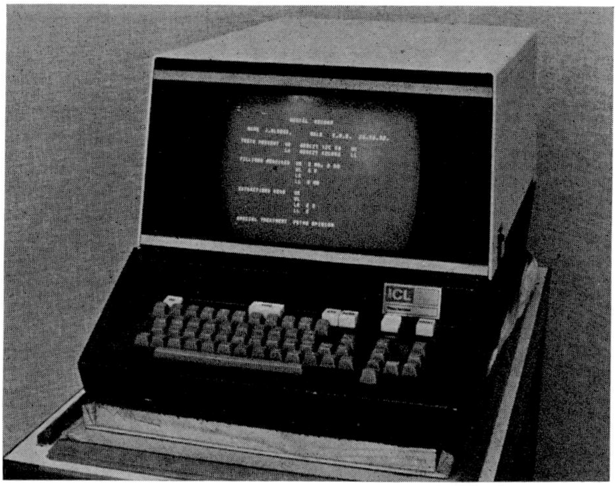

Fig. 25. A visual display unit showing how the computer might be used to present clinical dental information.

experiments have shown that the computer can also be used for patient records and patient administration and some local authorities are at present using these machines for their medical records and for operating a recall system for vaccination and immunization (*British Medical Journal*, 1968).

Much of the administration and routine returns can also be handled in this way.

Modern techniques are such that it is not necessary to be close to the computer in order to use it. Data can be transmitted over a telephone line and one can foresee the day when all the clinics in an area will be able to gain access to records stored centrally. The clinics would be equipped with a special type of input/output unit which has a typewriter keyboard for communication with the computer and either a television screen (*Fig.* 25) or a typewriter printer (right hand unit,

Fig. 22) for receiving messages. The operator would type in the name of the individual for whom the record was required and almost instantly full details would be transmitted back by the computer. This application is now being installed in some hospitals in this country and is very similar to the system at present being used by the major banks in this country.

The fields of dental epidemiology and dental public health have expanded and developed quite considerably over the past few years. If these subjects are to continue to expand at a similar rate then workers in the fields cannot afford to ignore the computer. They must be prepared to understand these machines so they can be used to their maximum effect and potential.

Acknowledgements I am most grateful to the staff of the Computer Unit of the United Birmingham Hospitals for their help and the use of their facilities. Thanks are also due to Mr. B. Scott, Operations Manager of the Unit, and Mr. R. Bettles of Leicester City Health Department for their assistance in reading and criticizing the manuscript. I am also grateful to Mr. R. Frazier for the illustrations and Miss J. Davies for clerical assistance, and, finally, I am most grateful to my colleagues for their advice and criticism.

REFERENCES

ANDERSON, R. J. (1967), 'The relationship between dental conditions and trace elements in soil and water', PhD Thesis, University of London Library.

—— (1968), 'Computer analysis of dental surveys', *Br. med. J.*, **4,** 124.

—— and BEAL, J. F. (1971), 'The analysis of dental surveys using the computer', *Int. J. biol. med. Comp.*, **2,** 309.

BRITISH MEDICAL JOURNAL (1968), 'Medicine and the computer', *Br. med. J.*, **2,** 823; **3,** 51, 116, 180, 247, 309, 367, 426.

BRITISH STANDARDS INSTITUTION (1962), *Glossary of Terms Used in Automatic Data Processing*. B.S. 3527.

CHRISTOPHER, A. (1967), 'The role of computers in dentistry', *J. Am. dent. Ass.*, **74,** 720.

CLARKE, C. D., MAYCOCK, G. J., and PRICE, D. A. (1973), *A System for Monitoring Child Dental Health*, County Health Dept., Shirehall, Shrewsbury.

EHRLICH, P., JONES, C. F., and BRITTON, K. (1969), 'Computerised student evaluation system', *J. dent. Educ.*, **33,** 336.

GLASS, R. L., ALMAN, J. E., and FLEISCH, S. (1965), 'Punch card method of recording student clinical achievement', *Ibid.*, **29,** 260.

— — — — — —, KAPUR, K. K., and EPSTEIN, H. D. (1969), 'Automated record system for computer programming of dental treatment', *J. Am. dent. Ass.*, **78,** 997.

HOUSTON, W. J. B. (1970), 'Automated measurements of photographs and radiographs', *Dent. Practnr dent. Rec.*, **21,** 100.

JACKSON, D., JAMES, P. M. C., and SLACK, G. L. (1963), 'An investigation into the use of indices devised for the clinical measurement of caries degree', *Archs oral Biol.*, **8,** 55.

JAMES, E., O'BRIEN, F., and WHITEHEAD, P. (1970), *A Fortran Course*. London: Prentice Hall International.

JAMES, F. D., GOOSE, D. H., and MOORE, G. E. (1968), 'The use of computers in dentistry', *Br. dent. J.*, **125,** 306.

KLEIN, H., and KRAMER, M. (1948), 'A dental record form for statistical machine tabulation', *J. dent. Res.*, **27,** 170.
—— and PALMER, C. E. (1940), 'Studies on Dental Caries. X. A procedure for the recording of dental examination findings', *Ibid.*, **19,** 243.
McCRACKEN, D. D. (1961), *A Guide for Fortran Programming*. New York: Wiley.
—— (1965), *A Guide to Fortran IV Programming*. New York: Wiley.
McLACHLAN, G., and SHEGOG, R. A. (1968), *Computers in the Service of Medicine*, Vols. I and II. London: Oxford University Press.
MARTHALER, T. M. (1963), 'Experimental design in epidemiological research', *J. dent. Res.*, **42,** 192.
MOORE, G. E. (1969), 'The use of computers in North American hospitals and dental schools', *Br. dent. J.*, **127,** 231.
ROSE, J. (1969), *Computers in Medicine*. London: Churchill.
SOLOW, B. (1964), 'A method of computer analysis of epidemiological malocclusion data', *Trans. Eur. Orthod. Soc.*, **40,** 391.
WORLD HEALTH ORGANIZATION (1971), *Oral Health Surveys, Basic Methods*. Geneva: WHO.

Chapter 12

An Approach to Dental Health Education for Schoolchildren

H. Colin Davis, FDS, RCS
Director, Oral Hygiene Service and Lecturer, Community Dentistry Unit, The London Hospital Medical College Dental School

Dental health education has already been described as an integral part of any dental public health programme, for it is generally accepted as a means of influencing consumer attitudes towards the service being provided. There have, however, been few instances where the traditional type of dental health education has been shown to influence significantly attitudes or behaviour, and fresh approaches to the subject are now being sought.

Mr. Davis outlines some of the motivational forces which influence behaviour, and how programmes of dental health education must be shaped to utilize them. He goes on to describe one particular approach, which shows promise, recently applied in Britain. Mr. Davis concentrates on education in schoolchildren, as it is likely that positive attitudes can be most readily shaped in this group.

No matter how comprehensive and efficient the dental care programme for a community may be, it cannot achieve its full potential unless it is based on mutual understanding between those who provide it and those to whom it is directed. The objective of dental health education is to enhance this mutual understanding, for community dental care is only of significance in the context of a community that cares.

A community is made up of individuals and in the context of dental care they will fall into three categories:

1. Those to whom the preservation of the natural dentition throughout life is essential to their well-being.

2. Those who are prepared to take reasonable care, but who accept the ultimate loss of all their teeth, and their artificial replacement as likely or inevitable.

3. Those who through fear, ignorance, poverty or lack of treatment facilities merely seek the relief of intolerable pain and gross disfigurement, or reject the possibility of treatment altogether.

The ratio between these three categories will vary greatly in different communities and will be dependent on many factors: social, economic, geographical and psychological. It is the responsibility of the members of the dental team through their social and professional behaviour, through the quality of the service they provide, and through the

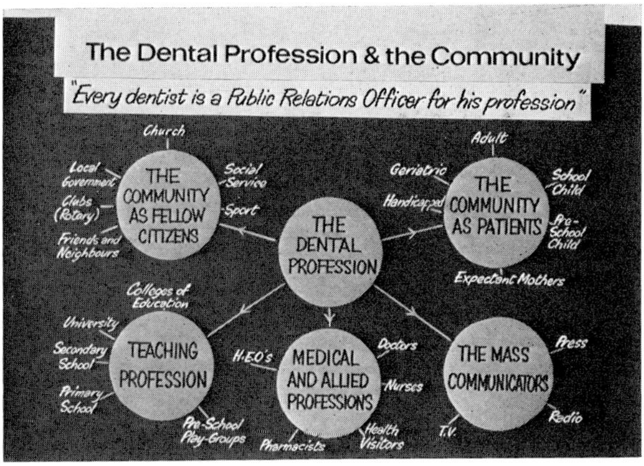

Fig. 1. Diagram to show the interrelationships of the dental profession with the community.

information about dental health which they disseminate to the various groups which make up the community (*Fig.* 1), to present themselves so effectively that mutual understanding will be achieved. Then more and more people will be drawn from category 3 to category 2 and from category 2 to category 1.

Education for dental health has as its first function to *transmit information*, information which will lead to a better understanding of the problems of dental disease, of the possibilities of early preventive action, and of the advances that are being made in dental research and clinical practice. An informed public can then be instrumental in furthering public health measures such as fluoridation (Knutson, 1970), and dietary modifications whether by manufacturers or outlets such as school tuck shops (General Dental Council, 1970; Journal of Dental Research, 1970). It is also encouraged to seek routine dental care, to appreciate and if necessary to pay for the more sophisticated treatments which the profession is trained to provide.

With the high level of dental disease in almost all parts of the world, the task is a formidable one (World Health Organization, 1970). Most countries have limited resources of manpower and derisory sums of money available to wage a campaign against a disease which the public accepts as inevitable, knows is not a killer, but the cure of which it still regards all too often as worse than the disease. Ranged against them is the vast machinery of manufacturing, importing, exporting, advertising and distributing a high sucrose, over-processed, plaque-conducive diet, aimed at an adult population which complacently accepts it and promiscuously passes it on to its equally eager off-spring.

But it is a pointless waste of time and effort to wage such a campaign at all unless it brings about a change in the public's attitude to prevention, the ultimate yardstick of its success being to bring the individual patient into the individual surgery, into the 'one-to-one' situation in which the responsibility for the motivation of the individual to form sensible oral hygiene habits is taken over by the dentist and the members of his team.

PRIMARY FUNCTION OF DENTAL HEALTH EDUCATION

It is only possible in one short chapter to deal in a little more detail with the primary function of dental health education which has been well defined as: 'the provision of dental health information to a total population in such a way that people *will apply it in everyday living*' (Young and Striffler, 1969); i.e., 'a person will change his behaviour only when he sees the action as a means to an end *which he himself desires*' (World Health Organization, 1954).

Furthermore that person will not take action *voluntarily* to achieve health and to avoid disease unless four requirements are satisfied (Kegeles, 1963; Kirscht et al., 1966):

1. He feels himself susceptible to the disease.
2. He thinks there will be serious consequences if affected by it.
3. He feels that the desired action will be effective and lasting.
4. He regards that action as less unpleasant than the disease itself.

The role of the dental health educator is to see to it that the four specific requirements for voluntary dental health action are satisfied by bringing home to people that:

1. Their susceptibility is such that the prevalence of dental caries and periodontal disease is virtually 100 per cent at some point in the life span of all people in present day communities regardless of their social or economic status.

2. The consequences are serious in that delay or failure to seek treatment leads to discomfort, pain, disfigurement, loss of function, impairment of general health, and unnecessary waste of money, manpower, and time.

3. Action is effective in that early regular dental care can prevent these things happening; and conversely that artificial replacements are a poor substitute for a healthy natural or conservatively treated dentition.

4. Action is not unpleasant in that preventive measures require simple commonsense and diligence; and that modern advances in training, equipment, materials, and anaesthetic methods can now remove the barriers of panic, fear, and pain and make dental treatment tolerable.

Furthermore if its advocacy is to be effective the maintenance of good dental health must be shown to be reasonable, practical, economic and desirable, offering positive rewards beyond a mere absence of ill-health.

Its code of practice may be summed-up in the mnemonic TASK:

T. Take a personal pride in your health, appearance, and social acceptability in all of which the mouth plays a key role.

A. Adopt sensible eating habits:
   1. Regular meals and a balanced diet. Ideally this should include fluoridated water, and, failing this, the appropriate fluoride additives.
   2. A minimum of between-meal eating and drinking of substances with a high sucrose content and sticky consistency.

S. Seek regular dental care, so reducing the time, cost and discomfort of treatment.

K. Keep up good mouth hygiene habits throughout life.
   1. Brush regularly once every twenty-four hours to remove all possible plaque from the tooth surfaces and gingival crevices (therapeutic cleaning).
   2. Brush after meals when practicable or finish with a naturally scouring food, or rinse vigorously with water to remove superficial stains and debris (cosmetic cleaning).

This basic 'pre-clinical' information, adapted to the age, intelligence, and status of the specific group in the community at which it is being aimed may be imparted through two possible channels, the mass media and the small group media (Rosen, 1966; Young, 1967).

THE MASS MEDIA

Television and radio programmes, whether commercially or professionally sponsored, the press, and the cinema can be used in a great variety of ways in arousing interest and conveying information about all aspects of dentistry and dental health. The preparation and presentation of effective material requires skill and imagination (Davis, 1966, 1967) and its acceptance depends on the goodwill of editors and producers, since dental disease has to take its place in the queue for honourable mention in competition with the more dramatic facts of venereal disease, lung cancer, and drug addiction.

It would be euphoric to suggest that dental health education through the impersonal mass media has any influence in reducing dental disease. On the other hand the enormous power of television in particular to create an informed public has not yet been harnessed as it might be in furthering the public's knowledge of dental health and disease.

THE SMALL GROUP MEDIA

The small group media of personal communication may be used in one of two ways based on the two broad conceptual models of health education (Steuart, 1969). First, the traditional authoritarian concept with its sharp dividing line between the professional who knows the facts about health and disease and who communicates them to the passive recipient, a one-way communication flow from the expert to the layman accompanied by exhortations to act appropriately for the benefit of his health. It is this didactic method supplemented by vast quantities of visual and audiovisual aid material of varying quality which is still for the most part blindly accepted and followed in most countries. Its main targets are the captive audiences of the schools system, of adult groups such as Parent/Teacher Associations, in antenatal clinics, and collectively in community dental health campaigns, the design of which will depend on the socio-economic situation of a specific community (Davis and Land, 1962; Sundrum, 1967).

There is ample evidence to show that all this activity, especially in the classroom, leads to a greater knowledge of the facts of dental health and disease as was demonstrated by the St. Albans Study (Davis et al., 1956) and in many subsequent ones. There is very little to suggest that with a continuing shortage of dental manpower it can bring about any lasting change in health behaviour or improvement in the health of the dental tissues (Parfitt et al., 1958) except in a quite exceptionally favourable situation such as that reported by Williford et al. (1967), or even when carried out as intensively as the 10-year comprehensive dental health programme in the town of Askov (Jordan et al., 1959) in the United States.

If the members of the dental team are going to make a significant contribution to the improvement of dental health through health education, if they really believe that 'it's not what people know about health, but what they do about what they know' (Cohen and Lucye, 1970) that matters, they must move forward as the teaching profession has to accept the second two-way conceptual model in which the professional and the client are co-operative and equal partners in a joint enterprise. In the nursery and junior school systems, where it is easier to instil habits in childhood rather than change them in adolescence, learning should be a creative process in which the role of the teacher has been aptly described as 'learning with each child instead of instructing a passive class—to be a well of clear water into which the children can dip all the time rather than a hosepipe dowsing them with facts' (Marshall, 1966).

This 'project' learning, which stems from the work of such pioneers as Montessori and Froebel, is in the primary school essentially 'a scheme of work from which children embark either singly or in groups for varying periods of time based on a topic which interests each child to such an extent that he or she wants to discover more about it' (Kent, 1968).

Furthermore, 'the theme can be chosen from almost any field of human activity—an incident from history, a description of a shark-fishing expedition in the South Seas, a cathedral, a scientific discovery, an archaeological dig' (Marshall, 1968).

AN APPLICATION OF PROJECT LEARNING

It was in fact an archaeological dig of an Iron Age settlement on the outskirts of a village in the west of England, undertaken by the teachers and children of the local school and also the children's parents which sparked off the idea of a pioneer project on teeth described by Maddick and Downton (1970), which has since been widely followed. During the dig the skeleton of a man in his thirties was discovered with thirty-two completely caries-free teeth still intact in the skull. The project began to evolve from the interest aroused in the dental condition of this ancient Briton and the ensuing discussion between the teachers on the one hand who had been trained to teach and who knew the foibles and capabilities of their pupils; and on the other the dentist who had been trained to practice dentistry and who was visiting the school as an 'expert' concerned with the dental health of the children.

Too often the 'expert' while fully supplied with the facts of his speciality lacks the gift of imaginative communication and may even do more harm than good by making such a notoriously difficult subject as dental health either boring, distasteful, or totally unrelated to the rest of life. On the other hand the busy teacher is tempted to use the arrival of an 'expert' as an excuse for abandoning his pupils in order to devote himself to some more pressing task.

But both parties forget that: 'The emphasis must be on the children learning, not upon an expert teaching his own subject however well he may be able to do so. But how welcome would such people be contributing each his own particular strength to a team of teachers all working along a line of discovery and creativity' (Marshall, 1968).

The joint undertaking which evolved from the discussion in the village school was a project on 'the human mouth' which was started by the 9–11-year-old children. In it, they would discover for themselves the major facts of oral hygiene, and the project would act as a centre of interest providing opportunities for them to develop work linking up their normal class-room learning in such subjects as English, mathematics, science, geography, and art.

The basis of the project was a controlled experiment to test the effectiveness of various ways of cleaning the teeth.

The parents were informed of the project and asked to co-operate by sending their children to school on the appointed day with a toothbrush and some toothpaste.

The children were divided into groups of five seated round a table and each one was given a chocolate biscuit; an article of food which would be tenacious, cariogenic, and easy to identify in the mouth. The first child acted as the control and simply ate the chocolate biscuit; the second ate the chocolate biscuit and then brushed the teeth with toothbrush and water, while the others timed it with a stop watch for the

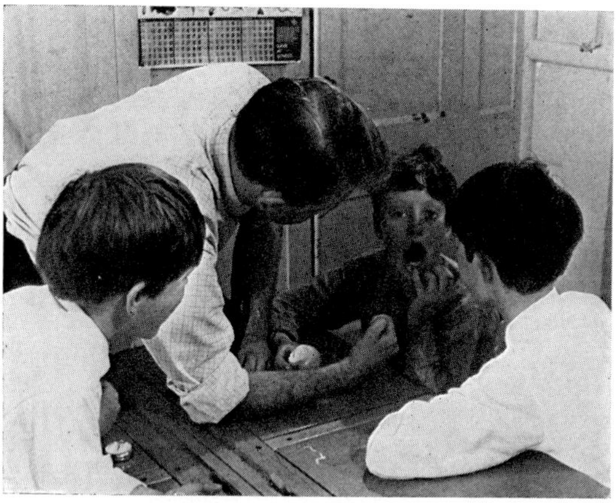

Fig. 2. The dentist assists the children in a classroom oral hygiene project.

visible clearance of all debris; the third then brushed with toothbrush and toothpaste; the fourth ate an apple or raw carrot; the fifth swished and swallowed water. Each method was timed for its relative effectiveness and compared with the very slow clearance from the uncleaned mouth of the control. Each child then wrote his own account of the experiment, thus learning to observe and to record his findings in lucid English.

The children became thoroughly absorbed in the experiment and they were all now proud possessors of a toothbrush and toothpaste which they may not have been before. They had seen in each other's mouths the results of carbohydrate stagnation, and how to avoid it (*Fig*. 2). Under the friendly guidance of the dental officer, who with the school teacher was now an integral part of a joint adventure in discovery, they saw the stages of dental development quite naturally in each other's mouths. They observed the transitional stages of a mixed dentition, real overcrowding and apparent overcrowding, what a filling looks like, why six-year molars are important, where the toothbrush fails to reach and a whole lot more.

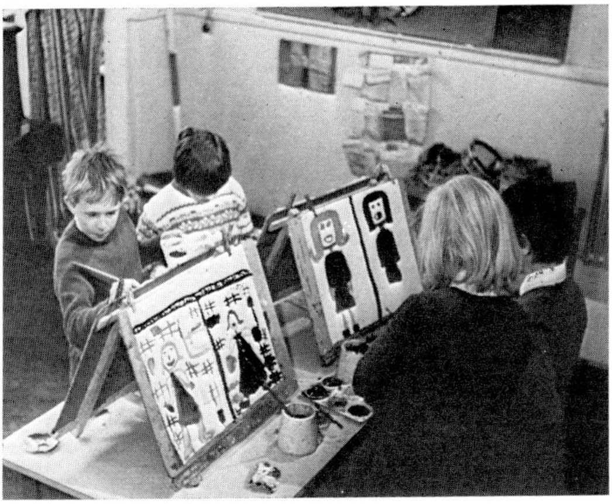

Fig. 3. Projects prepared by younger children.

With this controlled experiment their interest in their dental apparatus was roused, the facts made sense, their attitude was transformed, and their oral hygiene habits improved. A follow-up survey showed that many of the children had changed their brushing routine from once to

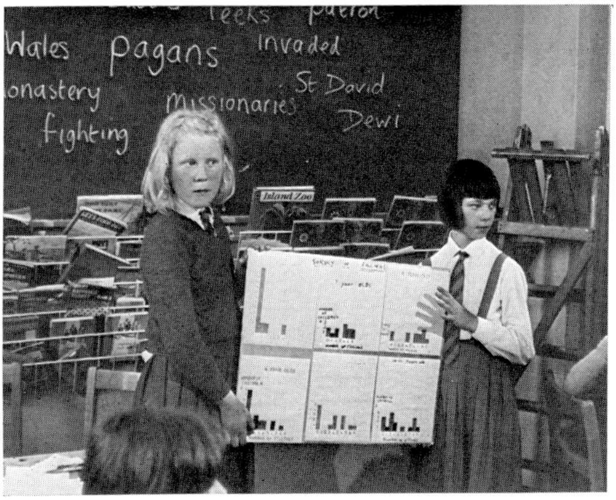

Fig. 4. A more detailed project from the older children.

twice a day and that all the children involved in the project now cleaned their teeth whereas prior to it 16 per cent never cleaned them.

Once the project is under way, it can be extended and developed in innumerable ways to include all the children in the school down to the very youngest, and they themselves come up with new ideas.

Furthermore the tangible results of the project: the notebooks, posters, histograms, maps, models, mimes, playlets, and puppet-shows, can be proudly shown to the parents at the school's Open Day (*Figs*. 3, 4).

ROLE OF THE MOTHER

It has been shown that mothers' dental health practices are one of the most influential factors in determining the nature of their children's practices (Rayner, 1970). The first priority for the dental health educator must then be to explain to mothers the facts of the developing dentition, and the need for good oral hygiene practices both for themselves and their offspring during the earliest formative years.

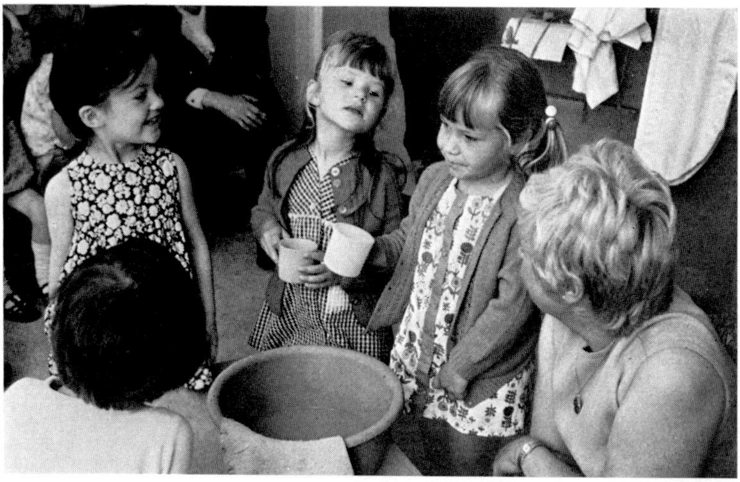

Fig. 5. Oral hygiene instruction in a preschool playgroup.

But it is in the preschool play-groups (*Fig*. 5), nursery and primary schools (where the links between the teachers, the parents, and the children are still so close) that the mother can be further educated through her children whether it be in helping her to confirm the habits which she has installed in the home, or in helping her to establish them when she has failed to do so.

If the appropriate members of the dental team are an added link they can do much towards achieving the primary objective of dental health education, that mutual understanding between those who provide a dental care service and those to whom it is directed.

REFERENCES

Cohen, L. K., and Lucye, L. (1970), 'A position on school dental health education', *J. Sch. Hlth*, **40**, 361.

DAVIS, H. C. (1966), 'Date with a dentist (Radiotalk)', *Dent. Hlth*, **5,** 5.
— — (1967), 'Date with a dentist (Radiotalk)', *Ibid.*, **6,** 19.
— — JAMES, P. M. C., and PARFITT, J. G. (1956), 'A controlled study into the effect of dental health education on 1,539 schoolchildren in St. Albans', *Br. dent. J.*, **100,** 354.
— — and LAND, D. (1962), 'Good teeth for Guildford. A study in civic enterprise', *Ibid.*, **112,** 430.
GENERAL DENTAL COUNCIL (1970), 'A suggested list of foods recommended for sale in school tuck-shops', Typescript.
JORDAN, W. A., SNYDER, J. R., PETERSON, J. K., and JOHNSON, R. A. (1959), 'The Askov dental demonstration; final report', *NW. Dent.*, **38,** 444.
JOURNAL OF DENTAL RESEARCH (1970), 'Supplement: The Role of human foodstuffs in caries', **49,** 6, part 1.
KEGELES, S. S. (1963), 'Some motives for seeking preventive dental care', *J. Am. dent. Ass.*, **67,** 90.
KENT, G. (1968), *Projects in the Primary School.* London: Batsford.
KIRSCHT, J. P., HAEFNER, D. P., KEGELES, S. S., and ROSENSTOCK, I. M. (1966), 'A national study of health beliefs', *J. Hlth Hum. Beh.*, **7,** 248.
KNUTSON, J. W. (1970), 'Water fluoridation after 25 years', *Br. dent. J.*, **129,** 297.
MADDICK, I., and DOWNTON, D. (1970), 'Project work in teaching dental health', *J. Sch. Hlth*, **40,** 197.
MARSHALL, S. (1966), *An Experiment in Education.* London: Cambridge University Press.
— — (1968), *Adventures in Creative Education.* London: Pergamon.
PARFITT, G. J., JAMES, P. M. C., and DAVIS, H. C. (1958), 'A controlled study into the effect of dental health education on the gingival structures of school children', *Br. dent. J.*, **104,** 21.
RAYNER, J. F. (1970), 'Socio-economic status and factors influencing the dental health practices of mothers', *Am. J. Publ. Hlth*, **90,** 1250.
ROSEN, B. J. (1966), 'Mass media: Effectiveness in education for dental health', *J. Publ. Hlth Dent.*, **26,** 256.
STEUART, G. W. (1969), 'Planning and evaluation in health education', *Int. J. Hlth Educ.*, **12,** 65.
SUNDRUM, C. J. (1967), 'Developing a dental health education programme in a less developed country', *J. dent. Aux.*, **5,** 17.
WILLIFORD, J. W., MUHLER, J. C., and STOOKEY, G. K. (1967), 'Study demonstrating improved oral health through education', *J. Am. dent. Ass.*, **75,** 896.
WORLD HEALTH ORGANIZATION (1954), *Health Education of the Public.* Geneva: WHO Tech. Rep. Ser. No. 89.
— — — (1970), *Dental Health Education.* Geneva: WHO Tech. Rep. Ser. No. 449.
YOUNG, M. A. C. (1967), *Review of Research and Studies Related to Health Education (1961–1966). What People know, believe, and do about Health.* Health Education Monographs No. 25. Society of Public Health Educators, 104, East 25th. Street New York 10010.
YOUNG, W. O., and STRIFFLER, D. F. (1969), *The Dentist, his Practice, and his Community*, 2nd ed. Philadelphia: Saunders.

ADDITIONAL INFORMATION

Some Sources of Information and Materials about Dental Health Education in the English Language:

The American Dental Association, 211 E. Chicago Ave., Chicago 60611.
The British Dental Association, 64 Wimpole Street, London W.1.
The General Dental Council, 37 Wimpole Street, W.1.
The Oral Hygiene Service, Hesketh House, Portman Square, London W.1.

In addition to conventional visual aid material the Oral Hygiene Service has prepared a teaching film and hand-book for teachers, and a film and source book for children for use in developing a dental project in primary schools.

Details of materials in other languages and organizations throughout the world concerned with dental health education can be obtained from The Secretariat, Federation Dentaire Internationale, 64 Wimpole Street, London W.1.

Chapter 13

Dental Education

Roy Duckworth MD, BDS, FDS, FRCPATH
Dean of Dental Studies, The London Hospital Medical College Dental School

The quality of health care in a community reflects to a large extent the education and training received by its practitioners.

In this chapter, Professor Duckworth considers a number of principles of dental education. He discusses its role in the delivery of care to the community, problems of recruiting and selecting students, and the development of the dental team within the dental school. The need for planned change is clearly stated; change when the objectives and priorities of education have been defined. Professor Duckworth also indicates some developments in curriculum organization which are required to produce the type of dentist which future social developments will demand.

The chapter is completed with a short section on postgraduate education in the United Kingdom.

The presentation and discussion of current philosophies and practices in dental education around the world is necessarily a large subject and cannot be attempted here. Overall approaches to dental education and guidelines for the development of curricula are provided in various World Health Organization Reports (1962, 1968, 1970), in a monograph by Durocher (1970), and much factual data describing curricula and their constituent courses in different countries are available in the World Health Organization Directory of Dental Schools (1967). Therefore, no attempt will be made to review these facets of dental education. Instead, this essay, which is concerned primarily with the United Kingdom, and one school's philosophies and practices in particular, will deal with those aspects of dental education which encompass community dental care and dental public health.

DENTAL EDUCATION AND THE COMMUNITY

The degree to which a community develops a system of dental education is a useful indication of the importance that community places upon the attainment of dental health. This development of dental education is sustained or retarded by inter-related promoting and limiting pressures which are generated within the community.

Historically, the dentist has always been the principal promoter of dental education and he must continue to be its most important advocate. Directly or indirectly, he has the opportunity to promote dental education whenever he persuades his individual patients, his community, and government that dental health is not only attainable and desirable but that it is an essential component of total health. When the dentist attempts to educate individuals and alter their attitudes and behaviour, those who respond and demand dental care promote the need for the education of dentists. Similarly, when communities make attempts to cope with unfulfilled demands and latent needs, the provision of new or improved systems of dental education is stimulated.

Faced with these pressures from society for more dental care and, by implication, for more dental education, governmental response is conditioned by the current availability of adequate resources. The development of dental education always faces competition from other national priorities which limit the flow of finance and the recruitment of manpower. Ideally, the diversion of these precious national resources into dental education should be related to the need and demand for dental care; but in reality, the ability to provide and to develop dental education is more often a function of the flow of resources into all forms of higher education. At this level, despite competition between different academic disciplines, substantial support is usually provided for the education of those who will serve the health professions, although, within the budget for this kind of education, dentistry all too often occupies a place of relatively low priority, even in countries with well developed economies.

The balance struck between opposing factors which promote and limit the development of dental education is not constant. From time to time cultural, social, and political pressures within the community may so alter this balance that the development of dental education is enhanced, retarded or arrested. It follows that if dental education is not to be static, but is to react to changing needs, dental educators must at all times be sufficiently flexible in their attitudes to adapt to these changes. For the good of dental health it is essential that advantage be taken of favourable changes and, when limiting forces are in the ascendency, educators must be prepared at least to maintain standards appropriate to the community's requirements.

To date, competing priorities for each nation's finance and manpower have led to a world-wide failure to develop dental education to the point where it can provide competent personnel to supply all the care which would be required if need came to be matched by demand. Although dentist–population ratios are known to vary from approximately one per one thousand to one per one million (Federation Dentaire Internationale, 1970), in no country has dental education been able to provide the skilled manpower required to satisfy the current demand for the prevention and treatment of dental diseases. Alas, if present policies in dental education, which, at least in the United Kingdom restrict teaching mainly to the education of the dentist, continue to be pursued there would seem to be little likelihood that the additional manpower resources required to meet future demands will become available.

In order to obtain the personnel to man a dental service, and to narrow the gap between demand and availability of services, most of the finance for dental education is provided by the community. Dental education must then be accountable to the community which will require it to fulfil certain major objectives. Society will endeavour to ensure that dental education is sufficient in quantity and quality, that it is efficient in execution and that it will lead to the provision of a high quality preventive and treatment service which will function economically (Chaves, 1969a).

A measure of the sufficiency of dental education is the production of adequate numbers of dentists and ancillary personnel educated to levels appropriate to the demands and needs of the community. Estimates of the demand for dental services, both quantitatively and qualitatively, are essential to the proper planning of dental education. In the past, high quality dental education has often been confused with education and training for the practice of elaborate technical dentistry. However, communities are now becoming more concerned that dental education should aim to maintain healthy oral tissues by prevention. Clearly, if there is a failure in dental education to reach the minimum levels of quantity and competence this aim will not be attainable and the dental health of the community will suffer.

However, it does not necessarily follow that there is benefit to the community if all dentists and their ancillaries are educated to levels far beyond those dictated by the demands of the community. If this is done those additional skills acquired in longer and more expensive education may atrophy through disuse in dental practice. In the long term, this atrophy of skills may lead to job dissatisfaction, consequential recruitment problems and a real decline in the overall quality of dental care. To prevent this it is important to relate dental education to the profile of demand for dental treatment in the community to be served (Chaves, 1969b).

Society demands that dental education should be an efficient process. This implies that the duration of dental education, and hence its cost, should be the minimum compatible with the attainment of the appropriate quality in the performance of its products: the dentists. Once educational objectives have been defined and methods of achieving them determined, the curriculum should be planned to prepare the student for dental practice in the shortest possible time, without needless repetition of course work. This community requirement for efficient dental education also demands that student selection should be based upon predictions of performance likely to minimize the failure of students.

As yet, the requirement of the community that dental education should lead to the economic delivery of dental services cannot be properly met. This situation obtains because the results of research have not fully defined what is economic and what is uneconomic. There are few useful data on cost–benefit analyses of preventive and therapeutic procedures carried out by the dentist. There is an even greater lack of data on the economic aspects of utilizing auxiliary personnel in one of the several ways currently under evaluation.

When data become available from many different studies currently in progress in different parts of the world, there will be greater understanding of the possible ways in which more economic use could be made of both professional and auxiliary manpower, whilst at the same time improving the standard of patient care. Then, it will be possible to make substantial progress towards the development of a form of dental education which will engender not only the delivery of quality services but their delivery in an economic manner.

PERSONNEL PROVIDING DENTAL SERVICES

DENTAL EDUCATION AND MANPOWER CONSTRAINTS

In most countries the only recipient of dental education is the future professional man or woman; the dentist, dental surgeon, or stomatologist who prepares for dental education by high attainment during secondary education and is, therefore, with the exception of a few countries, in relatively short supply. Dental education is long and expensive and, after graduation, the somewhat costly services of the dentist are, in many countries, available in full to only a relatively small proportion of the population.

In those parts of the world where this problem is recognized attempts are being made to overcome the manpower shortage. For example, in both the United States and the United Kingdom there have been proportionately large increases in the recent provision for dental education. Despite this expansion, however, there is evidence that the gap in the United States between population growth and increases in the number of dentists is widening rather than narrowing (National Advisory Commission on Health Manpower, 1967). If increased provision for dental education is to be the solution to the manpower problem it will need to be larger than is at first apparent from consideration of simple ratios expressing the relationship between dentists and population. Assessments of this kind, giving the present position and predictions for the future in such terms do not take into account the probability that, with improved socio-economic status and increased general and health education, a greater, and still greater, proportion of the community will probably seek more and more dental care of better and better quality.

Dental education for so long has been concerned almost exclusively with the education of the professional man or woman, but the wisdom of attempting to solve the manpower problem by the graduation of more dentists to practise in the traditional manner must be questioned, for the cost of creating new student places in dental schools is enormous. In the United States it has been estimated by Bohannan et al. (1972) that construction and other costs incurred before a new student place is occupied, lie between $250,000 and $275,000. If this scale of investment is necessary to augment the number of dentists in a community it would seem to be better to initiate the most effective preventive programme possible and then to evaluate alternative systems of education for the various types of personnel who might help the dentist to meet the changed requirements of community dental care.

It seems improbable that a country wishing to provide comprehensive treatment for its population will be willing to spend its available resources entirely upon the education of dentists without a careful look at the use of ancillaries. The education and training of the whole dental 'team' now demands attention as to its feasibility. If the best use is to be made of the dental team it is of paramount importance that all those who will work in it to deliver services should be educated and trained together. This objective will not be met simply by allowing courses for dentists to proceed side by side, in the same institutions, with courses for operating and non-operating ancillaries. On the contrary the curricula for these different members of the future dental team must be integrated in such a way that the dental students and trainee ancillaries of today become the members of the dental team of tomorrow.

RECRUITMENT TO DENTISTRY

The above presupposes an adequate supply of suitable applicants for places as dental students and trainee ancillaries, but the availability of suitable personnel varies from country to country. In the case of the dental student international differences in the numbers of applicants are quite large. Similar differences in the general level of academic attainment of applicants are said to exist, although it must be noted that international comparisons are difficult to make with any accuracy because of varying cultural influences. The availability of potential professional manpower in sufficient quantity and quality seems to depend upon complex cultural factors which have been reviewed by Fusillo and Metz (1971). They include the applicant's assessment of dentistry in relation to other careers which he might choose, the status in the community the recruit to dentistry sees himself enjoying, and the role in dentistry he thinks he will play after graduation.

In Scandinavian countries, where the dental profession is held in high esteem, the quality of entrants to dental school is high and recruitment of professionals seems not to be a problem. A similar situation exists in the United States where surveys have shown that 2–3 per cent of teenagers with high academic performance expected to be dentists (Lefcowitz and Irelan, 1962; Hood, 1963; Wertz, 1967). Although careers in engineering, medicine, and law attracted considerably greater proportions of the same age-group the flow of students to the places available in American dental schools was judged to be adequate.

In contrast, in the United Kingdom only one per cent of those who applied to enter a university in 1970 chose dentistry, whereas the corresponding figures for engineering, medicine, and law were approximately 15, 5, and 7 per cent respectively (University Central Council on Admissions Report, 1970). Even this small figure may overscore those who were so keenly interested in dentistry that no other career choice was entertained, for before application a school-leaver may be advised that he has no chance of entering a medical school and he may then choose dentistry as a more realistic alternative career. Consequently, at least 17 per cent of students currently entering British dental schools do so after failing to gain admission to study the university discipline for which they first applied and it is thought that most of these would have preferred admission to a medical school (University Central Council on Admissions Report, 1970). Only in this way are the available dental school places in the United Kingdom filled with adequate students.

Recruitment problems may also exist among those emerging from secondary schools who would be suitable for education and training in duties ancillary to the dentist. With the exception of the proportionately large numbers of dental hygienists in the United States and dental nurses in New Zealand, no country has attempted to educate vast numbers of ancillaries, therefore, the possible constraint placed upon dental education at this level, by competition from other careers, cannot be assessed. However, experience with relatively small schemes of education for ancillaries suggests that in many countries potentially serious manpower limitations will exist.

SELECTION OF DENTAL STUDENTS

The level of scholarship, community and practical interests, qualities of leadership, maturity, and motivation should all play a part in the selection of dental students. This tends to suggest that there are precise methods of selecting students for entry to dental education whereas, more often, the methods used appear to be traditional rather than rational.

In the United Kingdom most dental schools base selection upon biographical data, largely, performance in school examinations in a narrow range of subjects and the head teacher's report, supplemented by an interview conducted by experienced dental school teachers. Formal psychological assessment is not attempted, nor is use usually made of aptitude testing. In the United States selection methods are different. Many dental schools employ the Dental Aptitude Test (DAT) in the selection of their students. This test has manual and academic components which give rise to 13 test scores. Studies of the predictive value of the DAT and other forms of assessment have been reviewed by Kreit (1971) who concludes that there are low but significant correlations between the manual component of the test and subsequent grades in practical tests and that DAT academic scores, in conjunction with pre-professional college grades, give useful predictions of academic performance in a dental school.

Studies of psycho-social factors relating to the recruitment and selection of dental students have been reviewed by Fusillo and Metz (1971) who evaluate the relative importance to be attached to personality characteristics, interests, and role orientations from data obtained principally in the United States during the period 1955–70. Although this is a long period, during which the characteristics of dental students may well have changed, it does appear that the average members of the groups of students who were assessed: 'tended to be pragmatic, conforming, conservative, and not very academically oriented toward knowledge for its own sake. Dental students had outstanding ability to work at a task until it was finished, but were low in traits of leadership. They tended to have considerable interest in prestige and earning money' (Fusillo and Metz, 1971).

If the characteristics of conservatism, lack of leadership, and wish for autonomy exhibited by these students persist throughout the dental education of current and future students they may restrict the ability of new graduates to involve themselves in the provision of community care through the activities of the dental team.

It seems clear, therefore, that selection for dental education must now aim to identify and give preference to those with concern for community dental health who see themselves being involved in its provision and to those of outstanding managerial/executive potential who will be able to direct the delivery of dental care.

Notwithstanding the criticisms that biographical data indicate more about a prospective student's past performance than his potential after entry to a dental school, that aptitude tests have only limited predictive value, and that the role of psychological assessment in selection remains uncertain, experience shows that 'outstanding graduates' are most likely to result from the selection of 'outstanding applicants'. However, the definition of the 'outstanding applicant' and the uncovering of reliable methods for his early recognition still require further consideration.

SELECTION OF ANCILLARIES

The selection and training of ancillary workers throughout the world of dentistry is also a confused area in which there are even greater variations, both nationally and internationally. On the basis of low academic requirements, ancillaries have in some centres been trained in a very few days to perform relatively simple tasks, such as the application and removal of orthodontic bands. At the other end of the scale many highly educated girls have been recruited for extensive courses in dental hygiene which may lead to university first degrees and masterships after periods of from 2 to 6 years of education. If the dual pitfalls of both under and over-education are to be avoided it is essential to determine the clinical remit of ancillary workers, to accept a predental standard of education appropriate to their future tasks and to select, train, and educate accordingly. There is considerable danger in accepting trainees with school education well above that which will adequately fit them for their future occupation, for, if this is done, dissatisfaction may result and eventually, recruits may be few.

ASPECTS OF THE CURRICULUM

There are three traditional components which usually form the core of most present-day curricula: the preclinical or basic sciences, the study of general and oral diseases, and the theory and practice of clinical dentistry. To these there are now being added courses in the behavioural sciences and substantial allowances of time for the students' elective activity.

BEHAVIOURAL SCIENCES

Courses in those aspects of behavioural sciences which relate to the provision of dental care still need to be introduced in many schools. Teaching in behavioural sciences may range from basic courses in psychology and sociology, with or without direct application to dentistry, to behavioural topics relevant to community dentistry and dental health education. In North America, where such teaching has begun, recent experience suggests that the exposure of dental students to the teaching of behavioural science is not necessarily a rewarding exercise, unless the teaching is closely applied to problems in dentistry. This indicates the need to make teaching programmes of this type a conjoint effort between dentists, who will present the dental problem, and those in other disciplines who will bring their different skills to bear upon it.

COMMUNITY DENTISTRY

Community dentistry teaching is often neglected completely or left until relatively late in many present curricula. The argument has been advanced that the student can understand little of his responsibilities to the community until he knows something about dentistry. Nothing could be more fallacious. Teaching in community dentistry, with emphasis upon preventive aspects, should form the very hub of dental education around which its biological, clinical, and technological spokes should revolve. Many students and some of their teachers, probably conditioned by their own experiences as patients and as students, find it difficult to think beyond the narrow confines of the mouth of the individual patient they are called upon to treat. This is especially true if teachers ask students to refocus their attention upon their community responsibilities late in the curriculum. In consequence, many dental students are still highly individualistic on graduation, for they have been trained as lone operators, who are very competent technically, knowledgeable biologically, but capable mainly of providing a high quality repair service. These behavioural patterns, which fail to include real concern for community care and prevention, stem mainly from shortcomings in curriculum design.

It would seem preferable to begin dental teaching with emphasis upon community and preventive dentistry and those sociological topics germane to community care. To this end, dental educators must establish departments of community dentistry in each dental school if real emphasis is to be given to these subjects. Then, and only then, will it be possible to teach the biological, clinical, and technological aspects within their proper context.

INTEGRATION OF COURSES

There is an absolute division between basic science teaching and clinical teaching in British dental schools with the result that complete correlation (integration) of teaching throughout the curriculum has not yet been possible, but the need for it, especially in influencing student motivation, is slowly being realized. At present, because of this division, early course work often seems to lack relevance to a student who had hoped to make immediate contact with patients and, as a result, his motivation and the meaningfulness of his education often appears to suffer. The intention that this 'logical' presentation of basic information before clinical teaching is started will encourage the student to assimilate new ideas and understand clinical concepts is not necessarily fulfilled. It is perhaps worth remembering that 'logical' arrangement of course work in a linear fashion may be logical only to the teacher who has a grasp of the whole curriculum. Without knowing the final educational goal a student may find this system highly illogical.

How much better it would be if, from the outset of dental education, whole problems, community or individual, were to be presented to the student and subsequently broken down into their basic components which could then be taught side by side with relevant clinical concepts. This would seem likely to create greatly enhanced student motivation.

In the United Kingdom, the barrier to this complete integration of dental teaching is largely created by regulations which require a student to pass important examinations in anatomy, physiology, and biochemistry, often only nine months after entry to the dental school. It is deemed that a student cannot be permitted to begin clinical studies of any kind until he has passed these examinations. No doubt the intention behind this restriction is to ensure that students are fit to care for patients, but experience in other countries suggests that this safeguard is not essential. Better preclinical-clinical integration of teaching could be achieved, in the first instance, without the sacrifice of time by either group of teachers, if the timing of the preclinical examination was reconsidered. The same preclinical teaching could then be extended over a longer period, thus allowing some teaching of clinical topics to be brought forward into the early part of the curriculum. A 'diagonally integrated' curriculum, broadly of this type, is in operation at the University of Kentucky (Bohannan and Morris, 1970).

CLINICAL EXPERIENCE

Much of the time in current dental curricula is spent by the student in gaining experience in the care of patients. The profitable use of undergraduate time demands a student/patient-centred approach if there is to be efficiency in teaching and the creation of a suitable environment for learning. The curriculum should be structured so that patients benefit by the provision of the best possible service; and students benefit from the opportunity to provide total care and to follow the effect of this through a series of recall consultations. The serially arranged block courses, those that are supposed to follow each other in a 'logical' order, which are still used in many dental schools, operate against the principle of full patient care, for a student's clinical experience is fragmented in a way dictated by the immediate needs of his current subject teaching. Total patient care is thus excluded or made difficult. This can be remedied if tuition in different disciplines is integrated and planned to progress at approximately similar rates throughout the curriculum. Then, with careful matching of patients' demands to students' skills, it is possible for total patient care to be provided from the outset. A curriculum of this type has been in operation for a number of years at the London Hospital Medical College Dental School (Allred and Slack, 1968).

SMALL GROUP TEACHING/LEARNING

The process of dental education demands the interaction of students with teachers so that an environment for learning is created in which the teacher presents principles to the student, cultivates attitudes in him and attempts to alter his behaviour by encouraging him to apply these principles in finding solutions to clinical problems. It is in this way that a secondary school-leaver, or college graduate, is converted into a dentist. Unfortunately, this environment is not always created for much present teaching of dentistry still depends mainly upon the transmission of facts to large groups of students by one teacher in the lecture situation. This teacher-centred tuition appears to do little to develop the talents of the student, whose teachers would be more usefully employed in creating an environment appropriate to student-centred learning. This philosophy has important implications when teaching methods are chosen, for, although a dental student has the benefit of one-to-one teaching (at the chairside) probably to an extent greater than that experienced by a student in any other university discipline, this in itself is not enough. It should be heavily supplemented by student-centred small-group learning in which the student can practise his skills in handling newly acquired data.

For this purpose a small group is defined as a teacher with about 5–7 students in face-to-face contact, so that all can interact with each other, not just with the teacher. At this size, teaching in the group can be both subject-centred, by which it is meant that a body of knowledge can be covered and student-centred, that is, a student can receive special help with problems of understanding. Experience has shown that the term 'teaching' must really mean this and not just the delivering of information by the teacher, which is of no value to the student without learning. The imparting of knowledge must be followed by understanding, with subsequent synthesis by the student so that he can relate the new knowledge gained to that body of knowledge he already possessed. Above all, in dentistry, teaching is not complete until the student has converted knowledge gained into new attitudes and new behaviour of practical benefit to a patient and/or community afflicted by dental disease.

Although this method of teaching is not necessarily of demonstrable value in terms of examination results it does appear to enhance the interests of students, to increase their involvement and it may produce attitudes and behaviour after graduation which commit them to a greater community service role. In addition, possibly because small-group teaching systems usually create a heavy commitment for all available teachers, there appear to be benefits for the teacher which could be reflected in his teaching and the progress of his students (Duckworth, 1970).

THE WORLD OUTSIDE

Hitherto, dental education has been largely confined to the dental school building. The engagement of students in extramural dentistry, under the guidance of dental school teachers or specially recruited teaching associates, in dental practices, health centres, school clinics, and hospitals which are not teaching institutions, is a highly desirable development beginning to emerge in North America. In this way the dental school is making an attempt to introduce a student to his community and to the rigours of his professional career beyond all that protects him in the dental school environment.

The argument has been advanced that this arrangement for broadening the students' experience has all the worst features of the now outdated preceptorship system but this can probably be offset by the counter-argument that such a learning experience makes a substantial contribution to increasing the motivation of students by exposure to real community problems.

ELECTIVE LEARNING

An important component of many recently introduced dental curricula is elective learning time. Whenever a new curriculum is planned time is usually earmarked for elective activity. In addition to being allowed time for reading, reflection, and the maturation of previously acquired knowledge the student may choose to spend some of this time on the study of one or more optional subjects which might range from additional or specialized clinical practice, through an investigation at the laboratory bench, to an extended visit to an overseas country learning about patterns of health care.

This arrangement, however, has not always proved to be successful because tight control has not been maintained to preserve elective time for its intended purpose. There is an ever present danger that students may spend too much of it upon endless repetition of clinical exercises and upon prescribed tasks set by teachers, who, in their otherwise admirable striving to enhance the skills of their students by reinforcement, heap more and yet more work upon them.

OBJECTIVES OF FUTURE DENTAL EDUCATION

The objectives of dental education have been discussed from the standpoint of the community and now need to be defined from the stand-point of the dental teacher. Reference has already been made to the community's wish to have a sufficiency of dental education and an efficient dental education leading to the economic delivery of services. These general, broad objectives of dental education are supported by more detailed and specific ones which were the subject of a review by a World Health Organization Expert Committee (1962) and were extended by Durocher (1970). These specific objectives stress the sociological, biological, clinical, and technological components of dental education, all of which are essential to the complete education of the dentist. It is the dental teacher's responsibility to turn these aims into detailed educational objectives which, when coupled with a consideration of methods for their achievement, will lead to the reform of future dental curricula.

Sensible modification of existing programmes of dental education and the proper planning of new curricula is impossible without detailed examination of the community's profile of needs and demands (Chaves, 1969b). Sadly, most countries lack this knowledge and must plan their dental education on impressions of demand which may be quite inaccurate. This can have extraordinary effects upon the design of curricula. For example, in developing countries, curricula have been known to follow 'classical' European or North American patterns, although the communities eventually to be served have had quite different problems of dental disease. Thus, it would seem more rational to design curricula with a view to the frequency with which various aspects of dental care will be required by the population to be served and the teaching time needed to achieve competence. Then, planned and co-ordinated changes in dental practice can stem from deliberate changes in dental education, for curricula can be designed to create awareness of newer methods of meeting community needs.

After identifying the dental needs of a community the next step in the determination of educational objectives is to decide on the nature of the manpower required to provide the necessary preventive and therapeutic services. An hypothesis, which seems appropriate to the United Kingdom, has been advanced (Allred et al., 1972) which suggests that dental care will be the responsibility of specially designed teams whose members will be trained together to combat dental disease on a community scale. The size and composition of each team will be determined by the needs of the community it will serve. The teams will be led by one or more dentists who will be educated and trained to exercise control of patient care, to diagnose, to prescribe treatment, to check and supervise simple procedures and to carry out only the more complex operations demanding their unique skill and training. It is an essential part of the hypothesis that personnel ancillary to the dentists will assist in providing care for individuals rather than themselves acting independently to care for groups of people within the community. This hypothesis, which needs to be tested, not only suggests an outline for the future form of dental practice but it also suggests some of the principal educational objectives that will have to be met.

Much dental care requires the application of high quality technical skills without recourse to judgement based upon detailed theoretical knowledge and long experience. The bulk of the teaching of those skills should, therefore, be directed at the trainee ancillary. However, when there is a need for sociological, biological, and clinical knowledge beyond that necessary for simple technical competence, or when complex technical skills depend upon this knowledge for their successful attainment, teaching should be directed at the undergraduate or postgraduate dental student. Thus, the different but complementary roles of the dental student and the trainee ancillary should be identified at every point in the educational process. On this will depend the appropriate distribution of teaching resources between the two.

At an early stage in the definition of objectives it is essential to decide upon the intended relationship the dental graduate will have with others in the health professions. In some countries, where, usually because of the limited availability of resources and the dimensions of the problem, dentistry is necessarily seen as a service only at the fringe of medical care, the biological and medical components of the dental curriculum may have to be very limited in scope. Conversely, if the principal objective in other countries with greater resources is the education of a dentist able to integrate responsibility for total patient care with particular responsibility for the management of oral diseases, the pattern of education and training should be different. Then, the aim ought to be to produce a dentist who will be as widely educated and be as capable of advancing knowledge within his own speciality as a person working in any other specialist medical discipline. Dental education would be designed to make the dentist capable of providing, against a background of broad medical knowledge, a complete oral health service equivalent to that provided by his colleagues in other specialities of medicine. In this way the risk of dentistry becoming a technological service isolated from medicine, with the possible consequent decline in the standard of patient care, would probably be avoided.

CURRICULUM ORGANIZATION IN THE FUTURE

If dentistry is to be accountable to the public and dental education is to meet defined goals set by the community, new and more flexible curricula will need to be conceived. The pressures created in the United States by manpower shortages, health insurance schemes, and the costs of dental education have led Bohannan et al. (1972) to recommend alterations in the pattern of dental practice and in the use of manpower. These must stem from greater flexibility in a dental curriculum which provides for individualized education. The knowledge explosion is such that it will not be possible to attempt to provide an all-embracing curriculum but rather that there should be a core curriculum with the emphasis upon the prevention of disease instead of the repair of damaged tissues. They foresee that the student will have to be permitted to complete the core curriculum at a rate determined by his own ability and application, that the number and character of electives he selects will vary according to his personal interests and needs, and that the time of graduation will be determined by his own rate of progress.

Although dental diseases do not challenge life itself their almost universal prevalence constitutes a serious public health problem. Nevertheless, the need for a dental profession, with separate identity only at the fringe of medicine, to manage the two principal diseases of the teeth and supporting tissues and a relatively small number of other disorders of the mouth should not necessarily be perpetuated if it can be shown that another arrangement would make better use of available resources. It is the size of the dental problem, rather than its basic nature, which differentiates oral disorders from almost any other disorder in the rest of medicine. This similarity of disease processes, the now powerful influence of medical treatment upon dental management and the possibility of disturbing general disease states by local dental intervention are all reasons for advocating, in the section on the objectives of dental education, that it is desirable for dentists to have a broad basic education similar to that recommended for those in other medical specialities. Hence, the possibility of incorporating dental education and training in the United Kingdom into any future system of medical education needs to be examined. Attention should be given to the probable consequences of long-term developments in the prevention and treatment of the major dental diseases in so far as these might affect educational planning.

The idea that the dental team leader should work, at least in the United Kingdom, as a specialist within medicine, leads to a consideration of possible convergent developments in medical and dental education. In medical education there is concern that, as a consequence of the growth of knowledge in medicine, an individual should not be expected to become competent in more than a relatively small area of the whole subject. Many believe that present medical curricula are unable to provide both basic scientific education and wide vocational training. Recommendations have been made (Royal Commission, 1968) stating that the core of basic medical education, extending over three years, should include an increased content of cell biology, environmental studies, and behavioural sciences; as well as the traditional basic medical science subjects. To these might be added optional subjects providing limited courses, for example, in biophysics, computer science, or social anthropology, but the role of such subjects in the medical curriculum has yet to be evaluated. After a further two-year course in clinical methodology the graduate might hold a degree in medical sciences and would be a graduate in medicine fit for vocational training of a general or specialist kind. On this basis, the independent general or specialist practitioner would emerge, about eleven years after entry to a medical school, at approximately the age of twenty-nine, although he would have been serving his community, in salaried employment, from the sixth year.

It may well be that the recommendations of the Royal Commission will not be put into effect exactly in the form proposed. Nevertheless, it is evident that major changes in medical education, not too different from some of those recommended, are beginning to be implemented by several medical schools or are at the planning stage. Thus, account must be taken of these developments in so far as they may influence future dental education.

Although progress towards any new pattern of medical education in the United Kingdom will be slow, Allred et al. (1972) in anticipation that developments will occur, have argued that the dentist of the future should receive expanded basic education similar to that which might be provided for the future medical practitioner; in which case optional studies would include dentally orientated subjects. This does not mean that a dentist should be trained to be a medical practitioner any more than a medical practitioner should be trained to be a dentist, but that both require the same broad educational foundation. Indeed, the vocational training in dentistry, which would follow, would aim to convert the student with a basic medical education into a dental specialist within medicine. This dental training of more mature students would be integrated with the training of the ancillary personnel. From the outset, students and trainees would work to curricula with subject integration of the kind proposed earlier and in the more efficient environment of the dental team. Dental students would, therefore, be expected to complete their vocational training in dentistry in not more than three years, before entering a two-year period of supervised team general practice or specialist training in a particular field of dentistry. This new type of dental graduate would then be well equipped to lead teams of ancillaries in the provision of dental care and to prevent dentistry becoming a mere technology isolated from medicine.

This is just one concept of changes which might occur in dental education in only one country. It may well be unsuitable in other countries where, in order to meet urgent priorities, a short educational programme for the dentist and a brief period of training for the ancillary worker would be essential to satisfy immediate community requirements. This serves to emphasize, yet again, that it is the needs of society which must determine the form of dental education.

In several countries, the educational requirements for new types of ancillaries, both operating and non-operating are being explored. Thus, it is premature to speculate on the way in which the education of the dentist will be fused into an integrated whole with the training of the ancillary. It does seem, however, that, whereas a dental student on first contact with clinical studies will need the most skilled ancillary help available, there should be a time when his enlarging experience should fit him to become involved in contributing to the training of ancillaries. It is in this way that the foundation of the future team relationships could be laid.

POSTGRADUATE EDUCATION IN THE UNITED KINGDOM

Postgraduate dental education embraces the further education and training of the specialist, who would work both within and outside the hospital service; it covers the training of dental school teachers and research workers and the continuing education of all general practitioners. Numerically, this last group is the largest and the most important because its members are responsible for delivering most of the dental care to the community.

Undergraduate and continuing education of the practitioner should form part of a spectrum of activity, for it is neither possible, nor desirable, to separate postgraduate education from its precursor. Looked at in this way the new dental graduate is an incomplete product of the educational system who will require the opportunity to learn more through postgraduate experience immediately after graduation. Subsequently, he will need periodic embellishment of his knowledge and skills if he is to make available to the community the best possible service and derive maximum satisfaction from his chosen profession.

In planning curricula it is important to distinguish between that which should be taught to the undergraduate dental student, that which should be provided through immediate postgraduate training, and that which should be left for inclusion in programmes of continuing education. Hitherto, at least in the United Kingdom, there has been the philosophy that in order to produce a complete general practitioner most of every facet of dentistry should be taught to the undergraduate with the result, as knowledge has expanded, that dental curricula have become progressively more congested. In contrast, many dental schools in other countries have dealt with this problem by abandoning comprehensive education at the undergraduate level, leaving certain aspects of dentistry to be taught almost entirely as postgraduate disciplines.

No generalizations can be made about the allocation of teaching to the two sides of this interface between undergraduate education and postgraduate training. Much will depend upon community factors in different countries which will determine the types of preventive and therapeutic services demanded; the methods chosen for their delivery; the degree of specialization required; the degree to which the population is concentrated in urban areas and the stage of development reached by the hospital services. The end point chosen for undergraduate education must, however, be related to the availability of subsequent postgraduate training, in that curricula for undergraduate dental students have to be more complete if, later, they will have limited access to programmes of postgraduate education.

As well as providing for the continuing education of dentists, postgraduate dental education must also meet the quantitatively smaller demands for the education of the specialist practitioner, the teacher, and the research worker. If team work in dentistry assumes the greater proportions it should, and if there is to be delegation of many more tasks to ancillaries, the team leaders will be able to direct the provision of dental care and to provide most of the more complex services. In these circumstances, there may be a reduced need for specialist practitioners. However, the development of all that now exists in dentistry, and the discovery of new knowledge, depends mainly upon a continuing supply of teachers and research workers. Thus, because of their indirect but vital influence upon the dental care of the community, the education and training of teachers and researchers is a primary objective of dental education without which development would be retarded.

As yet in many dental schools in the United Kingdom arrangements for this development are somewhat haphazard. Few have at their disposal a complete series of graded posts which will allow selected new graduates to progress to career appointments in teaching and research. All too often aspirants have to be supported by a series of makeshift arrangements which are not necessarily in the best interests of their training. To overcome this and to provide long-term advantages to schools, priorities should be rearranged so that there can be created more established trainee academic posts giving logical progression to staff appointments.

REFERENCES

ALLRED, H., DUCKWORTH, R., JOHNSON, N. W., and SLACK, G. L. (1972), 'Proposals for planned change in dental education and practice', *Br. dent. J.*, **133,** 173.

— — and SLACK, G. L. (1968), 'The changing pattern of dental education', *Ibid.*, **125,** 187.

BOHANNAN, H. M., and MORRIS, A. L. (1970), 'A case study in dental curriculum change: University of Kentucky', *J. Am. dent. Ass.*, **82,** 13.

— — ROVIN, S., PACKER, M. W., and COSTIN, E. R. (1972), 'The flexible dental curriculum', *Ibid.*, **84,** 112.

CHAVES, M. M. (1969a), 'The objectives of dental education', *Int. dent. J.*, **19,** 430.

— — (1969b), 'Co-ordination of subjects in the curriculum', *Ibid.*, **19,** 455.

DUCKWORTH, R. (1970), *Teaching Methods in the Clinical Course of the Dental School of The London Hospital Medical College*. London: mimeograph.

DUROCHER, R. T. (1970), *Guidelines for the Development of Dental Curricula.* Washington, DC: WHO document, HP/DH/1.

FEDERATION DENTAIRE INTERNATIONALE (1970), *Basic Fact Sheets*. London.

FUSILLO, A. E., and METZ, A. S. (1971), 'Social science research on the dental student', in *Social Sciences and Dentistry* (ed. RICHARDS, N. D., and COHEN, L. K.). The Hague: Sijthoff and Federation Dentaire Internationale.

HOOD, A. B. (1963), 'Predicting achievement in dental school', *J. dent. Educ.*, **27,** 148.

KREIT, L. H. (1971), 'The prediction of student success in dental schools', in *Social Sciences and Dentistry* (ed. RICHARDS, N. D., and COHEN, L. K.). The Hague: Sijthoff and Federation Dentaire Internationale.

LEFCOWITZ, M. J., and IRELAN, L. M. (1962), 'Interests in dentistry: A pilot study of high school students. I. Effect of social status and academic ability', *J. dent. Educ.*, **27,** 48.

NATIONAL ADVISORY COMMISSION ON HEALTH MANPOWER (1967), *Report*, Vol. 1. Washington, DC: US Government Printing Office.

ROYAL COMMISSION (1968), *Report of the Royal Commission on Medical Education (Todd Report)*. London: HMSO.

UNIVERSITIES CENTRAL COUNCIL ON ADMISSIONS (1970), *Eighth report, 1969–70.* Cheltenham: England.

WERTZ, C. E. (1967), 'Career choice patterns', *Soc. Educ.*, **40,** 348.

WORLD HEALTH ORGANIZATION (1962), *Dental Education.* Geneva: WHO Tech. Rep. Ser. No. 244.

WORLD HEALTH ORGANIZATION (1967), *World Directory of Dental Schools, 1963.* Geneva: WHO.

——— (1968), *Undergraduate Dental Education in Europe; Conference report.* Copenhagen: WHO mimeograph.

——— (1970), *Postgraduate Dental Education in Europe; Conference Report.* Copenhagen: WHO mimeograph.

Chapter 14

The Future Delivery of Dental Care Services

G. H. Leatherman DMD, DSC, FDSRCS
Executive Director of the Federation Dentaire Internationale

A number of aspects of the present delivery systems for dental care have now been considered. But what of the future? In times of rapid social change will the present systems be maintained?

In this concluding chapter, a distinguished internationalist gives his views of how he sees dental services taking shape in the future. Dr. Leatherman sees the need for dentistry to develop more and more as a public health service. He considers some of the barriers to the delivery of care, and he describes how the education of dental students in the future must adapt to meet the requirements of a truly community-based service.

While the history of medicine as a whole can be traced back through many centuries, the concept of public health can only be traced back to the eighteenth century. Perhaps because dental decay and diseases of the gingivae and supporting bone are rarely direct causes of mortality, one has to wait another hundred years for the first reference to preventive dentistry which is the forerunner of dental public health services. Dentistry has generally been regarded as a limited service to the individual, aimed at preventing and treating diseases of the teeth and supporting structures. Its relationship to public health was not recognized until the early years of the twentieth century when the National Dental Association in the United States of America, now the American Dental Association, founded an oral hygiene committee, Professor Ernst Jessen founded the first municipal school dental clinic in Germany, and schoolchildren in Great Britain began to receive instruction in oral hygiene (Ennis, 1967). In 1900, the Federation Dentaire Internationale established a Commission of Oral Hygiene, which is now the well established Commission on Public Dental Health Services (Ennis, 1967).

Dental public health has been defined as 'the science and art of preventing and controlling dental diseases and of promoting dental health through organized community effort' (Young and Striffler, 1969). It was well into this century before the pattern of dental health care showed the first signs of changing from a problem for the individual and his dentist to one falling within the scope of public health, for modern research has shown that certain aspects of dental health cannot be approached on an individual basis. To be effective on a large scale preventive measures require public health programmes, for example the fluoridation of public water supplies (Leatherman, 1968).

There are basic social and scientific changes taking place all over the world, and any predictions about the future of dentistry as a public health service must take these changes into account. These changes have an increasing effect on our daily lives, and thus the dentist's ability to meet the challenge of how best to provide dental health for his community.

Every walk of life is now being examined by the social scientist. It is a present-day vogue of university disciplines to include ecology, which Webster's Third New International Dictionary defines as the study of reciprocal relationships between organisms and their surroundings. Every phase of modern living can be related to social science, including the delivery of dental services, the behaviour of the public in accepting such services, and their attitude towards dental health. In general the big social changes are in the nature of a move from ignorance to knowledge, from poverty to wealth, and from sickness to health, but the rate of these changes varies enormously in different countries. The development of any one of these changes is a prerequisite for the development of the others. As ignorance is eliminated, the standard of literacy is raised, a basic requirement for social development. With an increase in literacy and social consciousness there is an increase in productivity and wealth, factors which Dr. Willcocks described in Chapter 1 as the prerequisites for raising the standard of health in any country. The way in which social science research is becoming increasingly important is shown in the book, *Social Sciences and Dentistry* (Richards and Cohen, 1971).

The basic social problem in the world is the population explosion. The population is one of the basic resources for development and the people are also the consumers of the products of development. In many parts of the world the population explosion can be a barrier to social development. An example can be seen in the delivery of dental services where there are not enough qualified dentists to cope with the dental health demands of the world's population, let alone with their needs.

In addition to the population explosion, man is also faced with what is now referred to as the knowledge explosion, especially in the natural sciences. Any prediction as to the future of the dental profession must take these profound social developments into account, and must also consider the administrative and technological barriers to be eliminated before dental public health services can be delivered to meet the changing needs of the population.

A number of these barriers, so far as they apply to the development of dentistry as a public health service, will now be dealt with.

THE ATTITUDE OF ALMOST ALL GOVERNMENTS IN THE WORLD TOWARDS DENTAL HEALTH

This does not mean that dental health services are not provided by governments, but rather that few seem to consider dental health a necessary part of total health. One can only speculate on the reasons for this attitude as they vary from country to country, as naturally priority must be given to diseases which lead directly to disability and death. The experience of Great Britain has shown that a total and comprehensive dental health service is too costly, but there is a place for a priority dental service in the health services of every country. A major cause for the general neglect of dental services would seem to be ignorance, on the part of governments, of the importance of dental health in its relation to total health.

THE SHORTAGE OF MANPOWER IN DENTISTRY IN ALMOST ALL COUNTRIES AND THE CONSEQUENT HAPHAZARD DEVELOPMENT OF AUXILIARY SERVICES MORE BY PRESSURE FROM GOVERNMENTS THAN THE WISE PLANNING OF THE PROFESSION

The supply of manpower in dentistry is dependent upon education and it is this field that will have greatest influence on the future of dentistry as a public health service. Dental schools must change their curricula so as to produce dentists able to render the appropriate dental services required for the people in the country in which they wish to practise, and not a highly specialized service only for those individuals who can afford to pay high fees for it. There is a need for universally acceptable standards in dental education at ancillary, undergraduate, and graduate levels. Development of such standards would enable an international exchange of teachers, students, dentists, and ancillaries to take place freely, to the mutual benefit of the dental profession, ancillaries, and the recipients of dental services in all countries.

THE THIRD BARRIER TO BE OVERCOME IS THE FAILURE IN MOST COUNTRIES TO TEACH THE POPULATION WHAT IS ALREADY KNOWN ABOUT PREVENTIVE DENTISTRY. THIS MEANS THE DENTAL HEALTH EDUCATION FACTOR

A pattern of oral health care in any country or community must be largely influenced by what the government and the population in that country know about the delivery of dental services and the behaviour of the people in accepting such services and their own attitude towards dental health. The dentist and his ancillaries must organize, in conjunction with government and local authorities, health education campaigns to meet the conditions of the community in which they live and work. Manpower problems make it essential to motivate the population to make full use of preventive methods which can be implemented by the individual, such as:

1. A proper understanding of diet and nutrition as they affect developing teeth and contribute to dental disease.
2. The most effective methods of oral hygiene, bearing in mind the inadequacy of the toothbrush and toothpaste alone to completely remove and control dental plaque.
3. Early treatment from the dentist and regular subsequent visits.

FLUORIDATION

The single factor with the most profound effect upon the prevalence and pattern of dental caries is the ingestion of adequate amounts of fluorides. The World Health Organization has published a monograph entitled *Fluorides and Human Health* in which it is stated that:

> It has been shown that a certain level of fluoride consumption, especially when this is continuous from earliest childhood affords considerable protection for both permanent and milk teeth against caries without exerting any unfavourable influence on the appearance of the teeth or the periodontium. (World Health Organization, 1970.)

The most effective way to ensure adequate fluoride consumption is by fluoridation of drinking water. For districts without a piped water supply, there are other alternatives such as topical application to the tooth surface, enriched cookery salt, flour, and milk, fluoride tablets, toothpaste, and mouthwashes. McHugh has discussed all of these methods in Chapter 2. There is absolutely no evidence that a fluoride level of one part per million in drinking water has any harmful effects on the metabolism of food, the function of vitamins, or the activity of either hormones or enzymes. The whole problem of implementing fluoridation is a complex one and is considered fully by Burt in Chapter 3.

THE FOURTH BARRIER IS THE NEED FOR MORE AND BETTER CO-ORDINATED RESEARCH INTO ALL PHASES OF DENTAL HEALTH CARE

Socio-economics, community attitudes and behaviour, dental health materials and equipment are all subjects which must receive more attention. The major dental problems are the prevention of dental caries, the control of periodontal disease, the prevention of dentofacial anomalies, and the early detection of oral tumours. Research is being carried out in all these fields, but much greater co-ordination is required and the future must show a better co-operation between the research worker and the practising dentist.

There are other problems related to research. One is the need for using the internationally accepted World Health Organization standards of measurement for reporting epidemiological studies (World Health Organization, 1971) and the FDI two-digit system of tooth designation, enabling scientists and practitioners of any nationality to communicate with each other regardless of language barriers (Federation Dentaire Internationale, 1971). Another problem is the inability of most countries to deal with congenital birth defects, such as cleft lip and plate, largely because medicine and dentistry have no effective liaison in this field.

DENTAL EDUCATION

The problems surrounding dental education have been mentioned previously, but as a subject of such importance, dental education should be considered in more detail. It has been discussed in Chapter 13 by Duckworth; here are some further thoughts on future patterns.

A. Basic and clinical sciences must be taught side by side. The application of basic sciences to the systems within the body, and to the principles of clinical practice, must be clearly defined and demonstrated to the dental student during his preclinical studies. Dentistry must produce clinical teachers who have been trained to teach the basic sciences, and to close the gap between the scientist and the clinician. Both full-time teachers and part-time clinicians should be on the Faculty and both should have the privilege of clinical practice within the confines of the university.

B. Students need to regard dentistry in terms of a public health service, so that they are aware of the needs of the population in relation to prevention and early treatment, as well as to emergency treatment.

The major problems in dentistry which have a public health significance are dental caries, periodontal disease, both of which can be controlled, and dentofacial anomalies, including malocclusion and oral tumours.

The following should be the order of priority both for clinical training and treatment:

1. All children's treatment including orthodontics should be an absolute priority and taught and practised as a preventive and early treatment measure.

2. After the relief of pain, the condition of the supporting structures must be considered before the detection of caries. Students must learn the value of scaling and good oral hygiene prior to carrying out surgical intervention such as gingivectomy, gingivoplasty and curettage.

3. The early treatment of caries and the maintenance of a healthy pulp rather than the creation of root-filled teeth. Dental research, rather than industrial research, should develop better filling materials, and

should also place emphasis on the healing of an infected pulp rather than the creation of a germ-free root canal.

4. The teaching of oral surgical procedures to include extraction, pocket elimination, bone surgery, apicectomy, and the simple fracture and correction of dentofacial anomalies, but not maxillofacial surgery which requires postgraduate training leading to a higher degree. Oral surgery should also teach the study of local and general anaesthesia, as the latter is now being increasingly used for multiple restorative treatment.

5. The restoration of function by the insertion of partial, fixed, or removable prostheses and full dentures, and the study of occlusion in relation to the maintenance of healthy supporting structures.

6. A course of radiology and diagnosis including radiation hazards to the patient and the community.

C. Alongside the basic and clinical science teaching and practice, the student should be taking broad parallel courses in the social sciences and social services, which would include a study of:

1. Antisepsis and sanitation.
2. Public health and social welfare and the laws, functions, and objectives of health authorities.
3. Fluoridation as a community action.
4. The influence on physical and mental health of environment, economic circumstances, personal hygiene, and safety.
5. Health education methods.
6. The broader aspects of epidemiology and the preparation of statistical data.
7. Visits to centres and institutes of importance to public health, especially hospitals where the dental student must be familiar with procedure. With the introduction of national health services, insurance, and welfare programmes has come a vast expansion of hospital services. The public recognizes the hospital as a centre for health resources and treatment, hence treatment offered should include dental care.

This will necessitate in the future a much closer alliance between dental schools, dentists, and their hospitals if an adequate dental public health service is to be provided.

Young and Striffler (1969) summarize an analogy between procedures employed by the dentist and the public health worker in this way:

Patient procedures	*Community procedures*
Examination	Survey
Diagnosis	Analysis
Treatment Planning	Programme Planning
Treatment	Programme Operation
Payment of Services	Finance
Evaluation	Appraisal

They further write:

> Fundamentally, the procedures are identical, thus the training in procedural skills received by the dental student provides him with a basic pattern of approach to problems which should be helpful in enabling him to fill with confidence and distinction the role of advisor or counsellor on community health programme. (Young and Striffler, 1969.)

D. The dental student, as part of his training to provide a more complete community service, must be taught to practice as part of a team which will contain dentists and ancillaries. The dental health team is the future pattern of dental practice and will help the dentist to expand and improve his services to the world's population. The composition of the team will vary with its objectives, and the country in which it works, but basically it will be composed of two or more dentists and an appropriate number of ancillary dental personnel.

There are now several types of ancillary dental personnel which will influence the pattern of dental health care throughout the world. These have been discussed by Elderton in Chapter 9.

E. The dental student must be taught the relationship of his own health and economic success to the way he practises. This could involve a study of equipment, posture and office planning, type and location of practice, office procedure, taxation, banking, and investment.

The increasing inroads of social security make it evident, however, that dentistry is likely to be practised in the future either in large clinics, whether government or private, or in small rural clinics or mobile units. Well-trained ancillaries of the non-operating type can increase the output of the dentist, and the operating type can relieve the dentist of minor repetitive procedures. It must be remembered, though, that an increase in output increases the business administration problem, and the operating auxiliary requires supervision by a dentist whose own operating time is thus reduced. All clinics, government or private, mobile or static, will consist essentially of a number of dentists, possibly an anaesthetist, a surgeon and a consultant, together with a number of ancillaries and an administrative staff.

SUMMARY

The future of a profession in any country depends upon its education and research, its organization and practice, and an effective means of national and international communication. Every national dental association must be supported by all members of the dental profession, including ancillaries and their organizations, so that it can carry out its responsibilities, the most important of which are the establishment of sound principles and effective programmes which must contain as priorities:

1. The development of dental schools which will enable future dentists and ancillaries to render a dental health service to the community.

2. An effective public relations and health education programme reaching both the government and its people, including the medical, dental, and allied professions, with the accent on prevention.

Every dentist has an individual responsibility to:

1. Take continuing education courses.
2. Use modern equipment.
3. Support the training and use of auxiliaries and work with them as part of an effective health team.
4. Support his national organization and his international organizations, led by the Federation Dentaire Internationale.
5. Build his image as a member of his community supplying an essential part of health service.

The general dental practitioner the world over must be prepared to conduct a preventive dental practice, rendering the following services with his ancillary staff to child, adolescent and adult:

1. Accurate diagnosis and examination based on routine radiographs, study models, accurate history, nutrition studies, and mouth flora studies.
2. Education in sound oral hygiene practice, helped by disclosing solutions and instruction in correct dietary habits. Only the motivated patient using sound oral hygiene practices will control the progress of periodontal disease.
3. The maintenance of the dental arches by the control of:
   a. Mouth habits
   b. Malocclusion
   c. Space maintenance
4. Caries control by the use of:
   a. Appropriate fluoride therapy
   b. Good nutritional habits
   c. Early filling of lesions where the carious process has become established
5. Early diagnosis and treatment of:
   a. Occlusal disharmonies
   b. Dentofacial anomalies
   c. Oral lesions, after cytology tests
   d. Oral injuries in children, mainly on anterior teeth.

The future pattern of dental practice must develop with teams working in surgeries operated at first both by the government and privately, but the future may show that only the state will be able to build and maintain dental health facilities manned by a director, and staffed by administrators, specialists, general practitioners, and ancillaries all working together as a means of delivering dental care to a whole community.

The type of dentist that the future will demand has been described this way:

> The dentist of tomorrow will not be so much less a technician as more a physician. He will have to commit himself to the life of a continuous student with emphasis on basic knowledge that underscores prevention and away from techniques that change yearly, or face inevitable obsolescence. He will have to become aware of social obligation and not lose his humanitarian touch. (Nikiforuk, 1966.)

The broader base for dentistry of the future has been summed up by Sir John Walsh:

> Dentistry is a science and an art, but dental health is a state, a part of general health. The ultimate goal or purpose of dentistry is dental health for all people everywhere—world dental health. The responsibility for health is a shared responsibility between the government, the health profession, and the people both collectively and individually. (Walsh, 1970.)

REFERENCES

ENNIS, J. (1967), *The Story of the Federation Dentaire Internationale.* The Hague: Sijthoff and Federation Dentaire Internationale.

FEDERATION DENTAIRE INTERNATIONALE (1971), 'The F.D.I. two-digit system of tooth designation', *Int. dent. J.* **21,** 104.

LEATHERMAN, G. H. (1968), 'International patterns of oral health care', *Harv. dent. Alumni Bull.*, Special Supplement.

NIKIFORUK, G. (1966), 'Dental education in an innovative society', *J. Ont. dent. Ass.*, **43,** 7.

RICHARDS, N. D., and COHEN, L. K. (1971), *Social Sciences and Dentistry.* The Hague: Sijthoff and Federation Dentaire Internationale.

WALSH, J. P. (1970), 'Freedom—responsibility', *N.Z. dent. J.*, **66,** 310.

WORLD HEALTH ORGANIZATION (1970), *Fluorides and Human Health.* Geneva: WHO Monograph Series No. 59.

—— (1971), *Oral Health Surveys; Basic Methods.* Geneva: WHO.

YOUNG, W. O., and STRIFFLER, D. F. (1969), *The Dentist, his Practice, and his Community*, 2nd ed. Philadelphia: Saunders.

Appendix 1

The Dental Team: a Method of Research into its Maximum Effectiveness

H. Allred DDS, MDS
Professor of Conservative Dentistry, The London Hospital Medical College, University of London

The dental team is an important development in dentistry in recent years. More about its deployment needs to be known, and here Professor Allred describes one method of research into the most efficient utilization of the dental team.

INTRODUCTION

Dentistry has evolved through society's attempts to meet the demands made by those suffering from dental pain; from the ravages that dental disease has made to their appearance or, to a less extent, to their ability to masticate. Only the rich could afford other than the crudest kind of emergency treatment dispensed by any willing hands: the black-smith, cobbler, school teacher, or charlatan. However, the patronage of the wealthy, as in so many other fields, encouraged a few to develop the skills and to accumulate the knowledge that today we recognize as dentistry. Because of this historical background, dentistry is still considered by society at large as a service delivered by one person to another. Though materials and methods have been developed with corresponding increases in efficiency and effectiveness the delivery of dental care to the entire community is still dogged by a pattern imposed upon it by history. This pattern is characterized by the treatment of established disease and the repair of damage rather than its prevention and is aggravated by a general orientation towards the requirements of those sections of the community capable of meeting the financial implications of care rather than those best able to benefit by it.

The traditional methods of delivering dental care are, with increasing frequency, revealing their inability to meet the needs and demands of society. The realization of this along with the growing acceptance of the concept that health is a fundamental human right calls for a consideration of the problem from a different angle. The logical sequence of events would seem to be to first determine the needs and demands of a particular defined community with respect to dental care; then determine the most effective methods for fulfilling each stage of these needs and demands on a cost–benefit basis; and finally to determine the most appropriate level of such care that a society's resources are capable of providing for that community. Many countries however, possess established systems of delivering dental care which, no matter how ineffective they may appear to be in absolute terms, work and should not be disturbed, rather that new systems should be evolved based not merely upon ideas but also upon sound data. It is the means by which such data might be obtained that this chapter is concerned.

PRIMARY DATA REQUIREMENTS

Methods for accurate epidemiological surveys into the needs and demands of defined communities with respect to dental care have been developed in recent years. Though the picture, even in highly developed societies, is as yet very incomplete a start has been made. Only in the light of such information can the effectiveness of any measures of prevention or treatment be assessed, i.e. by comparing the needs and requirements of a defined community before and after the implementation of a system designed to meet them in whole or in part.

It is apparent that the effectiveness of any system must be related to its cost and the feasibility of it being established. Thus the cost–benefit characteristics of any proposed system has to be related to the financial and manpower resources of the society concerned. This cannot be achieved without an analysis of the types of personnel concerned in delivering dental care: the strata of society from whom they may be drawn; their availability; the cost and extent of their training; and the definition of their commitment.

THE DEFINITION OF PERSONNEL RESPONSIBLE FOR THE DELIVERY OF DENTAL CARE

The titles given to various groups of personnel vary from one country to another. Often the title and general commitment of a group, e.g., dental hygienists may be the same in one country as in another but the training considered to be necessary may be strikingly different in length even if not in content, and the length of training is a function of the cost of a service. In other cases, the title of dental assistant may be given to a dental graduate in one country and a surgery assistant in another. Indeed even the title of dentist is given to people with widely varying training in different countries. It is essential that precise definitions of personnel should include the remit of the commitment, the responsibility accepted and the education required of individuals within a given category. Without such definitions an exact analysis becomes impossible.

THE OBJECTIVES IN MEETING THE NEEDS AND DEMANDS FOR DENTAL CARE WITHIN GIVEN SOCIETIES

The development of a dental service within society may be examined through the achievement of a number of objectives. These objectives will be considered in what appears to be a logical sequence.

The most urgent demands made by society are naturally those related to the treatment of acute conditions invariably associated with pain. Thus, the establishment of personnel capable of diagnosing and treating such conditions of an emergency nature is of primary importance. Probably one of the best examples of a conscious decision being taken to provide care of this limited nature is in the case of expeditions to remote areas such as the Antarctic. Medically qualified personnel, accepting the responsibility for the whole care of the community, include such emergency treatment within their remit. By such means a man having training which fits him to diagnose a condition and to treat it in an unsophisticated but safe manner provides the care as a small part of an overall responsibility for the health of the patient. This is the starting point, and it is believed that no circumstances should evolve which remove the responsibility for the health of the patient from the personnel capable of accepting that responsibility. Evolution is, however, ideally seen to be acceptable in two directions: the evolution of ancillary personnel totally responsible to the principle, and secondly the evolution of the principle into a person still able to accept total responsibility for the health of a patient but tending to specialize his interest towards dentistry.

The second objective is, therefore, seen to be the development and training of ancillary personnel capable of carrying through such measures aimed at the prevention of dental disease as are known, are available and possible to implement. Such measures may be on a community or personal level, e.g., fluoridation of the public water supply or dietary and oral hygiene advice and training. It is only following these two steps that it is really logical to attempt to evolve a particular branch of the medical profession trained not only to care for the well-being of the whole patient but be specifically orientated towards diagnosing dental disease when it is present as distinct from when it produces symptoms demanding emergency treatment.

It is probably only at this stage that it is appropriate to begin to contemplate the employment of personnel capable of planning and providing the widest possible range of dental care, whilst accepting responsibility for the care of the whole patient. However, in view of the very wide variations in the nature of procedures within dentistry it is illogical to nurture the evolution of such personnel, who may now be called dentists, without giving comparable thought and finance to the personnel ancillary to them. Without such ancillary personnel the dentist becomes inefficient and therefore expensive, a state of affairs experienced in so many countries today.

To this point no mention has been made of the means by which such personnel as have been described might be produced. Though it is possible for a society to attain some level of dental care for its communities through the employment of personnel trained outside itself, it is unlikely that the last mentioned level could ever be maintained or even attained unless those capable of teaching dentistry were evolved. Finally, it becomes natural for a society to produce a limited number of individuals capable of advancing knowledge within dentistry.

THE DESIRE AND NEED FOR SOCIETY TO DETERMINE THE OBJECTIVES IT IS CAPABLE OF ESTABLISHING

Though the stages described may be debatable, they form a framework upon which discussion can be built. The attitude of societies to dental care varies and is influenced by many factors, from tradition to government and it is a common experience that the existence of a service does itself create a demand. The financial commitment of a society to dental care can, within certain limits, be determined at any particular time. This commitment can be rapidly changed by a conscious act of government, on the one hand directing financial support in dentistry's direction or on the other hand withdrawing it. It is the duty of the dental profession to provide society with a 'shop-window' with all the goods clearly priced, and to make certain that society gets value for whatever monies it finds itself able or inclined to devote to dental care. It would, for example, seem to be ill-advised to spend limited finances upon a dental school capable of producing only a small number of dental graduates in preference to fluoridating the water supply where indicated.

THE NEED FOR SMALL SCALE EXPERIMENTATION UNDER CONTROLLED CONDITIONS INTO METHODS OF DELIVERING DENTAL CARE

Within the last few years experiments have been carried out in an effort to define more objectively the roles of some of the individuals participating in the provision of dental care, and these have been ancillary personnel. But this is not enough. Experimentation is required to obtain data on the number and types of all personnel involved in providing dental care, the responsibilities, education and training of each type subjected to a cost–benefit analysis. It is clear that such information can only be obtained through an experiment of limited dimensions, rather than from the large scale implementation of unproved ideas. It is strange that in this most important field research is so rarely, if ever, carried out in the accepted pattern of a laboratory experiment. Indeed, few Research Laboratories of Clinical Dental Practice exist.

TYPES OF RESEARCH UNITS REQUIRED TO COLLECT AND ANALYSE THE NECESSARY DATA

EPIDEMIOLOGY

The form and function of a team or unit dedicated to the collection and analysis of data of dental epidemiological nature are discussed elsewhere. But the necessity for the establishment of such units within a society as a primary requirement to the provision of dental care cannot be over-emphasized. It is only in the light of such data that reliable further steps can be contemplated. Indeed it is not possible to assess the effectiveness of any system intended to meet the needs and demands of a given community unless its needs and demands are determined both before and after the implementation of such a system.

A RESEARCH DENTAL CARE UNIT

Nevertheless, whilst epidemiology can reveal the problem and assess the effectiveness of the solution it cannot itself evolve that solution. But this can be achieved through a research unit in which systems are created, data collected and analysed and conclusions drawn. Such would be a Research Laboratory of Clinical Dental Practice already mentioned, perhaps the most appropriate title is Research Dental Care Unit.

A research dental care unit is equipped and staffed so as to be capable of providing dental care to patients, yet being free of any specific service commitment to treat patients or to train personnel. Patients are treated and personnel trained only in so far as required for research purposes. The unit is dedicated to the collection, storage, and analysis of data.

The effectiveness of a service is ultimately a cost–benefit analysis: how much does it cost to provide what quality of care and to how many people. There are of course very many variables but the final assessments of productivity may be divided into two main groups: Quantity and Quality, e.g., How long will it take (i.e., how much will it cost) to restore a carious tooth through the use of amalgam and what is the life expectancy of a tooth restored in such a way, or again how long will it take to teach oral hygiene to a patient by a certain method and how effective is that method?

ASSESSING THE CARE PROVIDED

A Research Dental Care Unit will therefore concern itself with timing everything concerned with the provision of dental care. Thus, by the use of as simple and automatic methods as can be devised, every procedure is timed: the time a patient spends travelling to the unit, the time it takes to place a matrix band, insert an amalgam restoration, or carry out a prophylaxis. Through the accumulation of such data it is possible to determine if, for example, the additional cost of an extra dental surgery assistant is more than compensated for by increased production, or whether the use of a new type of more expensive amalgam alloy with improved handling characteristics results in such an increase in output that its use is financially advisable. Though the collection of such data is simple in principle it becomes complex in execution as a result of the very large number of items of data which have to be recorded. A single fact such as the presence of a carious lesion has to be related to one of thirty-two teeth in the permanent dentition and twenty in the deciduous dentition and to one or more of four or five surfaces on each tooth, i.e., 236 alternatives. It is not difficult to imagine how the recording and retrieval of this kind of data can become a complex matter.

The problems associated with the recording of quality are far more complex than those associated with quantity. Absolute objective methods of assessing quality are as yet undeveloped in most respects. It is assessed subjectively, with at best a few simple guiding criteria. Thus the quality of a restoration has been assessed as satisfactory or unsatisfactory through the subjective assessment of a few factors such as the contact point, adaptation of the restorations, etc. In this direction much work has to be done to develop objective methods of assessing quality which can be related to the long-term effectiveness of procedures. In a similar way the effectiveness of preventive measures of an individual character such as plaque control require careful and controlled assessment.

ASSESSING THE METHODS OF DELIVERING CARE

There is no problem in visualizing the very large number of facets to the provision of dental care that demand careful measurement and recording within the framework described, and yet this is but a part of the problem which concerns the services themselves. The other side relates the means by which these services are to be delivered.

Dental care can only be delivered by people, for people. Those who provide the care form a team of one or more individuals. Such a team may perhaps most appropriately be known as a Dental Care Unit and as it provides that care for a community as a Community Dental Care Unit. Comment has been made upon the variations in the type of care which might most appropriately be provided by society for its communities. Such variations cannot but be reflected in the composition of the teams which would most effectively fulfil these roles. Within a Research Dental Care Unit teams of personnel of varying composition and size should function and be compared with one another on a cost–

benefit basis. Data obtained under the circumstances existing within a Research Unit can, however, only be considered as the first stage to indicate the form of team which should be tested under more realistic conditions. Nevertheless a Research Dental Care Unit, having developed the mechanism would establish systems capable of recording data from as many types of systems as exist or could wisely be created.

To provide specific examples: data would be collected from established dental practices, both single handed practices and group practices, those employing ancillary personnel and those not doing so, etc. This type of data would be compared with that obtained from systems of dentists controlled teams of a more complex nature composed of numerous operating and non-operating ancillary personnel.

By such means, not only can the way in which dental care is provided be subjected to assessment but also the type of care provided. Data can be accumulated on the effectiveness of preventive measures; upon the development of early carious lesions, the cost-effectiveness of one type of restorative procedure compared with another; or of one method of plaque control against another. The potential of Research Dental Care Units is very wide indeed and can be the source of information to guide many developments in the provision of dental care. There is, however, another major part which a Research Dental Care Unit can fill, that is to obtain data which might indicate the sphere of responsibility and the appropriate training of the personnel composing the team.

THE DEVELOPMENT AND TRAINING OF PERSONNEL

Comment has been made about the historical evolution of the types of personnel concerned in the provision of dental care and the shortage of information relating to the effectiveness of the service they provide and training they receive. This is particularly so on a comparative plane for it is safe to assume that personnel trained in a particular way will provide a service for which they have been trained. It is quite another matter to determine if their training was more effective, and more economical than an alternative solution. It is necessary, therefore, to assess the effectiveness of not only various compositions of teams as described above but also the effectiveness of various types of personnel composing the team. Since the type of personnel can only be described with reference to their training and the remit of their responsibility within the team, a Research Dental Care Unit cannot but be concerned in education and training.

The effectiveness of established types of personnel: dentists, dental auxiliaries, dental hygienists, and others, forms a baseline for measurement. But new types of personnel, created by new and different training backgrounds should be compared with them. In addition, the efficiency of various ways of training personnel in clinical dentistry, particularly ways of training them together to work as a team, demands investigation.

The potential of training both the dentist and his ancillaries together is very great. Such a training team might well be termed a Training Dental Care Unit. It should be constructed according to the needs and demands of the patients attending for treatment, modified by the educational demands of those composing the team. But its function should be monitored by a Research Dental Care Unit so that changes can be brought about in the light of knowledge rather than only by imagination. Training through the functioning of a Training Dental Care Unit is potentially efficient and those forming the team, if trained as a team, will function more effectively than if they are trained remote from each other. If a team is to provide dental care then a team should be trained to provide that care.

The logical development of this theme sees such a Training Dental Care Unit as the *proforma* of the future clinical dental school, for the dental school is seen as the source of the whole team, not just of one or two constituent parts of that team. Experience in clinical dentistry is seen to be possible through the functioning of numerous Training Dental Care Units of different characteristics.

THE BASIC DESIGN OF SYSTEMS FOR PROVIDING TOTAL DENTAL CARE

Few dental procedures demand the full in-patient facilities of a hospital and yet the emergency treatment considered to be the first requirement of a dental service often needs them. It is therefore desirable to so organize the dental services to a community that access to a hospital service is attained. Care must be taken, however, to avoid using these expensive and limited facilities for care which could as safely and more efficiently be provided elsewhere.

The theme that has been developed throughout this chapter has been the employment of the team, under the direction of the dentist to provide dental care to a community. Dentists on their own initiative and through their own capital are increasingly developing the team approach within the limits that the law allows. However, the financial commitments required of a dentist to establish and house Dental Care Units are indeed considerable. The concept of Health Centres and the position of the dentist in relation to them has been examined in the United Kingdom. Many problems have been revealed but it is believed that many difficulties arise from an attempt to graft the traditional methods of delivering dental care into a strange and inappropriate environment.

The ideal composition, size, and design of a Dental Care Unit will vary with the community served and the level of service provided, but again ideas must be tested. There is an increasing acceptance within medicine of the idea of a larger unit replacing the single-handed practitioner and dentistry is following the same pattern. The Dental Care Unit will almost certainly evolve as a larger unit having a dramatically different ratio of dentists to ancillary staff than is at present experienced. The managerial, supervisory, and expert role carried out by the dentist himself will, it is believed, prove to be more attractive and rewarding than that experienced by the majority of dentists at the present time. The removal of mundane and repetitive procedures from the hands of the dentist will enable him to accept responsibility for more patients, so that a larger population of the community may benefit from his knowledge. Not the least benefit will be the ability of the dentist to devote a greater part of his time to those procedures and aspects of dental care which demand his special knowledge and skills. It is believed that most aspects of dental care are within the capability of one individual and the relief which the greater utilization of ancillaries will provide will enable him to employ and develop these skills to a maximum extent.

This does not mean that there will be no place for the specialist, for a Dental Care Unit may well have more than one dentist one or more of whom may develop particular interests and skills. In addition, within a group of Dental Care Units, possibly orientated around a Hospital, specialists or consultants in various disciplines could rotate on a sessional basis between the units.

The brief outline which has been given is necessarily inadequate and great problems are seen in its evolution, particularly within established systems. It is inevitable that with increasing commitments and increasing costs some such organization and evolution of dental care must come about. But the evolution and change should be guided by the dental profession in the light of knowledge.

THE SELECTION OF SYSTEMS ACCORDING TO A SOCIETY'S ABILITY TO MEET THE NEEDS AND DEMANDS WITHIN ITS COMMUNITIES

The necessity to consider the ability of society to meet the needs and demands would seem to be self-evident, and yet political considerations often overshadow the decisions. Society has a right to demand an account of the needs and demands balanced against the cost of each level of care, so that it may decide how most appropriately to spend such funds as it can make available. An essential priority therefore within any society today is to establish the means by which the needs and demands for care within its communities may continuously be assessed, and the means by which these may most appropriately be met.

Appendix II

Reorganization of the National Health Service

D. H. Norman, BDS, LDS, DDPHRCS
Chief Dental Officer, London Borough of Hounslow

The administration of the British National Health Service was described by Renson in Chapter 7. He concluded with some allusions to the organizational changes in the Service which were expected to take place. Since that was written, some developments have become clarified, and many firm decisions have been made.

The reorganized National Health Service is scheduled to come into operation in April, 1974. Mr. Norman here provides an outline of the pattern of change, though it will be appreciated that further modifications are likely at a later time.

The United Kingdom introduced a National Health Service in July 1948 providing free health care for all, irrespective of means.

Political considerations had dictated that the Service should be based on a tripartite system, with General Practioner, Hospital, and Local Authority services functioning side by side, but nevertheless remaining substantially autonomous. It was a framework well suited to the immediate needs, in particular the reorganization of hospital and specialist services (Ministry of Health, 1968).

The National Health Service is generally considered to be an improvement on the previous health care system, but problems have arisen. One is that the cost of the Service soon exceeded early estimates, resulting in the introduction of patient charges for some dental treatment, ophthalmic services, and prescriptions. Another is that the tripartite system has tended to produce artificial barriers between the three divisions of the Service. The resulting loss of co-operation may have lessened the quality of patient care; certainly it has tended to reduce job satisfaction among the providers of care.

This latter problem has been recognized for some time, for fourteen years after the National Health Service began a report from the Medical Service Review Committee concluded that: 'The most vital need is to unify and integrate in the widest sense all aspects of medicine in order to achieve the highest standard of medical care, and to avoid the sense of isolation and frustration to which we have drawn attention' (Medical Services Review Committee, 1962).

The earlier proposals for reorganization were described in the latter part of Chapter 7. These various proposals culminated in the National Health Services Reorganization Act of 1973.

At the time of writing the reorganization is planned for 1 October, 1973 in Northern Ireland, and 1 April, 1974 in England, Scotland, and Wales.

GENERAL ORGANIZATION

In England there will be three levels of planning: Area, Regional, and the Central Department. In Scotland, Wales and Northern Ireland, the regional planning level is omitted. The larger Areas will be further subdivided into Districts, which, while being important levels for the provision of health care, are part of the area and not a tier in their own right. This proposed structure is illustrated in Fig. 1.

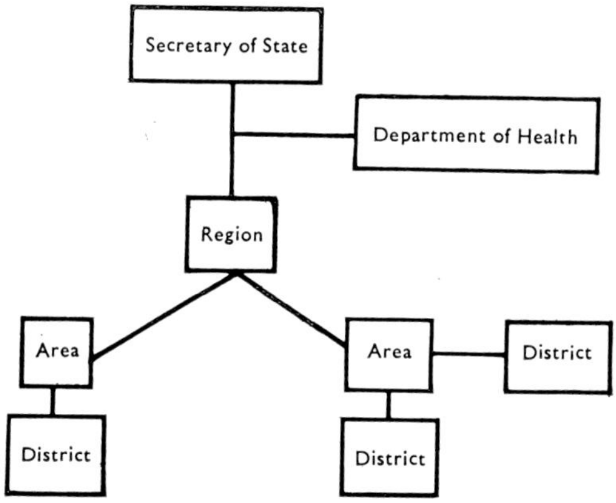

Fig. 1. Proposed structure of the reorganized National Health Service.

TABLE 1

Total no. of areas in proposed reorganization

Country	*Total no. of areas*
England	90
Scotland	15
Wales	8
Northern Ireland	4

In England there will be 14 Regions and 90 Areas. Table 1 shows the number of areas in England, Wales, Scotland and Northern Ireland.

REGIONAL HEALTH AUTHORITIES

The Regional Health Authorities will form part of a chain of responsibility running from the Secretary of State to the Area Health Authorities. The Authority itself will consist of a Chairman, who will be paid a part-time salary, and a number of members who will be unpaid but entitled to expenses. The Chairman and all members will be appointed by the Secretary of State for Health and Social Services.

The Regional Health Authorities will develop strategic plans and priorities, based on a review of needs identified by the Area Health Authorities. They will control the allocation of resources to Areas within them, adjudicating on competing priorities.

The Authority will be advised by a team of officers, comprising a Regional Medical Officer, a Regional Nursing Officer, a Regional Finance Officer, a Regional Administrative Officer, and a Regional Works Officer. The duties of a Regional Dental Officer have not been fully developed at the time of writing, but there will be a Regional Dental Officer.

Each Region will have a university medical school within its boundaries, but only six will have a dental school.

Until 1979 medical and dental consultants and senior registrars (except in teaching Areas) will be in contract with the Region.

AREA HEALTH AUTHORITIES

The boundaries of the Areas will be generally co-terminous with those of local authorities. This is to facilitate co-operation in the spheres of education, social services, and environmental health, all of which will remain the responsibility of local authorities.

The Authority will be comprised of a Chairman, who will be paid a part-time salary and appointed by the Secretary of State in consultation with the Region, and approximately 15 other members who may be paid expenses. Four of these are to be appointed from the matching Local Authority. Where an Area has a dental school within its boundaries one member will be a dentist. Other members will be appointed following consultation by the Regional Health Authority with the main health profession and trades unions.

The Authorities will be advised by an Area Team of Officers composed of the Area Medical Officer, the Area Nursing Officer, Area Finance Officer, and the Area Administrative Officer.

The Area Dental Officer will not be a member of the team but will receive all minutes and agendas relating to the team's meetings. He will have direct access to the Area Health Authority, and have the right to attend team meetings when appropriate.

THE DISTRICTS

As previously mentioned the larger Areas will be subdivided into a number of Districts. Each District will have a District general hospital and will be managed by a District Team of Officers, accountable to the Area Health Authority.

The District Team of Officers will comprise a doctor, nurse, administrator, and finance officer. A peculiarity of the District management team will be the addition of two other members, representing the practitioners and consultants working in the District, who will not be accountable to the Area Health Authority. Most districts will have a District Dental Officer although in some instances this function may be performed by the Area Dental Officer in addition to his other duties. The District Dental Officer, when appointed, will be accountable to the Area Dental Officer for his administrative duties.

The District (or District/Area in smaller zones) is the principal unit of health care. Approximately twenty-four English Area Health Authorities will contain only one District, and the maximum number of Districts in one Area will be six.

HEALTH CARE PLANNING TEAMS

Health Care Planning Teams will be set up at District level to consider specific health problems and patient groups such as children, the aged and the handicapped. From time to time transient health care teams may be set up to consider special problems.

It will be essential that the Area Dental Officer or District Dental Officer makes a full and meaningful contribution to the work of these teams.

THE FAMILY PRACTITIONER SERVICE

The practitioner services will continue as before reorganization, except that the Executive Council will be replaced by the Family Practitioner Committee at an Area level. The services will be founded directly from the Central Department. The Administrator of the Family Practitioner Committee will be attached from the Area Administrator's staff, but must be acceptable to the Family Practitioner Committee which will function with a considerable degree of autonomy. In Scotland there will be no separate Family Practitioner Committee and the services will be administrated directly from the Area Health Authority.

ADVISORY MACHINERY

Strong advisory machinery will be built into the National Health Service at all levels. Regional and Area Dental Advisory Committees will represent all fields of dentistry. At District level, there will be two dental representatives on the District Medical Committee, representing Consultant and General Practitioner Services.

COMMUNITY HEALTH COUNCILS

These will represent the consumer and will function at a district level, although it will be the duty of the Region to establish such councils. Half the members will be appointed by the matching local authority and the remainder by voluntary bodies and similar organizations. The councils will have wide powers of entry to premises, except in the case of the surgeries of general practitioners.

LONDON

In some respects minor variations will occur in the London area; the ambulance services for example will be administered as a single unit in Greater London irrespective of Regional and Area Boundaries.

LIAISON WITH LOCAL AUTHORITIES

Joint Consultative Committees will be set up to ensure adequate co-operation between Area Health Authorities and the matching local authority. Such co-operation will be particularly important in relation to school health services and the social services.

TEACHING HOSPITALS

In general, teaching hospitals will not retain the traditional Board of Governors, but Areas containing teaching hospitals will have medical and dental members on the Authority. A limited number of post-graduate hospitals will retain the old style of Governors for an experimental period of five years. In Areas with a medical or dental school consultants and senior registrars, will, contrary to the general practice, be in contract with the Area.

CONCLUSION

Reorganization of the National Health Service encompasses a series of major changes, and the challenge it presents to all those involved should not be underestimated.

It is natural that some disappointment has been expressed concerning the place of dentistry in the reorganized service. Despite this, the Area Dental Officer, with support from his colleagues, may yet have the freedom to develop potentially more effective services than have previously been offered in Britain.

REFERENCES

MEDICAL SERVICES REVIEW COMMITTEE (1962), *A Review of the Medical Services in Great Britain* (*Porritt Report*). London: HMSO.

MINISTRY OF HEALTH (1968), *The Administrative Structure of the Medical and Related Services in England and Wales* (first Green Paper). London: HMSO.

ADDITIONAL READING

Apart from the formal documents published by the Department of Health and Social Security, there are also many circulars issued by the Department. These circulars have been sent to interested sections of the existing health services. They are intended to be of only temporary interest, to be replaced at a later date by more permanent documentation. They have been published as Health Re-organisation Circulars (H.R.C.s) and in the future are likely to be difficult to obtain, though a few libraries, notably that of the British Dental Association, have maintained files of these. The reference numbers and the date of issue of the more important circulars are listed below, together with some other texts relevant to the reorganization.

TEXTS

Department of Health and Social Security (1972a), *National Health Service Reorganisation: England*. Cmnd. 5055. London: HMSO (The White Paper).

— — — —(1972b), *Management Arrangements for the Reorganised National Health Service*. London, HMSO. This document, frequently referred to as the 'Grey Book', gives details of management structures together with role specifications of key officers. Some details have been modified in later circulars.

Norman, D. H. (1973), 'National Health Service Reorganisation; a Bibliography', *Br. dent. J.*, **134,** 506, and **135,** 230.

CIRCULARS

H.R.C. (72) 2. Details of the boundaries of the fourteen English regions.

H.R.C. (72) 7. Guidance on the preparation of an area profile.

H.R.C. (73) 3. An important circular updating proposals for management arrangements in the re-organised service.

H.R.C. (73) 8. Proposals for forward planning.

H.R.C. (73) 17. Summary of the recommendations from the working party concerning collaboration of Local Authorities and Health Services.

H.R.C. (73) 19. Management arrangements in two districts areas.

H.R.C. (73) 26. Statutory Provisions within the framework of the re-organised service.

H.R.C. (73) 27. Arrangements for securing continuity of statistics of health service activity after 1974.

Index